# new choices in NATURAL HEALING

## FOR DOGS & CATS

# new choices in
# NATURAL
# HEALING
## FOR DOGS & CATS

Over 1,000 At-Home Remedies for Your Pet's Problems

HERBS ❧ ACUPRESSURE ❧ MASSAGE

HOMEOPATHY ❧ FLOWER ESSENCES

NATURAL DIETS ❧ HEALING ENERGY

By Amy D. Shojai and the Editors of

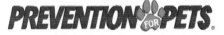

Medical Advisor: Susan G. Wynn, D.V.M.,
Executive Director of the
Georgia Holistic Veterinary Medical Association

RODALE

© 1999 Rodale Inc.
Illustrations © 1999 Randy Hamblin and Jim Starr
Cover photograph © Tim Davis/Stone

Printed in the United States of America
Rodale Inc. makes every effort to use acid-free ∞, recycled paper ♻.

**Library of Congress Cataloging-in-Publication Data**

Shojai, Amy, 1956–
    New choices in natural healing for dogs and cats : over 1,000 at-
home remedies for your pet's problems / by Amy D. Shojai and the
editors of Prevention for Pets.
      p.    cm.
    Includes index.
    ISBN 1–57954–057–0  hardcover
    ISBN 1–57954–461–4  paperback
    1. Alternative veterinary medicine.  2. Dogs—Diseases—
Alternative treatment.  3. Cats—Diseases—Alternative treatment.
I. Prevention for Pets (Rodale Press).  II. Title.
SF745.5.S48  1999
636.7'08955—dc21                          99–15692

**Distributed to the book trade by St. Martin's Press**

        8  10  9  7        hardcover
2  4  6  8  10  9  7  5  3        paperback

Visit us on the Web at www.rodalebooks.com, or call us toll-free at (800) 848-4735.

## OUR PURPOSE

We help you give your pets all the good health and loving care they deserve. In our books, you will find the latest information along with the wisdom and practical advice of the country's top veterinary experts. From behavior and training tips to improving quality of life, we will help you achieve the greatest reward of all—a lifetime of love and commitment.

**PREVENTION✦PETS.**

## New Choices in Natural Healing for Dogs and Cats Staff

**EDITOR:** Matthew Hoffman

**WRITERS:** Amy D. Shojai with Janine Adams; Laura Dearborn; Susan Easterly; Leah Flickinger; Phil Goldberg; Joanne Howl, D.V.M.; Susan McCullough; Lynn McGowan

**ART DIRECTOR:** Darlene Schneck

**INTERIOR DESIGNER:** Diane Ness Shaw

**COVER DESIGNER:** Leanne Coppola

**ILLUSTRATORS:** Randy Hamblin, Jim Starr

**COVER PHOTOGRAPHER:** Tim Davis/Stone

**ASSOCIATE RESEARCH MANAGER:** Jane Unger Hahn

**BOOK PROJECT RESEARCHER:** Leah Flickinger

**EDITORIAL RESEARCHERS:** Lois Guarino Hazel, Elizabeth Shimer, Nancy Zelko

**SENIOR COPY EDITOR:** Karen Neely

**PRODUCTION EDITOR:** Marilyn Hauptly

**LAYOUT DESIGNER:** Donna G. Rossi

**ASSOCIATE STUDIO MANAGER:** Thomas P. Aczel

**MANUFACTURING COORDINATORS:** Brenda Miller, Jodi Schaffer, Patrick T. Smith

### Rodale Active Living Books

VICE PRESIDENT AND PUBLISHER: Neil Wertheimer

EXECUTIVE EDITOR: Susan Clarey

EDITORIAL DIRECTOR: Michael Ward

WRITING DIRECTOR: Brian Paul Kaufman

MARKETING DIRECTOR: Janine Slaughter

PRODUCT MARKETING MANAGER: Kris Siessmayer

BOOK MANUFACTURING DIRECTOR: Helen Clogston

MANUFACTURING MANAGERS: Eileen Bauder, Mark Krahforst

RESEARCH MANAGER: Ann Gossy Yermish

COPY MANAGER: Lisa D. Andruscavage

PRODUCTION MANAGER: Robert V. Anderson Jr.

OFFICE MANAGER: Jacqueline Dornblaser

OFFICE STAFF: Julie Kehs, Suzanne Lynch Holderman, Mary Lou Stephen, Catherine E. Strouse

# Foreword

It wasn't long after starting practice that I found myself getting frustrated. Some pets, even those with seemingly simple problems, never seemed as healthy as they should be. They were getting all the right treatments, but the treatments were often causing symptoms of their own. And when I gave pets their yearly vaccines, I kept noticing that they often had dry, smelly coats or were scratching or their energy wasn't good—things that most veterinarians considered fairly normal.

After a while, my frustration turned into a plan. When my patients weren't getting better, I decided that I would look beyond the standard practices and expert opinions. I became a scout for emerging therapies.

I was amazed how many there were. Some I'd heard of, but others were entirely new to me. I had to remind myself—as doctors should—that these unfamiliar (to me) therapies just might work, even though I hadn't tried them yet. And often they did.

I'm still a great believer in mainstream veterinary medicine. But along with other veterinarians worldwide, I have learned that although modern medicine offers many miracles, it can't do everything. I have found from years of experience that dogs and cats don't always need the strongest drugs or the most invasive surgery. Even when they do need mainstream help, treatments such as nutritional supplements, massage, and perhaps even energy therapies can provide them with the extra fuel they need to get well and stay well.

You may be told that these remedies are not scientifically proven. This is usually true. And you may be told not to bother with them because they cannot possibly work. This is not true. Not every remedy in this book will work for every pet. Some of these remedies I use every week, and some I have never tried. The point is that pets—and their owners—are individuals, not bound to live by statistics. I say give these remedies a try. In many cases, they could make a world of difference.

*Susan G. Wynn DVM*

Susan G. Wynn, D.V.M.

# Contents

## PART 1: A New Approach

## PART 2: The Best Choices in Natural Healing

# PART 3: Common Health and Behavior Problems

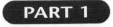

# PART 1

# A New
# Approach

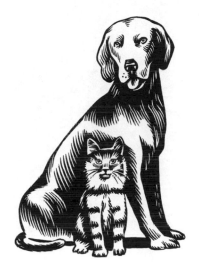

# CHAPTER 1

# Healing the Natural Way

Veterinary medicine used to be a lot simpler. Without a lot of equipment to lug around, vets made house calls, dispensing medicines along with the wisdom of years of experience. They got to know the families they worked with and had special insights into pets' lives—what they ate, how they spent their days, and what their usual energy was like. They looked at symptoms, too, but only as one part of a larger picture.

As technology advanced and veterinarians got more sophisticated, some of this personal touch was lost. Most vets stopped making house calls, and you almost never see them take pills or mysterious liquids out of a battered black bag. As with human doctors, modern vets still depend on good old-fashioned horse sense but rely more on the latest tests and techniques, like magnetic resonance imaging, keyhole surgery, and computer-designed medications.

For pets with serious injuries, this modern approach is hard to beat, says David H. Jaggar, D.C., M.R.C.V.S. (member of Royal College of Veterinary Surgeons, a British equivalent of D.V.M.), a holistic veterinarian and chiropractor in Boulder, Colorado, and a founder of the International Veterinary Acupuncture Society. It has limitations, however. Some veterinarians don't have time anymore to get to know their patients very well. When owners take their pets into the office, some vets will focus mainly on the symptoms in order to prescribe a specific treatment. For instance, a dog with hip dysplasia might be given steroids to relieve swelling and perhaps have surgery done to repair or replace the damaged joint. This relieves the immediate symptom, but it may not resolve the underlying problems that made the joint vulnerable in the first place, says Dr. Jaggar. And the treatments themselves may cause additional problems.

Veterinarians who specialize in holistic medicine feel that there is a better way. Without rejecting the many advances of modern medicine, they have shifted their focus to an older style of care. They may spend more time with pets in order to understand their personalities and lifestyles. More important, they look at physical and emotional problems as pieces of a larger puzzle. Illness is rarely caused by something as obvious as a weak joint, bacteria in the body, or pollen. In the holistic view, pets get sick because something happened that allowed external factors to cause illness. Unless you strengthen the body, dogs and cats will continue to get sick.

Consider cancer. Veterinarians fight it with drugs, radiation, or chemotherapy, and these treatments can be very effective. But the immune system has the ability to locate and destroy cancer cells before they spread. This is why holistic veterinarians often use herbs, diet, acupressure, and other natural treatments to strengthen the immune system. The idea is to help the body heal itself, whether or not your pet is undergoing other treatments, says Allen M. Schoen, D.V.M., director of the Veterinary Institute of Therapeutic Alternatives in Sherman, Connecticut, and author of *Love, Miracles, and Animal Healing*.

This approach isn't limited only to cancer, Dr. Schoen adds. Most illnesses, including such things as allergies, arthritis, and diabetes, can be partly controlled—and prevented—by harnessing the body's natural healing powers.

## The Search for Answers

Most holistic veterinarians started out as mainstream practitioners. Dr. Jaggar, for example, was on the faculty as a veterinarian at the College of Medicine at the University of Cincinnati. But he, along with many of his colleagues, found himself getting frustrated because the conventional focus on symptoms didn't seem to work as well as it should. "I knew there had to be other ways of dealing with things, so I started looking into other systems of health care," he says.

Along with his colleagues in holistic health, Dr. Jaggar discovered that many natural therapies used in human medicine, like herbs, flower essences, and homeopathy, work just as well for dogs and cats. Unlike drugs, which target specific symptoms, these and other natural remedies tend to have wider-ranging effects—on the emotions, various organs, and even on the personality, Dr. Jaggar says.

Some alternative therapies look a little strange to Western eyes. It is hard to believe that inserting a needle or pressing a point on one end of your pet can treat a problem at the other end. Doctors had a hard time believing it, too, until research showed that it works. Using a diagnostic technique called magnetic resonance imaging, experts have discovered that certain parts of the brain light up during acupuncture. Needling the outside of the foot—an area associated with the eyes—causes exactly the same reaction as if the eyes saw a flash of light. In other words, stimulating these points can affect ailing eyes by goosing the brain. Other studies have shown that acupuncture and acupressure stimulate the release of endorphins and monoamines, natural chemicals that block pain without the side effects of medications.

Not all alternative treatments are thousands of years old or come from the ends of the Earth. Holistic veterinarians also use traditional homegrown cures, such as Kaopectate for diarrhea or peppermint tea for an upset stomach. Herbs often contain the same active ingredients as modern drugs, minus the side effects.

Even though natural care is a new concept, at least among modern veterinarians, the evidence has clearly shown that it works: Changes in diet that clear up skin allergies. Simple movements that lubricate the joints and reduce arthritis pain. Herbs that stimulate the immune system and stop infection. The list goes on and on.

## Intensive Training

Veterinarians usually study for 8 to 10 years before receiving their D.V.M. (doctor of veterinary medicine) or V.M.D. (veterinariae medicinae doctoris) degrees. For holistic veterinarians, that is just the beginning. They continue their education by studying such things as acupressure, chiropractic, and homeopathy.

Some veterinary schools and universities offer classes and lectures on alternative medicine, but many of these treatments are still so new that academic instruction may not be available. Holistic veterinarians get most of their training from professional associations, such as the Academy of Veterinary Homeopathy or the International Veterinary Acupuncture Society. Or they apprentice themselves to experts in various fields. For instance, veterinarians interested in acupuncture may go to China to learn what the therapy does and how to use it, says Mary Rose Paradis, D.V.M., associate professor in the department of clinical sciences at Tufts University School of Veterinary Medicine in North Grafton, Massachusetts.

## Blended Care

Holistic veterinarians usually specialize in one or more alternative therapies, but they are well-versed in conventional medicine as well. This means that dogs and cats get the best of both worlds—the latest advances in mainstream medicine combined with the safety and effectiveness of natural treatments.

"Holistic care sometimes works better than conventional medicine. Sometimes it works best as a complementary treatment, and sometimes it doesn't work as well but has fewer side effects," says Dr. Schoen.

Dogs and cats with serious illnesses and injuries often receive a blend of treatments—surgery or transfusions, for example, combined with a flower essence like Bach Rescue Remedy to keep the body stable during the trauma. Pets with chronic conditions such as hip pain often do better with holistic care alone. They might receive acupressure to relieve pain, along with exercises and supplements that help the joint heal.

This blended approach is the reason many people take their pets to holistic veterinarians. They know that they will get the benefits of the latest research, along with time-tested natural treatments. Veterinarians appreciate this versatility as well. They may use conventional medicine to diagnose a bone fracture or detect cancer, then turn to holistic care to help pets recover more quickly. "I once treated a cat with homeopathy before surgically removing a piece of corncob that was stuck in the intestine," says Christina Chambreau, D.V.M., a holistic veterinarian in Sparks, Maryland, and education chairperson for the Academy of Veterinary Homeopathy. "I expected to see severe damage, but the homeopathy helped the abdomen stay healthy, with no inflammation at all."

# CHAPTER 2

# Why Your Pet Gets Sick: The Alternative View

It is almost a miracle the way veterinarians can diagnose, often in minutes, thousands of health problems, from minor infections to heart disease. From a single drop of blood, they can tell when dogs and cats have liver problems or if they have been exposed to bacteria. Urine screens quickly reveal problems with the bladder or kidneys. And sophisticated tests like ultrasound and magnetic resonance imaging make it easy to pinpoint problems deep inside the body.

This precision doesn't end with the diagnosis. The hallmark of modern medicine is that there are very specific treatments for specific problems. Once you understand the physical causes of illness, the thinking goes, all you have to do is "fix" the problem, and the illness will go away.

As we know, however, it doesn't always work like this. Suppose that two cats have been exposed to the same germs. One cat may get sick, while the other stays in the pink of health. Or suppose that two dogs have been exposed to the same cancer-causing chemicals. One dog may get grievously ill, while the other is unaffected. Why, given the same situation, do some pets get sick and others don't?

That's a question holistic veterinarians have been asking for a long time. Even though they recognize that certain things, such as bacteria, can cause illness, there are clearly other factors that determine whether or not pets get sick. Many of these factors, it seems, can't be seen through a microscope or detected with standard medical tests. And yet they appear to have a tremendous impact on your pet's health.

## The Power Within

Just as the world is filled with disease-causing organisms, the body is filled with defenses to resist them. In fact, no matter what your pet is confronted with, her body is well-designed to fight back. Studies have shown, for example, that cats that have suffered serious nerve injuries can recover complete muscle function. When pets take medications (or eat poisons), the liver produces extra enzymes to detoxify them. Even something as minor as a pulled muscle is swiftly addressed with an increase in blood flow, which brings additional oxygen and nutrients and carts off wastes. The main reason a pet gets sick, according to holistic veterinarians, is that something is interfering with the body's natural healing powers.

The key to self-healing is a strong defense system, which protects dogs and cats from everything from flu germs to cancer cells, says Deborah C. Mallu, D.V.M., a holistic veterinarian in private practice in Sedona, Arizona. More than their mainstream counterparts, holistic veterinarians believe that a weak immune system plays a key role in causing disease. Antibiotics fight infections, but they don't affect whatever weakened the immune system in the first place, she says. This is why holistic veterinarians focus less on things that cause disease and more on those that affect the body's defenses.

For instance, some veterinarians believe that there is a type of energy, or life force, that surrounds and flows into every living thing. You are not aware of this energy. You can't see it or hear it, and scientists still don't know how to measure it. But it is every bit as real as the invisible germs that surround us, says Dr. Mallu.

When this energy is flowing freely, dogs and cats have a superb ability to resist disease. But when the energy is blocked or unbalanced due to such things as stress or injuries, pets become vulnerable to illness. And once they get sick, the energy becomes even more unbal-

## ALTERNATIVE SUCCESS

## HEALTH FROM THE HEART

You wouldn't think that dogs have a lot of interest in their owners' private lives, but they notice a lot more than we give them credit for—and sometimes they react in ways that can literally make them ill.

Zack, a 100-pound German shepherd, was undergoing training to be a service dog when he started getting sick. His eyes were glassy, his jowls were moist and swollen, and he had a sore on the end of his nose that wouldn't heal. His owner, Deborah Sanders of Tulsa, Oklahoma, discovered that Zack was seriously ill with lupus, an autoimmune disease in which the body begins attacking itself.

"The vet recommended giving him cortisone to suppress the immune system, but I was afraid that would only mask the symptoms and not make him better," Deborah says. Looking for options, she consulted a holistic veterinarian, who recommended giving Zack fresh fruits and vegetables, along with nutritional supplements and acupuncture treatments in order to dampen his overactive immune system. Zack got a little better, but not much, and Deborah was giving up hope.

At about the same time, she finally left a long-term—and perpetually unhappy—relationship. To her amazement, Zack's symptoms began to disappear. She immediately called her vet, who explained that dogs have an uncanny ability to sense their owners' emotions and be affected by them. "When the stress went away, Zack made a phenomenal recovery," she says.

anced, making it much harder for them to recover, says Russell Swift, D.V.M., a holistic veterinarian in private practice in Dade, Broward, and Palm Beach Counties in Florida.

Everything dogs and cats experience, from the quality of afternoon light to an upsetting afternoon, can affect the body's energy balance. But a few things in particular, such as diet, stress, and exercise, play the biggest roles in determining whether pets get sick or stay healthy.

## Nutritional Risks

Just as the wrong fuel causes car engines to knock and ping, certain diets make the body vulnerable to problems. Most pets eat commercial foods, which are often loaded with artificial dyes, preservatives, and additives, says Dr. Swift. Dogs and cats have spent eons eating "wild," natural foods, and that is what their systems are designed for. It is only in the last several decades that they have been exposed to commercially prepared foods as well as the chemicals these foods contain—chemicals that their bodies simply aren't meant to handle, he says. In addition, artificial ingredients can trigger an immune response that can, quite literally, make pets sick.

The immune system is designed to attack foreign invaders while ignoring "natural" molecules, such as those found in foods. The chemicals in foods certainly aren't natural. If the immune system perceives them as threats, it will mount a defense. A meal of dry kibble can unleash a flood of basophils and other immune-system cells, which, in turn, release chemicals such as histamine. Unfortunately, these chemicals aren't entirely benign. In some cases, they can trigger a rash of itching, vomiting, or diarrhea, says Dr. Swift.

Diet affects the immune system in other ways as well. Among the most important components of immunity are antibodies. Antibodies are nothing more than specialized, germ-fighting proteins. The only time your pet can make enough antibodies is when she is healthy and well-fed, says Dana Eugene Waer, D.V.M., a holistic veterinarian in private practice in Fair Oaks, California.

In addition, the digestive tract has evolved to digest and process certain kinds of foods, says Dr. Swift. Extra ingredients such as food additives put a strain on the whole body as it works to break them down. It is especially hard on the kidneys and liver because these organs cleanse the body of impurities and unnecessary nutrients, he says. After years of being perpetually "on," they start wearing down, he explains.

Holistic veterinarians believe that diet—more specifically, a diet consisting of highly processed foods of questionable nutritional quality—is the main reason pets get sick. This is why holistic care nearly always involves changes in diet, regardless of other treatments your vet may recommend.

## Feelings and Health

When you go to the doctor, the first question that you are likely to hear is, "How are you feeling today?" Unless you are seeing a psychologist, you know that this is really a way of asking how you feel physically. But when you take your pet to a holistic veterinarian, the question is meant literally. One of the tenets of alternative care is that the emotions, in pets as much as in people, are intimately connected with health. Emotions don't necessarily cause disease, but they can weaken the body to such an extent that illnesses have the opportunity to creep in, says Lori Tapp, D.V.M., a holistic veterinarian in private practice in Asheville, North Carolina.

Research has shown, for example, that stress suppresses the action of antibodies and can delay wound healing by 25 percent. In fact, any type of negative emotion, such as fear or depression, can weaken the body and increase the risk of illness, says Dr. Tapp. And because the bond between people and pets is so intense, even your negative emotions can affect your pet, she says.

When it is time to give a physical exam, holistic veterinarians are just as thorough as their mainstream colleagues. They run many of the same tests and look for the same symptoms. But because emotional health has a such a strong impact on the body, they will delve much more deeply into your pet's behavior and personality. Has she been anxious or relaxed? Does she seem depressed or under the weather? When was the last time she seemed enthusiastic? The answers to these and other questions will help your vet understand all of your pet's risk factors, both physical and emotional.

Pets don't have to be nervous wrecks before they start suffering physical consequences, Dr. Mallu adds. Something as simple (and harmless) as a blast of thunder can leave them nervous for hours—and that may be all it takes to put a kink in their protective energy. That is why treating the emotions is sometimes the best way to treat the body.

## The Danger of Downtime

Dogs and cats used to be a lot more active than they are today. They chased mice and herded sheep. They climbed trees and explored acres of fields. They burned a lot of energy by padding after their owners when they went about their business. When people were active, their pets were busy, too.

Today, of course, pets and people spend more time cooped up in small yards and living rooms than exploring the great outdoors, and the lack of exercise is one of the main reasons they (and we) aren't as healthy as we could be. Holistic veterinarians believe that common conditions such as arthritis, constipation, and diabetes are directly linked to a slower-paced lifestyle, says Ihor Basko, D.V.M., a holistic veterinarian in private practice in Honolulu and Kilauea, Hawaii.

Pets that aren't active tend to gain weight, which strains the joints and can lead to arthritis, says Dr. Basko. Excess fat in the body contributes to metabolic diseases such as diabetes. And many of the body's natural processes work less efficiently when pets aren't active. Research has shown, for example, that exercise can improve the liver's ability to transport nitrogen wastes by 80 percent.

A lack of exercise does more than weaken the body. It also weakens emotional health, says Pat Zook, D.V.M., a holistic veterinarian in private practice in Stone Mountain, Georgia. Pets that don't exercise are much more likely to be bored, anxious, or depressed than those that stay busy, she explains. And when their emotions are weak, their bodies quickly follow suit.

Dogs and cats don't need a lot of exercise to keep their bodies' defenses working well, Dr. Zook adds. Getting as little as 20 to 30 minutes of exercise once or twice a day will stimulate all parts of the body, including the immune system. And that's exactly the edge they need to stay healthy.

# CHAPTER 3

# Making the Switch

Alternative, natural medicine has become one of the fastest-growing areas in veterinary care. More Americans are making the switch—not because they are dissatisfied with mainstream veterinarians, but because they feel that Western-style health care, with its emphasis on treating only physical symptoms, is too limiting. They also want to play a more active role in caring for their pets at home, and holistic veterinarians are more likely than their conventional counterparts to encourage this.

"Your veterinarian is just one part of the healing chain," says Deborah C. Mallu, D.V.M., a holistic veterinarian in private practice in Sedona, Arizona. You know your pet better than anyone, including your vet, she explains. You know when your pet is feeling a little off, when his energy is low, or when he is not eating with his usual enthusiasm. Your vet can draw blood, take x-rays, and run dozens of tests to diagnose physical problems, but you have a broader view because you know what is happening every day.

Switching to natural care requires more of a time investment because you aren't depending solely on your vet for the answers, adds George Carley, D.V.M., a holistic veterinarian in private practice in Tulsa, Oklahoma. Your vet will depend on you to notice things that she may not see in the office but that you notice at home. Even the smallest details—where your pet sleeps, whether he is more or less affectionate, even the light in his eyes—offer clues about his physical and emotional health that will help your vet decide which treatments to recommend.

## Choosing a Holistic Veterinarian

Veterinarians have been using natural remedies nearly forever, but holistic care is still a new specialty. There are about 60,000 mainstream veterinarians in the United States, but only about 1,000 veterinarians regularly practice holistic care. You may have to go a little further than the Yellow Pages to find a veterinarian who is right for you.

"Nothing beats recommendations from satisfied clients who have been there and had success," says Allen M. Schoen, D.V.M., director of the Veterinary Institute for Therapeutic Alternatives in Sherman, Connecticut, and author of *Love, Miracles, and Animal Healing*. You can also ask your regular vet for recommendations. Even if she doesn't practice alternative medicine, she will know people who do. Both holistic and mainstream veterinarians who belong to the American Veterinary Medical Association are listed in the same directory. In fact, many mainstream veterinarians like to team up with holistic vets because the collaboration provides additional options, says Mary Rose Paradis, D.V.M., associate professor in the department of clinical sciences at Tufts University School of Veterinary Medicine in North Grafton, Massachusetts. On page 434, you will find a listing of holistic veterinary associations, which can direct you to experts in your area.

Don't assume that your veterinarian doesn't practice holistic care just because you don't see it on her business card, adds Dr. Carley. Many conventional veterinarians have begun using alternative therapies even when alternative care isn't the main part of their practices.

Finding a holistic veterinarian is the just the beginning. You will also have to find out if the veterinarian you have chosen practices the types of therapy that you are interested in and whether you feel comfortable with the relationship. Most veterinarians welcome get-acquainted visits because they know that the best partnerships depend on trust. It is important that all of you—you, your vet, and your pets—get along well together.

## The First Visit

Dogs and cats hate going to the vet, no matter how many snacks or kind words they receive when they get there. There are unfamiliar sights and sounds. And dogs and cats can smell emotions such as fear that other pets at the vet's may be feeling. When they detect scary smells, they get frightened themselves, which is why many pets begin trembling before they walk in the door.

Holistic veterinarians strongly believe that emotions like stress and fear weaken the body and slow healing. That is why they make an extra effort to take some of the scariness out of the experience. Rather than using a metal examining table, for example, which has a cold, uncomfortable surface, Dr. Mallu uses one that is covered with flannel sheets and foam pads. She also has wind chimes and a small tabletop fountain because sounds from nature can reduce the body's production of stress hormones. And unlike most conventional veterinary offices, the examining room has a window. While she examines and treats pets, they can look outside, where there is a duck-filled pond and hummingbirds dive-bombing a feeder. "Pets that have always been nervous wrecks will even let me draw blood without anyone holding them," she says.

Veterinary offices are designed for efficiency, but holistic vets feel that they need to take a little longer in order to collect information about your pet's life and environment, such as what he eats, how much he is sleeping, and so on. Some visits last as long as an hour. You will also notice that your vet does a lot of touching, not only to probe for pain or stiffness but also to massage a muscle. Press an acupressure point. Do a quick spinal adjustment. Holistic veterinarians believe that the outside of the body provides very specific clues as to what is happening on the inside, so the physical part of the exam can be time-consuming.

After the exam, your vet will probably give detailed instructions about what you need to do at home. One of the guiding principles of holistic health is that your pet's physical and emotional environments play as much a part in sickness and health as internal factors do. Your vet will tell you what to look for, ways to keep your pet comfortable and relaxed, and how to do certain treatments.

Even though your visits may be longer than usual, in the long run you might spend less time at your vet's office than you did before because you will be doing certain procedures yourself. You won't feel abandoned, however. Most holistic veterinarians encourage people to call with questions. When you are not sure what to do or you see something that may be a problem, pick up the phone. Your vet will walk you through the process so that you can do it correctly and so that you don't have to put your pet through the stress of a trip to the office.

## A Strong Partnership

We are so accustomed to having experts—veterinarians as well as doctors—taking care of our families' health that it seems difficult or even unhealthy to do things at home. But owners know their pets exquisitely well and are uniquely qualified to perform many types of health care, says Dr. Mallu. You are not going to be doing brain surgery, after all. You will be watching your pet's diet. Giving him more exercise. Pushing an acupressure point or giving homeopathy. Little things that over a lifetime can be more powerful than drugs or surgery.

Consider diet, for instance. Veterinarians often recommend and sell commercial dog and cat foods. These foods work well for many pets, but they are generally more convenient than wholesome, says W. Jean Dodds, D.V.M., adjunct professor of clinical sciences at the University of Pennsylvania School of Veterinary Medicine in Philadelphia and owner of Hemopet, a national nonprofit animal blood bank in Irvine, California. Holistic veterinarians believe that the chemical additives and preservatives used in many commercial foods can cause a variety of health problems, including itchy skin.

One thing that your vet will recommend is that you switch to an all-natural food—or, better yet, that you prepare your pet's meals from scratch. "A homemade diet is best, but it is also the most difficult," adds Donn W. Griffith, D.V.M., a holistic veterinarian in private practice in Dublin, Ohio. You will have to spend time buying ingredients and cooking. And your pet will have to get used to the change, which also takes time, especially for dogs and cats that are set in their ways.

The extra time you spend, however, preparing the food and cajoling your pet to eat could easily add years to his life, says Roger L. DeHaan, D.V.M., a holistic veterinarian in private practice in Frazee, Minnesota.

Home treatment doesn't end with filling the food bowl. Your pet will also have to get used to home exams. The exams don't have to be any more complex than checking the shine on his coat, the light in his eyes, or the way he is walking or lying down, says Dr. Mallu. The goal of holistic health isn't for you to become a veterinarian but to be more engaged in how your pet is feeling and acting every day.

Don't underestimate the power of intuition, Dr. Mallu adds. It may not be scientific, but it is one of the best ways to discover when things aren't the way they should be. The closer your bond with your pet, the more often you will get "feelings" about his health. Consider these feel-

**ALTERNATIVE SUCCESS**

## REKINDLING THE SPARK

Veterinarians at Oklahoma State University had the worst kind of news: Teddy, a snow-white Samoyed, had a rare kind of lung cancer called malignant histiocytosis. They quickly removed part of Teddy's lung and put him on chemotherapy, but they doubted that he would live longer than six months.

Those weren't the kinds of odds that Teddy's owner, Vickie Cupps of Tulsa, Oklahoma, was comfortable with, so she kept looking for answers. She called George Carley, D.V.M., a holistic veterinarian in private practice in Tulsa, and asked about other options. In addition to Teddy's chemotherapy, Dr. Carley recommended giving him a healthier diet, along with vitamins to strengthen immunity and herbs to strengthen the liver and counteract the side effects of chemotherapy.

Over six months later, when Teddy's time should have run out, he was thriving. In fact, tests performed at Colorado State University showed that the cancer was gone. No one is sure what caused Teddy's amazing recovery. Vickie suspects that it was a blended success: cutting-edge medicine plus sophisticated holistic care. "It's so wonderful to see him playing with the other dog, having a big time," she says. "The spark is back in his eyes, and I never thought that would happen."

ings to be an early warning system, a way of discovering problems long before they show up on conventional tests.

Your vet will probably recommend that you stock up on basic medicines, such as homeopathic pills, herbal tonics, and flower essences. Some remedies are just for emergencies, and others you will use all the time. Health food stores often sell complete homeopathic home-care kits, or you can buy the remedies individually. "I'd never be without the homeopathic remedy Nux vomica, which calms vomiting and diarrhea, or the herbal remedy calendula (*Calendula officinalis*), which heals and soothes the skin," says Michelle Tilghman, D.V.M., a holistic veterinarian in private practice in Stone Mountain, Georgia.

## Evaluating Claims

Cats tiptoe into strange rooms, and dogs sniff everyone who comes in the door—it is their way of being cautious. You will want to follow their examples when you are choosing holistic treatments, says Dr. Schoen. There are many new, excellent therapies, but the popularity of holistic care has encouraged some companies to leap into the market with products that haven't been adequately tested or widely used.

It is never easy, even for veterinarians, to separate legitimate break-throughs from trendy but ineffective treatments. You don't want to dismiss odd-sounding remedies just because they are new and unfamiliar. Even penicillin had its doubters at first. But a little healthy skep-ticism—and a large dose of common sense—can keep you out of trouble, says Dr. Schoen.

When you hear that a new product is effective, look for the hard sci-ence and studies that back up the manufacturer's claim. The Internet, which is filled with responsible and authoritative Web sites—along with some that are dubious at best—is a great resource. And holistic veteri-narians will gladly cite by the pound when research is available. The National Institutes of Health conducts ongoing studies into a variety of alternative treatments for people, and many of these treatments, which are often reported in newspapers and scientific journals, work for pets as well. Veterinary journals also publish studies and measure the effects of different techniques. Pets have different needs than humans, of course, so you will want to review these resources with your veteri-narian before trying new therapies yourself.

Some therapies are so new or so unusual that there haven't been any conventional studies. In these cases, you will have to rely on anec-dotal evidence, firsthand experiences from pet owners or veterinarians, says Lori Tapp, D.V.M., a holistic veterinarian in private practice in Asheville, North Carolina. Not all anecdotal evidence is created equal. Someone trying to sell a product will make sweeping claims that you would be right to suspect. Veterinarians or pet owners with nothing to gain will provide more credible evidence.

One of the best things that you can do is trust your instincts, says Dr. Mallu. As long as you know a treatment can't hurt and your veteri-narian has given the go-ahead, you can feel comfortable giving it a try. It very well may help, and that is a gamble worth taking.

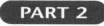

# PART 2

# The Best Choices in Natural Healing

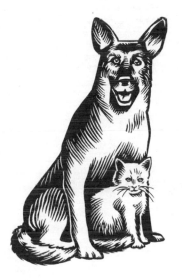

# CHAPTER 4

# Healing with Touch

Whether they are licking sore feet, rubbing a stiff shoulder into the grass, or swooning with delight as you rub their bellies or backs, dogs and cats know instinctively that touching feels good—and is good for them.

Holistic veterinarians have begun to recognize what dogs and cats have known all along—that touching keeps them healthy. Different forms of touch therapy, from massage to acupressure to the gentle application of a warm towel, can ease pain, reduce stress, and help injuries heal more quickly. There is even evidence that serious internal problems like asthma and heart irregularities respond to hands-on care, says David H. Jaggar, D.C., M.R.C.V.S. (member of Royal College of Veterinary Surgeons, a British equivalent of D.V.M.), a holistic veterinarian and chiropractor in Boulder, Colorado, and a founder of the International Veterinary Acupuncture Society.

The great thing about hands-on healing is that you don't have to be a veterinarian to get results. Many forms of touch therapy, like massage and acupressure, are easy to learn and safe to administer. And in some cases, they can reduce the need for drugs or risky (and expensive) medical treatments. The power to cure your pets, say holistic veterinarians, is literally at your fingertips.

Elderly pets with arthritis, for example, can often regain their mobility and play like youngsters again when their owners spend a few minutes a day massaging and stretching their tight muscles and joints. Applying a cold pack to a sprained leg or injured tail numbs the pain almost instantly while reducing swelling and inflammation. It is even possible to control epileptic seizures with acupressure, a simple technique in which you apply finger pressure to specific points on the skin, says Randy Caviness, D.V.M., clinical instructor of small animal acupuncture at Tufts University School of Veterinary Medicine in North Grafton, Massachusetts, and a holistic veterinarian in Concord.

"When you touch your pets, their heart rates decrease dramatically, which indicates that they are relaxing," adds Michael W. Fox, B.V.M. (bachelor of veterinary medicine, a British equivalent of D.V.M.), Ph.D., a veterinary consultant in Washington, D.C., and author of *The Healing Touch*. In fact, many holistic veterinarians use a technique called TTouch (pronounced "tee-touch") to calm pets before and after veterinary treatments. TTouch is thought to reduce stress and help pets heal more quickly.

As a bonus, the same touches that pets love are good for you, too. A number of studies have looked at the "pet effect" and found that animal owners who touch their dogs and cats lower their own blood pressure and stress levels. People with pets also get fewer colds and backaches and are less likely to have insomnia than those without a little furry comfort, says James Serpell, Ph.D., associate professor of humane ethics and animal welfare at the University of Pennsylvania School of Veterinary Medicine in Philadelphia.

## How Touch Heals

It is obvious that dogs and cats love being touched as much as we love touching them. When your dog leans into you with her shoulders and your cat does the Velcro-wrap around your ankle, you know exactly what they are asking for—and you are happy to oblige.

The benefits of touch, however, are more than skin-deep. Holistic veterinarians believe that every inch and aspect of your pet's body, from the muscles in her back to chemical reactions inside her cells, are interconnected. Touching the outside of your pet's body can change what happens on the inside, says Dr. Jaggar.

Veterinarians have found that massage and acupressure stimulate the production of endorphins, natural chemicals in the body that re-

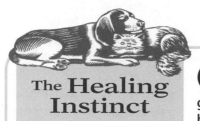

## The Healing Instinct

Cats love to be clean and will spend as much as four hours a day grooming their paws, faces, and bodies. But that licking tongue does more than keep them looking sleek. There is some evidence that daily grooming rituals—for dogs as well as cats—may help relieve stress, tone the muscles, and ease their aches and pains, says Michael W. Fox, B.V.M. (bachelor of veterinary medicine, a British equivalent of D.V.M.), Ph.D., a veterinary consultant in Washington, D.C., and author of *The Healing Touch*.

In fact, pets will "present" their owners with the part of the body that needs attention, says Dr. Fox. A dog with arthritis, for example, will sometimes back into people in order to solicit a rump rub or lean against your legs with her shoulders to get a neck massage. Cats will often butt you with their heads and arch their necks—it is their way of getting a quick massage in a place that is hard for them to reach, he says.

Of course, dogs and cats also get up close and personal simply because they appreciate the attention. "Some pets will become quite demanding," Dr. Fox says.

lieve pain and promote feelings of well-being. Massage also stimulates the lymphatic and circulatory systems, which can help flush away toxic compounds like lactic acid that cause pain, says Junia Borden Childs, D.V.M., a holistic veterinarian in private practice in Ojai, California.

One of the most important benefits of touch therapy is that it may cause subtle shifts in your pet's "energy flow." Just as thoughts are carried by electrical impulses in the nervous system, other forms of energy travel through the body, says Russell Swift, D.V.M., a holistic veterinarian in private practice in Dade, Broward, and Palm Beach Counties in Florida. When the energy flow is blocked or disrupted, pets can experience a variety of physical problems, from itchy skin to diarrhea.

Techniques such as acupressure may correct the body's natural energy balance, stopping problems at the source, says Christina Chambreau, D.V.M., a holistic veterinarian in Sparks, Maryland, and education chairperson for the Academy of Veterinary Homeopathy.

Holistic veterinarians aren't sure exactly how touch therapy works or what happens in the body when energy flows are stimulated, reduced, or redirected. "We don't understand how acupuncture and acupressure reduce nausea, benefit respiratory disease, or increase heart rate and blood pressure, but it is clear that stimulating certain points along the meridians does cause changes in the body," says Mary Rose Paradis, D.V.M., associate professor in the department of clinical sciences at Tufts University School of Veterinary Medicine.

What makes touch therapy so amazing and mystifying is that sometimes the benefits occur a long way from the area being touched. For example, pressing a point on the kidney meridian located on the ankle can be very helpful for pets with anemia or bone-marrow problems, according to Cheryl Schwartz, D.V.M., a holistic veterinarian in San Francisco and author of *Four Paws, Five Directions: A Guide to Chinese Medicine for Cats and Dogs*. This may be because the kidneys produce a hormone called erythropoietin, which stimulates bone marrow to make red blood cells.

## Putting Your Hands to Work

There are many forms of touch therapy. Each works in different ways and is recommended for different conditions. That's why it is important to talk to your vet and get a proper diagnosis before putting your hands to work at home.

Compared to mainstream treatments like giving drugs, most hands-on care is extremely safe. But it is not without risks, warns Dr. Jaggar. For example, even though range-of-motion exercises can strengthen muscles and help pets recover from injuries, stretching joints and muscles too far can make things worse. It is always a good idea to have your vet walk you through the treatment step-by-step before you do it on your own. And of course, you will want to call for help if your pet doesn't get better—or is getting worse—within a day or two after starting the treatments.

Touch therapy (along with holistic veterinary medicine) is still fairly new, so it is not always easy to find a practitioner. To make sure that you are getting the best advice and care, ask your vet (and your friends) for recommendations. Or you can write to one of the holistic veterinary associations. The Alternative Healing Resource Guide on page 434 will help you find experts in your area.

## STANDING TALL

Life wasn't easy for Dana. As sometimes happens with Great Danes, her enormous size—she was over 100 pounds—made it difficult for her to get around. Her hips hurt, and it was hard for her to stand up. It even hurt to wag her tail. Not surprisingly, she was cranky and short-tempered—so much so that her owner finally put her up for adoption.

Enter Patricia Whalen-Shaw, a registered massage therapist and owner of Optissage, an animal massage school in Circleville, Ohio. She knew Dana and her owner and was sure she could help. So she adopted Dana right away. Whalen-Shaw began massaging the painful areas—a little bit each night. She knew that massage would help loosen the muscles and tendons and improve blood flow to the sore spots. She expected to see some improvement but was amazed how quickly it occurred.

Every day, Dana got a little looser and more mobile. She got to the point where she could get up and lie down without any problem, and her pain essentially disappeared. The daily massage even brought the wag back into her life. "Dana went from being an aggressive dog to a happy one," says Whalen-Shaw.

## Massage

One of the most beneficial forms of touch, and one you can do right away, is massage. It is recommended for problems with the muscles, tendons, and other soft tissues. Massaging your pet increases blood flow and removes lactic acid from sore spots, both of which can help her recover more quickly. Holistic vets usually recommend massage for treating muscle spasms, strains, and sprains. It also helps loosen tight tendons and scar tissue from old injuries and is often used on pets with sore hips or a crick in the back.

"You will usually see improvement in two or three treatments," says Michelle Rivera, a certified massage therapist, a veterinary dental technician, and co-owner of the Healing Oasis Veterinary Hospital in Sturtevant, Wisconsin. Massage is also a great way to prevent injuries, she adds, because it loosens muscles and helps keep pets flexible.

Massage isn't only for muscles. It also reduces stress and strengthens the immune system, which can help pets with serious illnesses like kidney or heart disease, says Dr. Fox. For instance, cats that are sick often refuse to eat—and not eating makes them weaker. Giving them a massage can "get the juices flowing" and tickle their appetites back to life, he says.

And because massage helps rid the body of toxins as well as such things as anesthetic and medications, it is often recommended for helping pets recover after surgery, Rivera adds.

## Different Strokes

Every pet reacts differently to massage. Some like a soft touch with your palms or your fingertips, while others crave a deeper knead. You will soon discover your pet's "sweet spots" along with the "shy spots"— areas that she'd just as soon you left alone. Most cats enjoy cheek and chin attention, while dogs will lean on you to invite a back-of-the-rump rub or roll over on their backs for a little tummy attention. You will have to experiment a bit to find the touch and pressure your pet likes best. "If the muscle suddenly tightens, you might be going too hard," says Dr. Fox.

It is really impossible to give your pet too much massage. Dogs and cats with long-term problems, such as arthritis of the hip, will get the most benefits if their owners massage them once or twice a day, every day. Short-term problems, on the other hand, will often get better after one or two short sessions, says Dr. Jaggar.

"Generally, a 10- to 15-minute session is enough for most dogs and cats," says Dr. Fox. When you are ready to roll up your sleeves and go to work, here are a few massage techniques you will want to try.

**Relax them with effleurage.** This is a gentle type of massage in which you use long, slow strokes, moving your palm from the head down to the tail and feet. You can begin and end every massage session with effleurage or use it as a transition stroke when switching to a different technique, says Patricia Whalen-Shaw, a registered massage therapist and owner of Optissage, an animal massage school in Circleville, Ohio.

Effleurage helps move blood through the body and is the best way to help pets relax, Whalen-Shaw adds. She recommends starting with a soft touch, then gradually increasing the pressure. When your pet starts looking sleepy or you hear deep sighs or rumbling purrs, you will know that you have the pressure and pacing just right, she says.

While effleurage is usually used to help pets relax, it can invigorate them, too. This is important if your pet seems depressed, says Dr. Fox. It can also be helpful when you are trying to encourage an overweight pet to get her tail in gear and off the couch. When you are using effleurage to stimulate energy, all you have to do is reverse your strokes—moving up from the tail toward the head—and increase the tempo, he says.

Of course, many pets hate having their fur ruffled, so if this technique appears to be more aggravating than invigorating, you will want to back off.

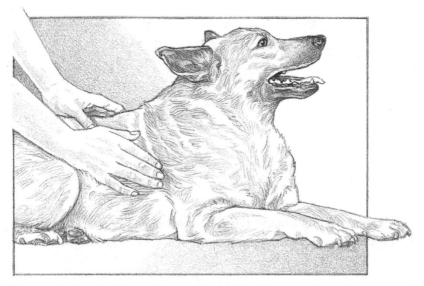

Effleurage, the gentlest form of massage, is used to help pets relax and to prepare the muscles and joints for more vigorous massage techniques.

**Touch away soreness.** Pets that have sore muscles after an overly exuberant run, for example, will appreciate a little fingertip massage. With your fingers extended and held together, rub your pet in small, circular patterns. Exert enough pressure so that you are moving the muscles under the skin and not just gliding over the surface, as with effleurage, says Whalen-Shaw. Continue massaging your pet until you feel the muscles relax.

Fingertip massage is particularly good for pets with sore hips, says Dr. Fox. For back problems, you can massage gentle circles on the back, moving from the neck down to the tail, putting pressure on either side of the spine. Don't press directly on the spine or other bones because that is often painful, he warns.

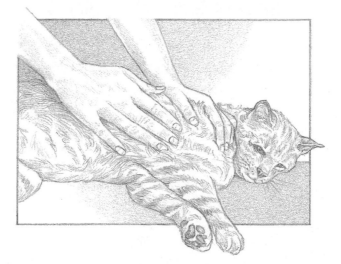

Fingertip massage, in which you use firm pressure to rub the skin and underlying muscles in small, circular patterns, helps relieve soreness.

**Stimulate the muscles with petrissage.** More vigorous than fingertip massage or effleurage, a technique called petrissage helps relax and stretch scar tissue, which is often a problem in pets with arthritis or old injuries, says Dr. Fox. The idea is to grip the muscles next to (but not on top of) bones and give them a gentle squeeze and roll, like kneading bread dough.

The kneading action of petrissage stimulates blood flow and helps the lymphatic system remove waste products from the muscles, says Dr. Fox. Since this technique is quite vigorous, it may be painful for some dogs and cats. He recommends beginning with effleurage to get your pet in the right mood for petrissage. If you don't relax her first, she won't sit still for all the pressure, he explains.

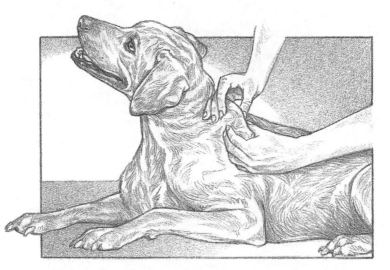

With petrissage, you gently grip the muscles and give them a simultaneous roll and squeeze, like kneading and rolling dough.

**Hit the trigger points.** When muscles are under stress, which often occurs in pets with hip dysplasia or other joint problems, they may form hard little spasms called trigger points. The best way to take the pain out of trigger points is with trigger-point massage. Pressing on trigger points pushes blood out of the muscle. Then, when you relax the pressure, fresh blood flows back in, bringing in oxygen and washing out toxins, says Dr. Caviness.

When your pet is suddenly limping or having trouble moving around, feel around the problem area. What you are feeling for are hard little knots within the muscles underneath the skin. Trigger points are extraordinarily sensitive—your pet will squirm when you hit the bull's-eye.

Using your thumb or forefinger, slowly and gently press down on the trigger point, without rubbing. Hold the pressure for about five seconds, then release it. "This technique is one of those things that hurts and feels good at the same time," says Dr. Caviness. One treatment at a time is enough for each trigger point. In many cases, the knot will disappear right away, and your pet will start moving more comfortably again.

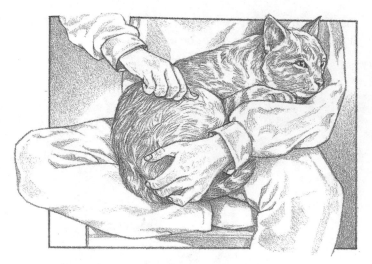

Trigger-point massage, in which you press sore spots with your thumb or forefinger, is used to break up muscle spasms. Your pet will let you know when the massage is too painful.

## Acupressure

Even though acupuncture—a traditional remedy in which long, thin needles are inserted into the skin—has been used for thousands of years, conventional veterinarians were never convinced that it worked. But in 1996, the American Veterinary Medical Association gave the thumbs-up to acupuncture, calling it an "integral part of veterinary medicine."

The problem with acupuncture is that it is not a do-it-yourself remedy—but acupressure is. Using nothing more than the well-placed pressure of your fingers or thumbs, acupressure can help relieve arthritis, diarrhea, and many other conditions.

According to traditional Chinese medicine, your pet's body is filled with a type of energy called *qi* (pronounced "chee") that flows along invisible pathways. These pathways, called meridians, link together every part of the body, including the skin, organs, and muscles. Many holistic veterinarians believe that pets get sick when this natural flow of energy is unbalanced or somehow interrupted, says Dr. Paradis.

Veterinarians have found that you can correct energy imbalances in the body by pressing certain places on the skin called acupressure points. There are hundreds of these points, most located along one of the body's meridians.

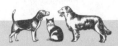

# Animal Magnetism

Holistic veterinarians have discovered that even small magnets may help relieve arthritis, epilepsy, and a variety of aches—with none of the side effects of conventional therapy.

Magnets are thought to promote healing by influencing the body's natural magnetic fields, says Randy Caviness, D.V.M., clinical instructor of small animal acupuncture at Tufts University School of Veterinary Medicine in North Grafton, Massachusetts, and a holistic veterinarian in Concord. All animals, including human beings, have tiny magnetic crystals in their brains, he says. When pets get sick, a little magnetic boost appears to accelerate the body's healing process. Veterinarians have found, for example, that broken bones and wounds heal more quickly when a magnet is placed nearby.

For pets with arthritis, holistic veterinarians will sometimes encourage pets to lie on a large magnet that resembles an electric blanket. For pets with more local problems, such as a broken leg, smaller magnet strips may be placed around the area. In some cases, magnets are fastened against one or more acupressure points. By affecting the body's energy flow, this can help prolong the effects of acupressure or acupuncture treatments. "The magnet stimulates the point in a very gentle but prolonged way," Dr. Caviness explains.

Practitioners who use acupressure identify each point by one or more letters and a number. The letters refer to the meridian the point is on and are an abbreviation for the organ that "rules" that pathway. For instance, an acupressure point with the letter L is the lung meridian, ST is the stomach meridian, and LI is the large intestine meridian. The numbers tell where on the meridian the point is located. So, the point ST25 refers to the 25th point on the stomach meridian.

In the traditional view, pressing an acupressure point either releases excess energy or brings more energy to areas where it is running low. Veterinarians often use a different vocabulary to describe this process, but they have found that the ancients had it right. Many traditional acupressure points are located above areas with concentrated packets of nerves and blood vessels. Pressing these areas stimulates the nerves, which can ease pain and promote healing, says Allen M. Schoen, D.V.M., director of the Veterinary Institute for Therapeutic Alternatives in Sherman, Connecticut, and author of *Love, Miracles, and Animal Healing*.

*(continued on page 34)*

# The Main Points

Thousands of years ago, the Chinese discovered that the body is criss-crossed with energy fields and pathways. They mapped out 14 energy pathways, called meridians, and 361 acupressure points. Every one of these points, alone or in combination with others, can be stimulated to change the flow of energy through the body.

Holistic veterinarians believe that pressing one or more acupressure points can relieve pain, prevent illness, and help the body recover more quickly. Every point affects a different area, of course, so you have to know which one to stimulate. These illustrations show the main points.

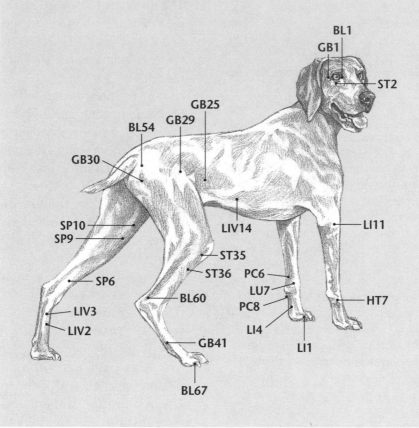

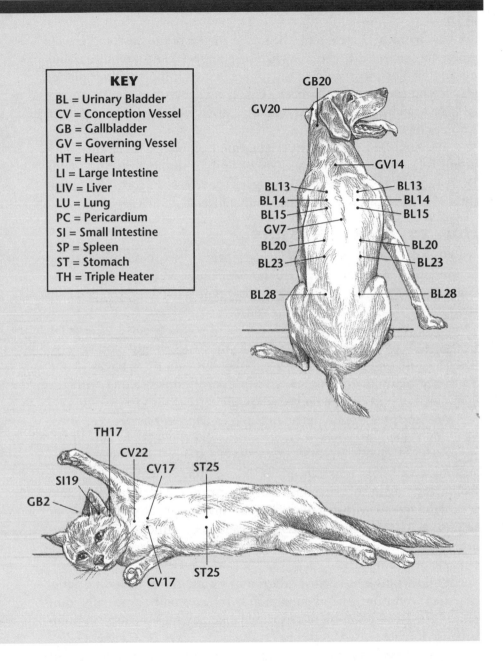

**KEY**

BL = Urinary Bladder
CV = Conception Vessel
GB = Gallbladder
GV = Governing Vessel
HT = Heart
LI = Large Intestine
LIV = Liver
LU = Lung
PC = Pericardium
SI = Small Intestine
SP = Spleen
ST = Stomach
TH = Triple Heater

Essentially, acupressure is like pressing the Off button on disease, he explains.

One pathway, for example, begins at the tip of the nose and travels along the spine to the tip of the tail. Pressing several acupressure points along this pathway—such as the points between the shoulder blades (GV14), at the base of the neck (CV22), and between the front legs (CV17)—can help ease coughs that are caused by bronchitis, according to Dr. Schwartz.

"Research has shown that the stimulation of certain acupressure points releases neurochemicals like endorphins that relieve pain," adds Dr. Paradis. Acupressure can also trigger the release of cortisol, an anti-inflammatory hormone produced in the adrenal glands.

## How to Use Acupressure

Holistic veterinarians spend an intense six months learning acupuncture techniques, but the basic principles are easy to understand. Once you know which acupressure points to target, you can help treat many of your pet's problems yourself.

"Most conditions need a combination of points to correct," says Dr. Caviness. Your veterinarian will show you which points you need to press for different conditions. Refer to the illustrations on pages 32 and 33 to see many of the common acupressure points, along with the symptoms or parts of the body each point corresponds to.

Most acupressure points are located in depressions between muscles and bones. As you stroke your pet, feel for a slight dip in the tissue—it is probably one of the acupressure points. Even if you are not sure exactly where a certain point is, you may be able to find it by feeling for a slight shift in temperature. "A warm point indicates an area where there is an acute energy blockage," says Nancy Zidonis, co-owner of Equine Acupressure in Parker, Colorado, and author of *Canine Acupressure*. "When you find a cold point, it means there is more of a chronic problem and the energy has been depleted from the area."

While acupressure is helpful for many conditions, including acne, diarrhea, vomiting, and asthma, it also relieves pain, especially joint pain. "The BL60 point on the rear ankle is known as the aspirin point because it relieves pain anywhere in the body," says Dr. Caviness.

Unlike many mainstream medical techniques in which a slight error can cause serious problems, acupressure is more forgiving. Even if you are not sure exactly where to press, coming close will still be helpful. If you are trying to relieve hip pain, you can often do it by pressing anywhere near the problem area, even if you are not exactly on the proper acupressure point, says Dr. Caviness. It is not likely that you will overstimulate a point using acupressure, and it is not dangerous to press the wrong point either, he adds.

Even though acupressure is extremely safe, it shouldn't be used for some conditions. Holistic veterinarians believe that pressing acupressure points on pets with cancer may stimulate tumors to grow. In addition, acupressure may be dangerous for treating wounds and infections because the pressure could cause the infection to spread, says Dr. Caviness. It is always a good idea to check with your vet before trying acupressure yourself, he adds.

In many cases, once you know what is causing your pet's problem, acupressure may help correct it. Here's how, says Susan G. Wynn, D.V.M., a veterinarian in Atlanta and co-editor of *Complementary and Alternative Veterinary Medicine*.

🐾 Use the illustrations on pages 32 and 33 to find the acupressure point (or points) that correspond with your pet's symptoms.

🐾 Place your index finger (or your thumb when treating a large dog) on the point and press straight down into the body—don't rub or make circular movements. You want to push hard enough to make an indentation in the tissue, but not so hard that it causes pain.

🐾 Hold the pressure for five seconds to one minute, then release. Repeat the treatment the next day.

You won't often see immediate results, but you should notice some improvement in your pet's condition in 24 to 48 hours, says Dr. Caviness. Acute conditions like a strained muscle will often get better after two or three treatments. But for long-term problems like arthritis, you will have to continue the treatments for some time. For example, your vet may recommend that you press the points once a day for two to three days in a row. After that, you might repeat the treatments every other day or every third day for a few weeks. Then you will probably continue the treatments once a week until the problem is under control.

## Hot and Cold Therapy

You will often see a cat snoozing in a warm patch of sunshine or a dog stretched out on a cool linoleum floor. Pets naturally gravitate to-

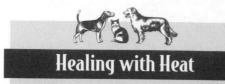

## Healing with Heat

It looks more like witchcraft than veterinary medicine, but science has shown that moxibustion—a technique in which heat is applied to one of the body's acupressure points—is very effective for easing arthritis and other types of long-term pain.

Moxibustion gets its name from *moxa*, the Chinese name for the herb mugwort. When this medicinal herb is wrapped like a cigar, set on fire, and passed back and forth over an acupressure point, the heat "wakes up" nerves underneath the skin, causing the body to release chemicals that help relieve pain, says Randy Caviness, D.V.M., clinical instructor of small animal acupuncture at Tufts University School of Veterinary Medicine in North Grafton, Massachusetts, and a holistic veterinarian in Concord.

Since moxibustion requires the use of "live" fire, it is obviously not something you would want to try at home. But in the hands of a skilled practitioner, moxibustion is quite safe, says Dr. Caviness. The heat quickly passes through the skin and into the nerves, and the healing effects will start right away.

ward warm or cool places—sometimes because they want to get comfortable and other times because they know the change of temperature is good for them. Pets with fever, for instance, may spend hours in a cool bathtub or on a tile floor to lower their body temperatures, says Dr. Schoen.

You can use the power of hot and cold to keep your pets healthy. Applying a cold pack to a bruise causes blood vessels to constrict, reducing blood flow and slowing the production of pain-causing enzymes and chemicals, says Dr. Caviness. Doing this right after an injury can stop swelling and help the area heal more quickly, he says.

For stiff joints, on the other hand, warmth is very helpful. Applying a heating pad or hot-water bottle to the sore spot increases circulation so that blood moves more quickly through the area. "This helps wash out some of the inflammatory enzymes and chemicals that cause the pain," Dr. Caviness says.

It is not always easy to know whether to apply heat or cold. "According to an old Chinese saying, you should heat the cold and cool the heat," says Dr. Schoen. "If you have heat and inflammation, you want to cool that down. If you have a knot and a cold area, you want to increase circulation."

It is not always an either-or situation, he adds. Veterinarians often recommend using a combination of hot and cold. After an injury, such as a sprained leg, you might apply ice right away to reduce swelling and ease the pain. After a day or two of cold treatments, you might switch to heat to improve circulation and speed healing. It is a good idea to ask your vet which treatment will be best for your pet.

## How to Use Heat

Dogs and cats naturally enjoy being warm, so treatments with hot-water bottles, hot packs, sun lamps, or warm baths can be very soothing. For older pets, especially, or those with hip problems, applying a hot pack will provide welcome relief.

When applying heat, here is what veterinarians advise.

**Distribute the heat.** Whether you are using a hot pack, hot-water bottle, or heating pad, start by wrapping it in a towel or a thick blanket. This will spread the heat over a larger area so that it doesn't burn the skin, says Dr. Schoen.

**Keep it low.** Veterinarians have found that a little bit of warmth applied for a long time—say, about 20 minutes—is more effective and safer than hotter applications for shorter periods, says Dr. Caviness. When using a heating pad, put it on the low setting. Fill hot-water bottles with warm, not hot water. If you are using a heat lamp, place it far enough away that it just delivers a spot of warmth—too much heat will make your pet uncomfortable and could cause a burn.

**Watch their signals.** Most dogs and cats enjoy warmth and will happily luxuriate as long as you will let them. When they are ready to walk away, let them go—they instinctively know when they have had enough. If they are seriously injured or can't get away from the heat, make sure that you stay with them so that you can remove the heat within 20 minutes or when they start looking uncomfortable. Pets with serious injuries may get burned if they can't readily move away from the heat.

**Use it sparingly.** While some heat is good, more isn't necessarily better. Dr. Caviness recommends applying heat no more than twice a day.

## How to Use Cold

While heat is usually used for easing muscle stiffness or sore joints, cold is excellent for reducing swelling and inflammation. It also numbs pain quickly, relieves muscle spasms, and helps stop bleeding.

Commercial ice packs work very well, but you don't really need them, says Dr. Caviness. A plastic bag filled with ice or even a sack of frozen peas works just as well. In fact, veterinarians often recommend using frozen peas because the bag will conform to the shape of the body where it is applied, he adds.

Unlike heat, which must be buffered to protect the skin, cold works best when it is in direct contact with the skin. The intense cold will ease pain very quickly and won't harm the skin because pets are protected with thick fur, says Dr. Schoen. In fact, pets with swelling and inflammation usually enjoy the cold sensation and will actually lean into the ice pack to get a little more of it.

Vets recommend applying cold for 15 to 20 minutes, two or three times a day until the swelling goes down. If you are not sure whether you should apply cold, feel your pet's body—you may discover warm areas that need to be cooled, says Dr. Caviness. In most cases, a day or two of cold therapy is plenty, he adds.

## Touching the Emotions

Dogs and cats don't fight with their bosses, fret about the stock market, or worry about crime. But there is a surprising amount of stress in their lives—from trips to the vet or unexpected visitors in the house to the crash of thunderstorms. They don't always understand what's happening, and changes in their routines can upset them and make them nervous. And when dogs and cats are stressed, they often develop behavior problems like missing the litter box or snapping at the man who delivers the morning paper. Stress can even cause physical problems, such as urinary tract infections.

One of the best remedies for stress—in pets as well as people—is a reassuring touch. Dogs that are upset and frightened will often push as close against you as they can—and may even climb into your lap if you will let them. Cats calm themselves with grooming—they will lick their coats for hours when their stress levels are high. But whether it comes from their own rough tongue or their owner's hand, touch is a very powerful remedy for anxiety.

Nearly any kind of touch can relieve anxiety, but a technique called TTouch is especially helpful, says Joyce Harman, D.V.M., M.R.C.V.S., a holistic veterinarian in private practice in Washington, Virginia. Developed by Linda Tellington-Jones, an animal trainer and consultant in Santa Fe, New Mexico, and author of *Tellington Touch: A Breakthrough Technique to Train and Care for Your Favorite Animal*, TTouch is often used to help treat pets with behavior problems that are prompted by stress, fear, or pain. In fact, it is routinely used by handlers at the San Diego Zoo to calm animals before they receive veterinary care.

Veterinarians have found that TTouch actually changes electrical activity in pets' brains. This can help them relax and learn new (and better) ways of relating to people or situations. TTouch is particularly helpful for aggressive or fearful dogs and cats. Even cats that never sat in their owners' laps before can be transformed into virtual love-cats in just a few sessions.

TTouch involves stroking your pet in small, circular movements. There is something about these patterns that appears to change brain activity and makes dogs and cats more receptive to learning. The touches are done all over the body, although the ears are often a favored location, especially for pets suffering from shock or other serious injuries, says Dr. Harman.

The basic technique is called Clouded Leopard TTouch. It is used to heighten a pet's awareness and takes her beyond her usual instincts. Another technique, the Raccoon TTouch, is used for relaxation and also to help wounds heal, says Dr. Harman.

Experts recommend beginning with light TTouches on the top of the head, stroking from the middle of the head out over the ear to the tip, or using light TTouches on the body. Even pets that are shy, aggressive, or in a lot of pain respond well to a little ear attention. But it really doesn't matter where you begin. TTouch anywhere on the body is very soothing, Dr. Harman says.

For large dogs, you can make the circle with all of your fingertips. For kittens and puppies, use one or two fingers. Moving in a small circle, push the skin in a clockwise direction, making sure to complete an entire circle plus a little more. The idea is to move the skin, not just slide your fingers over it. After completing the circle, move your hand an inch or two away to the next location without losing contact with the skin. Then form another circle, and then another, until you have made connected lines of circles all over the body. Using TTouch for 10 minutes a day for a week will often cause a noticeable change in your pet's behavior and stress levels.

# CHAPTER 5

# Using the New Natural Medicines

Modern veterinary medicine has made it possible for dogs and cats to live healthier lives than ever before. Conditions such as diabetes and thyroid disease can now be treated with inexpensive medications. Long-term problems like hip dysplasia are eased with over-the-counter drugs, and most infections can be cured almost instantly with antibiotics.

Conventional drugs, however, aren't perfect solutions. While they are very effective at targeting specific symptoms, they often cause additional problems at the same time. "Aspirin is great at relieving pain, but it can also lead to gastric ulcers and stomach bleeding," says Randy Caviness, D.V.M., clinical instructor of small animal acupuncture at Tufts University School of Veterinary Medicine in North Grafton, Massachusetts, and a holistic veterinarian in private practice in Concord.

A bigger problem is that modern drugs often treat symptoms rather than the underlying causes of disease, says Christina Chambreau, D.V.M., a holistic veterinarian in Sparks, Maryland, and education chairperson for the Academy of Veterinary Homeopathy. It is like giving an itchy dog a shot instead of getting rid of the fleas, she explains. You can relieve the symptoms temporarily, but sooner or later he is going to be scratching again.

Holistic veterinarians believe there is a better way.

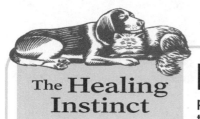

## The **Healing Instinct**

**M**other Nature did more than sprinkle the earth with healing plants. She gave animals the instincts to nibble those plants whenever they are feeling ill.

"When chimpanzees get sick, they will leave the group and go to a particular tree to eat the leaves," says David H. Jaggar, D.C., M.R.C.V.S. (member of Royal College of Veterinary Surgeons, a British equivalent of D.V.M.), a holistic veterinarian and chiropractor in Boulder, Colorado, and a founder of the International Veterinary Acupuncture Society. "Horses will do the same thing," he adds.

At one time, dogs and cats may have shared that healing instinct, says Teresa Fulp, D.V.M., a holistic veterinarian in private practice in Springfield, Virginia. "But they may have lost some of that ability when they became domesticated."

When your cat is demolishing the houseplants or your dog is grazing on the lawn like a sheep, he is probably not doing it because he is sick, she says. He is probably just having a salad for lunch.

Of course, some plants like philodendrons and dieffenbachias can be harmful for pets. So can grass that has recently been sprayed with chemicals. If you are not sure that your pet is eating what he should, ask your vet for advice.

Rather than seeking "cures" in the laboratory, they try to help pets heal themselves. They have discovered that natural medicines and techniques like homeopathy and flower essence therapy can strengthen the body so that it is more resistant to disease. At the same time, many of these "new" medicines will stop symptoms just as effectively as drugs—usually without the side effects.

It is not that holistic veterinarians don't use modern medications—most of them do. But by using natural remedies whenever possible, says Dr. Chambreau, you can keep your pets healthier so that they don't need drugs in the first place.

For instance, the traditional treatment for diabetes is to give dogs and cats injections of synthetic insulin, which allows the body's cells to take in glucose (blood sugar). This controls the symptoms of diabetes, but it doesn't correct the underlying problem. In some cases, however, a combination of natural remedies, including dietary changes and homeopathy, can treat the disease. "I've given diabetic cats homeopathic remedies, and they no longer needed insulin injections," says Dr. Chambreau.

## Getting Started

Natural medicines are very safe and easy to use, but they have to be used responsibly, says Michelle Tilghman, D.V.M., a holistic veterinarian in private practice in Stone Mountain, Georgia. Every pet responds differently to various remedies, she explains. In fact, two pets with exactly the same condition will probably need different remedies and doses because of other factors that may be affecting their health. That's why it is important to talk to your veterinarian before starting a natural treatment program at home.

Even though natural medicines have been around for thousands of years, it is only recently that they have been studied and widely used by veterinarians and pet owners. It is not always easy to find an expert who can help you choose the best natural remedies and provide instructions on using them safely. Ask your veterinarian (or friends who are already using natural remedies) to recommend an expert who is trained in homeopathic, herbal, and nutritional medicine. Or you can write to one of the holistic veterinary associations listed on page 434, which will point you to experts in your area.

## Homeopathy: Helping the Body Help Itself

One of the most exciting natural therapies—and one you can start using right away—is homeopathy. Homeopathic medicine is based on the concept that like cures like. The idea is to give pets minuscule amounts of substances that in larger doses would cause the same symptoms as the disease the pet already has. According to experts, this amplifies the original symptom and "wakes up" the body's defenses, allowing them to recognize the problem and gear up for the attack.

Homeopathic physicians have spent years identifying substances that cause certain symptoms. They do this by testing, or "proving" the substances in healthy people, who then describe what they are feeling. (Pets aren't used in provings because they can't describe their symptoms.) "There are more than 2,000 homeopathic remedies that have

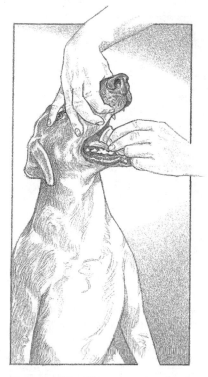

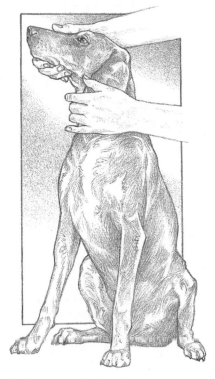

Homeopathic pills are easy to give to dogs. (Don't touch homeopathic pills with your fingers because this can reduce their effectiveness.) Grip the nose with one hand and point it upward. With your other hand, pull down the lower jaw and pop the pill toward the back of the throat.

Hold the mouth closed and massage the throat until you see your dog swallow. Then take a look in her mouth to be sure the pill went down.

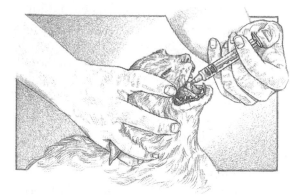

Cats don't like taking pills and will put up a fight when you attempt it. An easier way to get the benefits is to use a homeopathic solution. Draw the solution into a needleless syringe or a dropper, tilt the cat's head back, and squirt the medicine into the side of your cat's mouth.

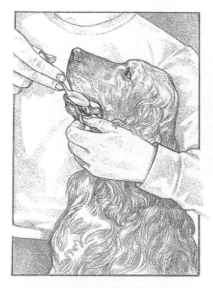

An easy way to give liquid medication to a resistant pet is to gently pull out the back corner of the lower lip, making a pouch. With the head tilted back, pour the liquid into the pouch with the other hand.

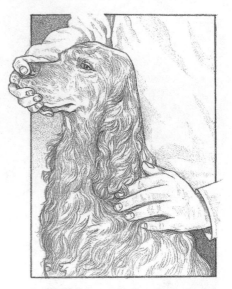

Gently hold your pet's mouth closed, and briefly put your thumb over his nostrils to make him swallow.

been proven," says Dr. Chambreau, "and they work just as well in pets as in people."

When you read the label on a homeopathic remedy, you will see a designation like "1X." This means that the remedy is diluted 1:10, or one part of the active ingredient to nine parts liquid (usually distilled water or alcohol). A dose of 3X means that a remedy has been diluted 1:10 three times. In homeopathy, this is a pretty concentrated dose. Many remedies are 1C, meaning they have been diluted 100 times, or 1M, which have been diluted 1,000 times. It is not uncommon in homeopathy for a remedy to be diluted so much that in a drop of medicine there might not be a single molecule of the active ingredient.

The extreme dilution of homeopathic remedies has led mainstream veterinarians to call the entire system into question. How, they ask, can a remedy with *no* molecules of the original substance possibly be effective? Homeopaths believe that the process of repeatedly diluting and shaking (or succussing) encodes the liquid with a "memory" of the original substance. "The more it is diluted and succussed, the more powerful the remedy becomes," Dr. Chambreau explains. That means the 3 potencies (10-times dilutions) are weaker than the M potencies (1,000-times dilutions). This runs counter to modern science, which holds that things get weaker as they get more dilute.

Homeopathic remedies made for use at home usually are the lower potency X-strength, while C- and M-strength remedies are typically used by veterinarians, says Teresa Fulp, D.V.M., a holistic veterinarian in private practice in Springfield, Virginia.

Some researchers speculate that the active ingredients in homeopathic remedies are so minute that they are able to slip through the body's blood-brain barrier, possibly influencing the nervous system in ways that can't be measured yet. In one study, researchers from the University of Washington and the University of Guadalajara looked at 81 children with diarrhea. They found that children treated with homeopathy got better 20 percent faster than those given an inactive (placebo) drug. And in one large study, in which scientists in the Netherlands reviewed 107 smaller studies, they found that 75 percent of the research showed homeopathy to be effective. What works for people, veterinarians say, clearly works for pets as well. "We can't explain exactly how it works, but it is powerful medicine," says Dr. Chambreau.

## Putting It to Work

Drugs are generally effective no matter who is taking them, but homeopathic remedies require more of an individualized approach. For instance, a remedy called Nux vomica is often used to treat diarrhea caused by eating rich food. When the diarrhea is caused by something else, the preferred remedy might be Arsenicum. It often takes some trial and error before matching the right remedy with each pet, Dr. Chambreau says.

Homeopathic medicines don't always work quickly, she adds. Short-term problems like diarrhea may get better after giving your pet just a few homeopathic doses. Long-term conditions like arthritis often require long treatments because it takes time for the body to mobilize its defenses.

You can buy books (called materia medica) that list all the homeopathic remedies. Dr. Chambreau recommends a book called *Organon of the Medical Art* by Samuel Hahnemann, the founder of homeopathy.

For simple problems like a sore paw or runny nose, it is perfectly safe to follow the instructions in this or other books and do homeopathy yourself at home, says Dr. Fulp.

"Even if you give the wrong remedy by mistake, it is not likely to do harm," adds Russell Swift, D.V.M., a holistic veterinarian in private practice in Dade, Broward, and Palm Beach Counties in Florida.

You can buy homeopathic remedies at health food stores and some pet supply stores. It is fine to use human homeopathic remedies for pets, says Dr. Fulp. "Your pet's size makes absolutely no difference in the amount you give," she adds. "All that matters is how frequently you give it. Giving it more often makes it stronger."

Homeopathic remedies can be expensive. But since the doses are very small and the unused portions last nearly forever, you get a lot of medicine for your money. A good way to begin is to pick up a "home kit," which will include several remedies, along with instructions on using them. When you are just getting started, here is what holistic veterinarians advise.

**Try one thing at a time.** Even though dogs and cats often have more than one symptom when they are ill, you should use only one remedy at a time. Using too many remedies may disrupt the "energy field" in the body and interfere with healing, says Dr. Fulp. This is especially true when you are using a remedy blend, she adds. Don't give your pet additional remedies—including non-homeopathic treatments like flower essences or acupressure—unless your vet tells you to.

**Watch for results.** While most short-term problems like vomiting or swelling will go away on their own, they may clear up more quickly when they are treated with homeopathic remedies. "If your pet isn't feeling better within two to three days, you have probably chosen the wrong remedy, and you will want to call your vet," says Dr. Fulp.

**Give less instead of more.** Unlike drugs, which are designed to knock out symptoms entirely, homeopathic remedies are only meant to help the body heal itself. In most cases, you will give the remedy for a day or two, then stand back while your pet's natural healing powers go to work. "You want to try a remedy and then stop to see what happens," says Dr. Chambreau.

**Handle them carefully.** Homeopathic remedies can lose their power when they are exposed to electromagnetic fields, such as those produced by television sets or even your body. Touching the medicine with your hands can reduce its potency or, if it is absorbed through your skin, affect you more than your pet, says Dr. Fulp. You don't want to hide homeopathic remedies inside treats either. They must be given without any "sugar coating," she explains. And don't feed your pet within 15 minutes of giving a remedy.

**Keep them pure.** Homeopathic remedies may lose their effectiveness when they are exposed to heat or sunlight or if they are stored near strong-smelling substances like coffee or perfume. When stored carefully—preferably in a dark, cool place—they will retain their potency just about forever, says Dr. Fulp.

## Herbs: Nature's Drugs

Drugstore convenience hasn't always been around the corner. Long before scientists began putting medicine in capsules and pills, veteri-

## Call the VET

Herbal remedies are often much safer than their pharmaceutical counterparts, but they still contain powerful compounds. You should always check with your vet before starting herbal treatments at home, especially if your pet is taking other medications, says Allen M. Schoen, D.V.M., director of the Veterinary Institute for Therapeutic Alternatives in Sherman, Connecticut, and author of *Love, Miracles, and Animal Healing*.

Pets with heart problems, for example, are often treated with a drug called digitalis. An herbal remedy for heart problems is hawthorn (*Crataegus laevigata*). When the two are given together, they can amplify each other's effects, essentially causing an overdose, says Dr. Schoen.

Another potential problem is that herbs aren't as precisely regulated as drugs. An herb from one manufacturer may be two or three times stronger than an identical herb from another manufacturer. The only way to be sure that your pet is getting the right herb and the right dose is to check with your vet first.

# The 15 Top Herbs

The U.S. Department of Agriculture has cataloged more than 80,000 herbs, many of which are thought to have healing powers. For the majority of health problems, however, you only need to use a few herbs. Here are the herbs veterinarians often recommend. To be safe, you'll want to talk to your vet before using them at home.

| Herb | Used to Treat |
| --- | --- |
| Aloe (*Aloe vera*) | Constipation, skin irritation |
| Calendula (*Calendula officinalis*) | Skin injuries |
| Chamomile (*Matricaria recutita*) | Skin irritation (topical), stomach problems, mild stress |
| Comfrey (*Symphytum officinale*) | Skin injuries (topical only) |
| Dandelion (*Taraxacum officinale*) | Water retention |
| Echinacea (*Echinacea angustifolia* or *Echinacea purpurea*) | Infections, inflammation |
| Eucalyptus (*Eucalyptus globulus*) | Nasal congestion |
| Ginger (*Zingiber officinale*) | Nausea, motion sickness |
| Ginkgo (*Ginkgo biloba*) | Old age, mental dullness |
| Goldenseal (*Hydrastis canadensis*) | Infections, bronchial inflammation |
| Hawthorn (*Crataegus laevigata*) | Heart irregularities |
| Milk thistle (*Silybum marianum*) | Liver problems |
| Red clover (*Trifolium pratense*) | Bronchitis |
| Slippery elm (*Ulmus rubra*) | Diarrhea, constipation, coughs |
| Valerian (*Valeriana officinalis*) | Stress, pain, aggression |

narians were carefully harvesting herbal remedies. Today, we often think of herbs as being old-fashioned, but, in fact, a large percentage of today's medicines are actually derived from their herbal counterparts.

Even when herbs contain almost the same chemicals as modern drugs, they are sometimes more effective because they haven't been whittled down to a single component. Willow bark (*Salix alba*), for example, contains a chemical very similar to aspirin, making it an effective pain remedy, says Dr. Caviness. And other things in the willow bark help protect against gastric ulcers, a major side effect of aspirin therapy, he says.

Holistic veterinarians have found that most herbs, from dandelion (*Taraxacum officinale*) to marigold (*Calendula officinalis*), contain veritable pharmacies of active ingredients within their seeds, roots, leaves, and bark. This means that one herb may be used for many conditions. For instance, slippery elm (*Ulmus rubra*) contains natural compounds that can help stop diarrhea, says Dr. Tilghman. It also contains substances that will ease a sore throat.

Holistic veterinarians rarely use herbs alone, Dr. Tilghman adds. They often combine herbs with conventional medicines, giving your pet the best of both worlds. Dogs and cats with an infection might be given antibiotics to knock out the bacteria and an herbal tonic containing astragalus (*Astragalus membranaceus*) to strengthen the immune system. "Tonics can increase white blood cells, which boost the immune system and make pets more resistant to disease," she explains.

Herbal remedies can be confusing at first. There are dozens of common healing herbs, and they come in many forms—fresh, dried, concentrated, or packed into capsules. Here are a few tips for making the right choice.

**Pick the right form.** Even when the active ingredients are the same, herbs have different effects, depending on how they are prepared and packaged, says Susan G. Wynn, D.V.M., a veterinarian in Atlanta and co-editor of *Complementary and Alternative Veterinary Medicine*.

🐾 Bulk herbs. These can be fresh and green or dry, crumbly, or powdered. Bulk herbs are usually prepared by mixing them into food or steeping them in hot water, which releases the active compounds. The resulting teas and decoctions work quickly because they are absorbed very readily by the body.

🐾 Extracts and tinctures. These are liquid, concentrated forms of herbs. As with herbal teas, they pass quickly through the intestinal wall and are often recommended when pets need fast relief, such as from pain. Extracts and tinctures can be mixed a drop or two at a time in a glass of water and poured on your pet's food. Or you can put them straight in your pet's mouth. Some tinctures are made by soaking herbs in alcohol, which may be dangerous—as well as unappetizing—for cats. Other tinctures are glycerin-based, which may be better for some pets.

Extracts and tinctures can be quite powerful, and doses vary widely, so it is important to talk to your vet before using them.

🐾 Tablets and capsules. Nothing is more convenient than giving herbs in pill or capsule form—assuming that your pets don't mind taking them. Herbal tablets and capsules are just as effective as fresh herbs as long as you use them before their expiration dates.

**Know your supplier.** Unlike drugs, which are produced and packaged with scientific precision, the strength of herbs can vary from batch to batch, depending on such things as climate, soil conditions, and which fertilizers were used. The only way to be sure that you are getting the best quality is to ask your vet to recommend a reputable supplier, says Nancy Scanlan, D.V.M., a holistic veterinarian in private practice in Sherman Oaks, California.

**Read the label carefully.** Many herbs have similar-sounding names—for example, bitterstick, used to strengthen immunity, and bitterroot, used for asthma and breathing problems—so it is easy to choose the wrong one. Some manufacturers list both common and scientific names on the label, which helps prevent confusion.

**Shop for freshness.** Fresh and dried herbs don't last forever, says Dr. Tilghman. When buying packaged herbs, look for expiration or harvest dates on the label. When buying them in bulk form, put your nose to work. Fresh herbs should smell fresh. If they smell dry or musky, they have probably given up their essential oils and won't be as effective.

**Store them carefully.** Herbs quickly lose strength when they are exposed to light and heat, so be sure to store them in a cool, dark place. Some herbs will react with chemicals in plastic containers, so it is better to store them in glass instead.

## Flower Essences: Good Vibrations

Dogs and cats enjoy life best when things are calm and predictable. Sudden changes in their routine—anything from a move to a new house to an incoming thunderstorm—can make them anxious and insecure. And any kind of emotional turmoil can lead to health and behavior problems later on.

One of the best ways to soothe nervous pets is with flower essences, says Dr. Fulp. Made from the essential (and greatly diluted) oils of wild

# Essential Essences

Holistic veterinarians often recommend flower essences for healing the emotions. The essences can be quite expensive, so you don't want to buy more than you need. Here are 12 flower essences that veterinarians recommend.

| Essence | Used to Treat |
| --- | --- |
| Aspen | Fear of the unknown |
| Beech | Intolerance |
| Centaury | Excessive submission |
| Larch | Lack of confidence |
| Mimulus | Fear of the known |
| Rescue Remedy | Mental or physical trauma |
| Rock rose | Terror |
| Star-of-Bethlehem | Shock |
| Vervain | Overenthusiasm |
| Vine | Dominance or aggression |
| Water violet | Aloofness |
| Willow | Resentment |

plants, trees, and bushes, flower essences such as Bach Flower Remedies are known as vibrational therapy, meaning that they help return the body's emotional energy fields to a proper balance, she explains.

Holistic veterinarians usually use a single flower essence to treat specific types of emotional stress. The essence mimulus is good for soothing fears. "Vervain calms nervous energy, vine helps stop aggression, and rock rose helps with terror," says Dr. Fulp. In some cases, several flower essences are combined into one remedy. The essence called Bach Rescue Remedy contains the essences impatiens, star-of-Bethlehem, cherry plum, rock rose, and clematis. "Rescue Remedy is good for any kind of stress because it helps make pets more mellow," she says.

Flower essences are harmless, and accidentally using the wrong one won't cause problems, Dr. Fulp adds. They usually work quickly,

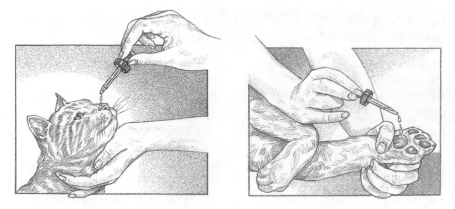

Holistic veterinarians recommend flower essences for many different emotional and physical problems. The essences are very easy to administer. You can either squirt the proper amount in your pet's water bowl, or you can put a few drops on the bridge of her nose or the pads of her paws, where they will quickly be absorbed into the body by licking.

and your pet should start feeling better within a few days. You can use flower essences by themselves or in combination with other therapies. In most cases, however, it is best to keep things simple, she says. "Using three or less at a time will usually give the best results."

Flower essences are very easy to use. "For cats, put a couple of drops in their water bowls so that they sip it all day long," says Dr. Fulp. "For dogs, drip the essence directly into their mouths or put it on their noses to lick off. Veterinarians usually advise giving one to three drops a day until your pet is feeling better. When giving the drops directly, don't let the dropper touch their skin or mouths. Otherwise, the bottle will become contaminated, she explains.

You can buy flower essences in most health food stores, and some pet supply catalogs are carrying them as well. They are usually sold near a chart or list that explains which essences are recommended for different conditions. As with most natural remedies, flower essences should be stored in glass bottles away from direct sun, microwaves, or heat.

## Aromatherapy: The Power of Scents

Dogs and cats have phenomenal senses of smell; they can read odors the way people read Post-it Notes. But odors do more than communicate messages, as any cat worth his catnip knows. Holistic veterinarians have discovered that certain scents act like medicines, affecting the body on a biochemical level. But rather than being absorbed from the stomach, as with pills, the fragrant scents used in aromatherapy are absorbed by the mucous membranes in the nose. The chemicals of the aromas go straight to the brain, explains Dr. Fulp.

Holistic veterinarians have found, for example, that the scent of lavender oil causes temporary sedation and helps pets relax. Other aromas can lower blood pressure, slow the heartbeat, and ease feelings of anxiety.

The oils used in aromatherapy are available in health food stores and some pet supply catalogs. The oils usually come from natural sources, although synthetic (and cheaper) versions are available. As with flower essences, you can buy single oils or oil blends. "I once treated a cat who was refusing to eat and was extremely ill with a respiratory infection," says Dr. Fulp. "Within 10 minutes after giving him a powerful decongestant blend, he was up, walking around the cage, and demanding food."

Holistic veterinarians have only recently begun working with aromatherapy and have just begun to document what these oils can and cannot do. Until more is known, says Dr. Fulp, it is essential to check with your veterinarian before using aromatherapy on your own—especially because some oils, like peppermint and pennyroyal, can be dangerous or even fatal when used on pets.

Once your veterinarian has recommended aromatherapy and given you the proper oils, here is how to put them to work.

**Dilute the oil.** The essential oils used in aromatherapy are much too strong to use straight from the bottle. "Dilute the oil half-and-half with a vegetable oil like peanut oil," says Dr. Fulp. This will prevent burning if it touches the skin. Use essential oils only where your pet can't lick them off—on his ears or the back of his neck. It may be safer to use a diffuser, which vaporizes the scent into the air.

**Aim for the ears.** When using aromatherapy, it is important to apply the drops where the scent will reach the nose and the oils will penetrate the skin. "Massage a drop or two on the inside of the ear tip where there is not much fur," says Dr. Fulp. "That's near the face so the pet breathes the scent, but he can't reach it to lick it off."

**Use it briefly.** Unlike drugs, which may be taken for days or weeks, aromatherapy usually works very quickly. "It's almost always a short-

## ALTERNATIVE

# 🐾SUCCESS

## TURNING BACK THE CLOCK

Starsky moved pretty well for a 16-year-old—once he got going. But getting up in the morning or climbing stairs had become increasingly difficult for the husky-shepherd mix, so his owner decided to get some help.

"I took Starsky to my conventional vet, and he just threw drugs at him," says Jim Grisanzio, a science and medical writer in Marlboro, Massachusetts. The drugs didn't really help, Jim recalls, and the side effects were making Starsky worse. "I tossed the medicine in the garbage and found a holistic vet."

His new veterinarian immediately recommended a new diet because Starsky had a little bit too much padding under his fur, which was putting extra strain on his sore joints. The vet also recommended that Starsky take alfalfa (*Medicago sativa*) mixed in a little applesauce for the hip pain.

This simple prescription made all the difference. Starsky started losing weight, and his limp went away. Within three months, the pain in his hips seemed to be gone, and Starsky was getting up and down the stairs without a hitch. "He was feeling great," Jim says.

term treatment," says Dr. Fulp. "The effects usually wear off in four to six hours, but one treatment is usually enough," she says.

When your pet doesn't get better right away, it is fine to use aromatherapy three times a day for one or two days. After that, you will need to call your vet, Dr. Fulp advises.

## Dietary Supplements: Nutritional Cures

Even when you give your pets an all-natural, high-quality food, there is still a possibility that they aren't getting all the nutrients they really need. That is why many holistic veterinarians recommend giving dogs and cats dietary supplements—not just for maintaining overall health but also for fighting disease.

There are diseases that have been linked to previously unrecognized deficiencies of certain nutrients, says Dr. Scanlan. "For instance, the recommended minimum amount of taurine in cat foods had to be increased in recent years because cats weren't getting enough and were developing blindness and heart disease."

While some dietary supplements are used simply to improve your pet's diet, they are being used more often to treat specific conditions. Pets with arthritis are sometimes given supplements made from green-lipped mussels. They contain compounds called glycosaminoglycans, which can help heal and rebuild damaged cartilage. "And using omega-6 and omega-3 fatty acids together in the right ratio can reverse skin problems like dandruff and reduce itching caused by allergies," adds Dr. Scanlan.

Nearly all holistic veterinarians and an increasing number of mainstream vets are now recommending that dogs and cats be given vitamin C and E supplements. Both of these nutrients are powerful antioxidants that help reduce the effects of free radicals, harmful oxygen molecules that are naturally produced by the body. Supplementation with these nutrients can help slow the aging process so that pets live longer, says Dr. Scanlan.

Dietary supplements don't give fast results, she adds. Fatty-acid supplements may take a month or more before they cause noticeable improvements in skin conditions. Other supplements, like vitamin C, work slowly over a lifetime. You may not notice any difference at all in how your pet is acting or feeling. But at the cellular level, changes will be happening—changes that will help keep your pet healthy and strong for the rest of his life.

Even though many dietary supplements are quite safe, they shouldn't be used indiscriminately. For one thing, supplements may interfere with other medications that your pet may be taking. More important, every dog and cat has different needs and will require different amounts of various substances. Don't assume that the human doses listed on labels are appropriate for dogs and cats. "Supplements are like any other medicine," says Dr. Scanlan. "You shouldn't use them without talking to a veterinarian who is knowledgeable about nutritional therapy."

## Water: The Liquid of Life

Water is so common that it is strange to think of it as medicine. But holistic veterinarians believe it is one of the best "drugs" for protecting your pet's health. Water does much more than quench his thirst. It regulates his body temperature, aids in digestion, and lubricates his tissues. More important, it is the body's mass-transit system. It is constantly transporting oxygen and nutrients to cells throughout the body and carrying away the wastes.

Holistic veterinarians don't write prescriptions for water, but it is an essential part of many treatment plans. Pets with constipation are often encouraged to drink more because water lubricates the digestive tract and helps stools move smoothly, says Carin A. Smith, D.V.M., a veterinary consultant in the state of Washington and author of *101 Training Tips for Your Cat*. Water can also flush away bacteria that cause urinary tract infections, and a high-water "diet" is often recommended for pets with urinary stones. For pets with arthritis or hip pain, using water externally—in the form of a good swim—will strengthen the joints and help prevent pain.

You can't force your pets to drink more water. What you can do is make water more appealing. Here are a few tips veterinarians recommend.

**Buy bottled water.** Many pets dislike the smell (and taste) of chlorine and other substances in tap water, says W. Jean Dodds, D.V.M., adjunct professor of clinical sciences at the University of Pennsylvania School of Veterinary Medicine in Philadelphia and owner of Hemopet, a national nonprofit animal blood bank in Irvine, California. Bottled spring water is inexpensive, and most pets prefer it to tap water, she says.

**Add a little flavoring.** When you want your pet to drink more, try adding a little flavor to his water bowl by pouring in a small amount of juice from a can of clams, for example. "My dog loves the water that's left after boiling meat or chicken," Dr. Smith says.

**Put gravy on the menu.** One of the easiest ways to help your pets get more fluids is to moisten their dry food with a little water, says Dr. Smith. Or give them moist or canned foods, which contain a lot more water than dry kibble.

**Change the bowl.** Dogs and cats are extremely sensitive to odors, and plastic water bowls may develop "off" smells that discourage them from drinking more. Switching to glass or ceramic bowls will prevent odor buildups, Dr. Smith says.

## CHAPTER 6

# Natural Diets– The Advantages

They drool at the scent of a Thanksgiving turkey, come running at the "whir" of the can opener, or try to swipe bacon from your breakfast plate. For pets, eating is one of life's dearest pleasures—it is an instinct that once helped them survive.

Pets today fill their stomachs by begging for handouts or simply waiting for kibble to appear in their bowls. But it wasn't always so easy. Your dog's ancestors ate anything that didn't move faster than they did, from unwary birds or unattended eggs to ripe fruit or riper fish. Cats were more finicky, even in bygone times. They wanted food that was still wriggling and would swallow bite-size mousy morsels in one gulp—hair, skin, bones, and all.

"Wild" diets gave dogs and cats everything they needed to stay healthy. They got protein and fat from meat, calcium from crunching on bones, and vegetables from the digestive tracts of their prey. Gnawing on bones and chewing through tough skin even provided natural dental care by scrubbing their teeth clean.

Over the centuries, however, dogs and cats gradually moved from the barnyard into the backyard. Rather than hunting their own food, they waited for their humans to feed them. As a result, the menu changed. Rather than eating mice or fallen fruit, they feasted on ready-to-eat

*(continued on page 60)*

# "Bone Appétit"

Veterinarians have traditionally recommended keeping bones away from dogs and cats because the combination of sharp teeth and strong jaws can reduce some bones to splinters, which could damage your pet's insides.

According to holistic veterinarians, however, a little supervised bone chewing is very good for your pet's health. Chewing is nature's way of keeping the teeth clean. In some cases, regular bone chewing can virtually eliminate the risk of dental disease, says Allen M. Schoen, D.V.M., director of the Veterinary Institute for Therapeutic Alternatives in Sherman, Connecticut, and author of *Love, Miracles, and Animal Healing*.

Besides, it is not the bones themselves that cause problems, but cooking the bones, which makes them much more likely to splinter than when they are raw, says Susan G. Wynn, D.V.M., a veterinarian in Atlanta and co-editor of *Complementary and Alternative Veterinary Medicine*.

Of course, a big dog (or a determined cat) can reduce even raw bones to splinters. You need to pick a bone that is too big to swallow and too tough to break apart. Small dogs and cats enjoy raw turkey or chicken necks, says Dr. Wynn. For larger pets, she recommends raw lamb shanks or knuckle bones.

She advises blanching raw bones for 15 to 30 seconds in boiling water to kill bacteria. (The bacteria in meats is more likely to harm humans than pets.) It is also important to watch your pet chew. If he is reducing bones to splinters or is chewing hard enough to break a tooth, you will want to play it safe and give him chew toys, such as those made by Kong, instead. Your vet will help you decide whether bones or chew toys are best for your pet.

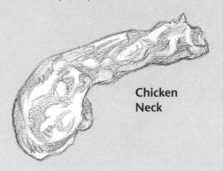

**Chicken Neck**

Turkey or chicken necks are best for cats and small dogs who chew lightly and won't crack the bones.

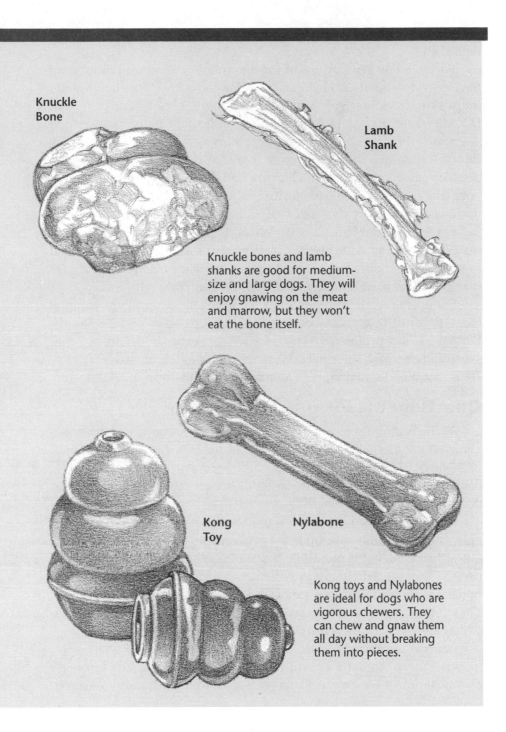

**Knuckle Bone**

**Lamb Shank**

Knuckle bones and lamb shanks are good for medium-size and large dogs. They will enjoy gnawing on the meat and marrow, but they won't eat the bone itself.

**Kong Toy**

**Nylabone**

Kong toys and Nylabones are ideal for dogs who are vigorous chewers. They can chew and gnaw them all day without breaking them into pieces.

packaged foods. And their health, say holistic veterinarians, may have paid the price.

Within a few generations of moving indoors, dogs and cats began having symptoms that they may not have had before, like bad breath, itchy skin, intestinal gas, and dull, dry coats, says Susan G. Wynn, D.V.M., a veterinarian in Atlanta and co-editor of *Complementary and Alternative Veterinary Medicine*. These symptoms appeared so slowly that veterinarians didn't realize at first that there was a problem. As decades passed, things like bad breath and dandruff came to be seen as normal. "But flaky skin isn't healthy," she explains. "To holistic veterinarians, it is an early sign that something is wrong."

Part of the problem, says Dr. Wynn, is that commercial pet foods may not always provide all the nutrients that some dogs and cats need to be healthy at different times in their lives. They also provide things that pets don't need, like chemical additives and preservatives.

Some chemicals in foods have been linked to problems ranging from dandruff or a greasy coat to liver disease, says W. Jean Dodds, D.V.M., adjunct professor of clinical sciences at the University of Pennsylvania School of Veterinary Medicine in Philadelphia and owner of Hemopet, a national nonprofit animal blood bank in Irvine, California.

## Questionable Progress

At the beginning of the twentieth century, technological advances changed the way that Americans ate and the way they thought about their diets. "Natural" foods came to be seen as old-fashioned, while packaged, processed, ready-to-eat foods became the norm not only for people but also for their pets.

Even when commercial foods are made with high-quality ingredients, they invariably give up some of their nutrients, along with their digestibility, during processing. And some commercial pet foods don't use the best ingredients in any event, says Nancy Scanlan, D.V.M., a holistic veterinarian in private practice in Sherman Oaks, California. They often contain meat by-products or vegetable sources of protein, which aren't always easy for pets to digest, she explains.

In order to replace some of the nutrition that processing takes out, manufacturers sometimes add nutrients to pet foods. But throwing chemicals into a bag or can isn't a great substitute for natural nutrition, says Dr. Scanlan. Nor does it always make a lot of sense. For example, pet foods are often sprayed with artificial flavors or dyed with artificial colors, even though dogs and cats couldn't care less what color their dinners are.

One preservative that has raised concern is propylene glycol, which has been used to keep moist pet foods fresh. Veterinarians have discovered that it causes a type of anemia in some cats and may lead to bloat in dogs. "This is another example of why those of us practicing holistic medicine are nervous about foods with artificial preservatives," says Dr. Scanlan. "We're afraid that if you use even tiny amounts long enough, they may cause problems."

Pet food manufacturers try to make their products safe and nutritious, of course. But even the best safety studies typically look at only one ingredient at a time, often for six months to two years. Holistic veterinarians worry that chemicals that may appear to be safe when they are studied for just a few years may turn out to cause long-term problems. And even if a chemical is safe by itself, it is difficult to tell what will happen when it is combined with other chemicals in the body, like those from flea medications, says Dr. Dodds.

## Back to Basics

Most holistic veterinarians are convinced that the single most important thing that you can do for your pet's health is to give him a more natural diet. A balanced natural diet gives cats and dogs shiny coats and healthy skin and keeps them lean, happy, and energetic, says Russell Swift, D.V.M., a holistic veterinarian in private practice in Dade, Broward, and Palm Beach Counties in Florida. "I've seen natural diets improve digestive problems such as chronic colitis, diarrhea, and constipation. And I've seen dramatic improvements in pets with kidney disease and liver problems."

Some national pet supply stores—and all stores specializing in holistic pet health—carry a wide range of natural foods, such as Innova, Wysong, Solid Gold, PetGuard Premium, and California Natural. Also available through mail order, these and other natural foods typically contain high-quality ingredients and don't use chemical additives or preservatives.

Even though commercial natural foods are preferable to their main-

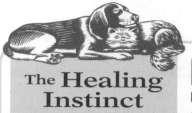

## The Healing Instinct

Pets aren't the most discerning eaters. They will snack on roadkill or live goldfish as enthusiastically as they down a bowl of fresh kibble. But there is some evidence that their tastebuds are guided by their bodies' needs.

Studies have shown, for example, that dogs have a large number of "sweet" tastebuds. In the evolutionary scheme of things, this caused them to seek out the ripest fruits and vegetables, which are usually the sweetest as well as the most nutritious and digestible, says Allen M. Schoen, D.V.M., director of the Veterinary Institute for Therapeutic Alternatives in Sherman, Connecticut, and author of *Love, Miracles, and Animal Healing*.

Cats don't go for sweets, but they do crave meaty flavors. This is important because cats, unlike dogs, are true carnivores. Their natural craving for meat makes it possible for them to get all the essential amino acids, which are found mainly in meats.

So the next time your dog noses up to your ice cream cone or your cat comes running when the steak's on the grill, don't assume it is because of bad manners. They are just doing what comes naturally.

stream counterparts, no processed, artificial food is perfect for every pet, especially pets with health problems. To get the most benefits, says Dr. Wynn, "you may want to feed your pets fresh foods as well."

Many holistic veterinarians, in fact, recommend bypassing commercial foods altogether and making all of your pet's food at home, using only the freshest, most wholesome natural ingredients. "A natural diet should duplicate as closely as possible what pets used to eat in the wild," says Dr. Swift.

This doesn't mean putting cans of "mouse mousse" on the pantry shelf. Nor does it mean turning your pets loose to forage in the field, where they will encounter harmful parasites along with modern-day traffic on country roads. What it does mean is trying to duplicate the balance of proteins, carbohydrates, fats, and other nutrients that dogs and cats were designed to eat, says Allen M. Schoen, D.V.M., director of the Veterinary Institute for Therapeutic Alternatives in Sherman, Connecticut, and author of *Love, Miracles, and Animal Healing*.

Every pet is different, of course. Dogs and cats need different amounts of protein and fat. Puppies and kittens need more calories than adults. Pets with conditions such as diabetes, kidney problems, pancreatitis, or food allergies can't always eat the same foods as other pets. So before starting your pet on a natural diet, it is essential to work closely with your veterinarian to plan the proper approach.

"For example, wild animals get their calcium from eating raw bones," says Dr. Scanlan. A natural diet consisting of raw or cooked meat won't provide this calcium. That's why most homemade natural diets include calcium supplements, often in the form of bonemeal. You will need to check with your vet about the proper amounts to add.

Dogs and cats might also benefit from fruits and vegetables, which, in nature, they got from consuming the stomachs and intestines of their prey, says Dr. Scanlan. Giving them vegetables is an acceptable substitute, she adds.

The most important step in planning a natural diet is to provide the right mix of nutrients. For dogs, this usually means one-third protein, one-third vegetables, and one-third grains, says Dr. Scanlan. "Cats have a higher requirement for meat protein, so they need roughly one-half meat, one-quarter vegetables, and one-quarter carbohydrates." Every pet has different needs, so it is a good idea to discuss these amounts with your vet.

Ripe vegetables and fresh meats contain the highest amounts of nutrients, so you may find yourself shopping a little more often, Dr. Scanlan adds. It is worth doing because dogs and cats have a nose for freshness—give them meat or produce past its peak, and they will likely turn up their whiskers.

It is also a good idea to shop for organic foods so that fewer pesticides or other chemicals find their way into your pet's diet, notes Dr. Swift.

Feeding your pet a natural diet isn't as convenient as tearing the top off a bag. But once you are in the habit, it only takes a few minutes a day—and the benefits can last a lifetime. Here is what holistic veterinarians advise.

**Pick the right protein.** Almost any kind of meat will provide plenty of protein as well as the necessary fat. Holistic veterinarians often recommend beef, chicken, turkey, lamb, pork, or venison. Seafood, eggs, and tofu are also good on occasion. Avoid using too

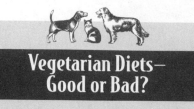

## Vegetarian Diets— Good or Bad?

More and more Americans are switching to vegetarian diets, either because of health concerns or because they have moral objections to eating meat. What's good for people, some owners believe, is also good for their pets.

But it's not that simple. While humans originally ate a "wild" diet consisting mainly of fruits, vegetables, and grains, dogs and cats have always included meat in their diets. Even though it is possible for a dog to survive—or even thrive—on a well-planned vegetarian diet, cats must have meat in order to survive.

Cats are "obligate carnivores," which means that they require certain nutrients that only meat provides, says Susan G. Wynn, D.V.M., a veterinarian in Atlanta and co-editor of *Complementary and Alternative Veterinary Medicine*. "Vegetarian diets are never appropriate for cats," she says.

much tuna, however, because many cats will become addicted and won't want anything else.

For older pets or those with dental problems, you may want to cut the meat before putting it in the bowl. "You can use ground or diced meat to help your pet adjust, but it is more natural and better for dogs and cats to eat larger chunks so that they have to chew or tear the meat," says Dr. Swift. Chewing larger pieces of meat will help keep their teeth clean, he explains.

**Add some carbohydrates.** Your pet's brain and muscles are fueled by sugars and starches, which they get from carbohydrates. Whole grains like brown rice and barley are excellent sources of carbohydrates. So are sweet corn, potatoes, and whole-grain breads.

Dogs and cats don't digest grains as readily as they do meats, so it is important to cook grains in order to unlock the nutrients inside. Simmer rice or other grains until they are soft. To add a little extra flavor, cook them in chicken or beef broth, which most pets find appealing.

**Add some vegetables.** We don't usually think of vegetables when planning our pets' diets, but vegetables are great sources of vitamins, minerals, and dietary fiber. Some of the best vegetables for pets include carrots, zucchini, broccoli, celery, parsley, cucumber, alfalfa or bean sprouts, and beets, along with leafy greens like spinach and chard. Giving your pet several vegetables with each meal will provide the widest range of nutrients, says Dr. Swift.

You don't need to cook or peel the vegetables, he adds. In fact, you don't want to because most of the nutrients are found in the skins. "The vegetables should be pureed, blended, or juiced to pulverize them the way they would be found in the wild diet," says Dr. Swift. You can add some extra flavor to the mix by adding a little bit of broth or garlic before blending. Don't use onions, however, which can be dangerous for cats.

**Add some innards.** "Organ tissue like liver, kidney, heart, spleen, and brain are a normal part of a carnivore's diet, but it is nearly impossible to find all of them in the grocery store," says Dr. Swift. He recommends supplementing a homemade, natural diet with a multiple-glandular supplement for pets, such as Pet G.O., available by mail order. Multiple-glandular supplements for humans can also be used. Give one-quarter of the human dose to cats and dogs under 15 pounds, one-half of the dose to those 15 to 30 pounds, and the full dose to dogs over 30 pounds.

**Give a digestive aid.** Since dogs and cats traditionally got their vegetables secondhand by eating their prey, the vegetables were easy to digest. When they are eating raw vegetables, however, they may need some extra help. "Supplementing their diet with digestive enzymes helps the process along," says Dr. Swift. He recommends giving them enzymes made specifically for pets, such as Vet-Zime, Prozyme, or FloraZyme, following the directions on the label.

**Plan ahead.** The one drawback to homemade natural diets is that they don't have a long shelf-life, so you will have to prepare them fairly often. You can store homemade natural meals for about three days in the refrigerator. Or you can freeze meal-size servings, which will last indefinitely.

Once you have put the food out, however, it will go bad fairly quickly. Dr. Swift recommends leaving the food out for no longer than 20 minutes. If there are any leftovers after that, throw them away. You can be sure that your pet will be a little hungrier by the time the next meal comes around.

**Make the change slowly.** Giving pets a new food—even one that is wholesome and homemade—may upset their stomachs at first. In ad-

**ALTERNATIVE**

## ☙ SUCCESS

### C. J. BOUNCES BACK

C. J. had always been a happy, enthusiastic dog whose greatest joy was his food. When C. J.'s appetite disappeared along with his energy, his owner knew right away that something serious had to be wrong.

It turned out that C. J., an eight-year-old mixed breed, had chronic kidney disease. His veterinarian offered medications, but not a lot of hope. C. J. only had about six months to live, the vet said.

His owner wasn't going to give up that easily, so he turned to alternative medicine. One of C. J.'s new doctors, Russell Swift, D.V.M., a holistic veterinarian in private practice in Dade, Broward, and Palm Beach Counties in Florida, found that compounds in the blood had accumulated to toxic levels—a common occurrence in pets with kidney disease. Making problems worse were the cooked-meat ingredients in C. J.'s food. Cooked meat isn't completely digested in the intestines, and the leftover waste products were straining C. J.'s kidneys to the breaking point.

Dr. Swift immediately put C. J. on a raw-food diet and sent him home. The raw ingredients would be easier for C. J.'s body to digest, Dr. Swift told his owner, which in turn would put less strain on the kidneys.

Two weeks later, the payoff was clear: Follow-up tests showed that C. J.'s blood-waste levels had dropped by 50 percent. His energy and his appetite had started returning as well. "The raw-food diet completely reversed the signs of disease," says Dr. Swift.

dition, some pets, especially cats, won't eat new foods unless they are just as pungent and intensely flavorful as what they were eating before. To make a successful transition to a natural diet, you have to introduce it slowly.

For the first few days, replace about one-eighth to one-quarter of your pet's usual food with the natural food, says Dr. Wynn. Every day, add a little bit more of the new food while taking away some of the old.

If you do this slowly, most dogs and cats will keep eating heartily without ever noticing the difference.

It is also a good idea to warm the food slightly before putting it out. Warm temperatures intensify the aroma, which is especially important for cats. In addition, anything that adds a strong flavor to the food will whet your pet's appetite. You can temporarily spike it with sardines, for example, or a little canned tuna juice. Or you can simply wet it with a little chicken or beef broth, says C. A. Tony Buffington, D.V.M., Ph.D., professor of clinical nutrition at the Ohio State University Veterinary Hospital in Columbus.

Fresh-food diets are typically more satisfying than commercial foods, and most pets will eat a little less than they did before. Some, however, will find their new diets so tasty that they will eat all day if you let them. Ask your vet how much you should be serving, and then stick with it no matter how much your pet begs for more.

## The Raw Diet

Each time your cat ambushes a bird or your dog snaps up a gopher, they are tasting life as their ancestors experienced it—raw. Many holistic veterinarians believe this is still the best approach to their diets.

Cooking can destroy vital nutrients and make meats harder to digest, says Dr. Swift. Raw beef, for example, has considerably more taurine, an essential amino acid for cats, than cooked beef does. In addition, heat may change the molecular structure of foods, he says, making it harder for enzymes in the body to break down proteins. This results in incomplete digestion, which puts strain on the entire body.

"We know that there are problems with things like *E. coli*, salmonella, and parasites in raw meat," adds Dr. Scanlan. To get the benefits of a raw-meat diet while reducing the risks, she recommends using only fresh meat, keeping it refrigerated before serving it to your pets. (Avoid using raw pork or fish, which may contain parasites.) You can also rinse raw meat with food-grade hydrogen peroxide, mixing a teaspoon of the peroxide in a quart of water. Or you can lightly steam or boil the meat, says Dr. Schoen.

"A healthy digestive tract has many natural defenses," adds Dr. Swift. "Remember, animals have been eating raw foods forever. The risks of processed foods are much greater."

# What's in It for Your Pet?

Holistic veterinarians recommend giving pets commercial natural foods because they contain whole foods without chemical additives and preservatives. Common pet foods found in supermarkets, on the other hand, contain ingredients that may be less than ideal. We asked Susan G. Wynn, D.V.M., a veterinarian in Atlanta and co-editor of *Complementary and Alternative Veterinary Medicine*, to analyze the ingredients in a popular supermarket pet food. Here are her impressions.

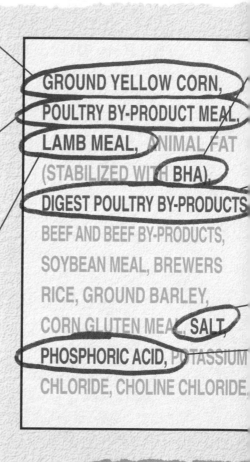

This is a good protein and carbohydrate source, but since most cats and dogs are meat-eaters, I would prefer to see it third or fourth on the list. That is where you will see it on most high-quality food labels, where meat is the first ingredient and reappears within the top three.

This is one of those terms that is hard to interpret. "By-products" could be organ meat, which is nutrient-rich. But they could also be necks and feet, which are fairly indigestible. Natural foods would probably use the highly digestible and nutritious whole chicken or chicken meal, which is what I'd rather see.

At least this is whole lamb and not by-products. Meal is essentially dehydrated meat and organs and is a good source of protein and other nutrients. But if this were first on the label instead of third, it would be a sign that this food contains more meat, which is better for our carnivorous pets.

GROUND YELLOW CORN, POULTRY BY-PRODUCT MEAL, LAMB MEAL, ANIMAL FAT (STABILIZED WITH BHA), DIGEST POULTRY BY-PRODUCTS BEEF AND BEEF BY-PRODUCTS, SOYBEAN MEAL, BREWERS RICE, GROUND BARLEY, CORN GLUTEN MEAL, SALT, PHOSPHORIC ACID, POTASSIUM CHLORIDE, CHOLINE CHLORIDE.

BHA is an artificial preservative, which is probably not safe to eat every day. Artificial preservatives aren't necessary if the food sits on the shelf less than two months. Most natural brands use safer natural preservatives like rosemary extracts, vitamin C (ascorbic acid), or vitamin E (natural mixed tocopherols).

Even the best pet foods lose some of their nutritional value during processing, so manufacturers routinely supplement them with extra vitamins and minerals, such as potassium and vitamin $B_{12}$. It is a reasonable way to ensure that pets get all the nutrients they need.

**ITAMIN SUPPLEMENTS**

**, A, $B_{12}$, $D_3$), COPPER SULFATE, ANGANESE SULFATE, NIACIN, ALCIUM PANTOTHENATE, IBOFLAVIN SUPPLEMENT VITAMIN $B_2$), THIAMIN MONONI-RATE (VITAMIN $B_1$), POTASS-UM IODIDE, PYRIDOXINE YDROCHLORIDE (VITAMIN $B_6$), ODIUM SELENITE, FOLIC ACID, IOTIN**

This is fairly meaningless, and you probably won't find it in natural foods. It is actually unidentified meat parts and fat that have been sprayed onto kibble to give it flavor. Given its location on the label, it probably doesn't contribute much in the way of nutrition. If it were higher up, I would be worried since by-products sometimes aren't the best source of nutrients.

Healthy pets aren't as sensitive as people to the effects of salt, so it is really not a problem. On the other hand, it doesn't add anything useful beyond taste.

This is a metallic-tasting ingredient that is typically used as flavoring in commercial food. When natural-food companies add extra flavoring, they use the real stuff—garlic or other spices.

## Cooking for Convenience

Even though a fresh-food, natural diet is very good for your pet's health, not everyone has the time (or the inclination) to cook from scratch. That's okay. You can combine the benefits of a natural diet with the convenience of commercial foods by giving your pets a little bit of each—a packaged pet food mixed with a few leftovers from your table.

"Many people are convinced that dogs and cats won't thrive unless they feed them very carefully, but that's simply not true, says Dr. Buffington. "If you are feeding your pet high-quality processed food and are also throwing in some broccoli or fish once in a while, you are not going to disrupt the balance."

Choosing the right commercial foods can be tricky, adds Michael W. Fox, B.V.M. (bachelor of veterinary medicine, a British equivalent of D.V.M.), Ph.D., a veterinary consultant in Washington, D.C., and author of *The Healing Touch*. One way to tell if the food you are buying is high-quality is to look at the label. It should say that the food has "passed feeding trials established by AAFCO." This organization, the American Association of Feed Control Officials, is responsible for regulating the quality of pet foods. Its seal of approval means that dogs and cats given the food stayed healthy and thrived during the testing period.

Of course, foods that carry the AAFCO label may still be filled with chemical additives and preservatives. "There are a few natural commercial foods out there that are quite good, but they are not always widely available or easy to find," says Dr. Wynn. Regardless of the food you are buying, it is worth taking a minute to read the label to make sure that you are getting the highest quality. Here is what to look for, according to experts.

🐾 Ingredients in pet foods are listed on the label in descending order. Those at the beginning of the list are more plentiful than those toward the end. For cats, choose a food that has meat as the first and second ingredients, says Dr. Wynn. Ideally, it should be the same in dog foods, she adds, but meat can be at least two of the top three ingredients.

🐾 The best pet foods will list meat, beef, chicken, or other whole foods on the label, says Dr. Scanlan. Avoid those that list food "fractions"—for example, wheat middlings or corn gluten instead of the whole grain—since these ingredients are often the leftovers from human food processing and don't provide the best nutrition. "You want it to say 'meat' or the next best thing, 'meat meal,'" she says. "You don't want anything that says 'by-products.'"

🐾 Some preservatives are necessary for preventing natural foods from becoming rancid. Just make sure that the preservatives are also natural, says Dr. Dodds. These include vitamin C (also called ascorbic acid), vitamin E, or mixed tocopherols. Watch out for synthetic preservatives such as ethoxyquin, BHA, BHT, propylene glycol, or propyl gallate, she says.

🐾 Quality foods get most of their flavor from the ingredients themselves but may use some natural seasonings as well, says Dr. Wynn. Look for seasonings such as spices or garlic. Avoid foods with artificial flavor enhancers like phosphoric acid.

🐾 Dogs and cats don't care what color their food is, but some manufacturers put colors in anyway. Some coloring agents, such as those made from carotenoids, are perfectly healthful. Others, like azo (a coal-tar derivative) and nonazo dyes, are pure chemistry and should be avoided. You should also stay away from color preservatives like sodium nitrite, says Dr. Wynn.

It is not always easy to find natural pet foods that meet all these criteria, says Dr. Wynn. "It takes some research to find everything out, but holistic vets have already done this work for you, so ask for their recommendation."

# CHAPTER 7

# Healing with Thoughts, Feelings, and Sounds

When you are sick, your cat keeps you company. Your dog hides during arguments with the kids. When you are feeling blue, your pets act depressed, too. Dogs and cats are so deeply influenced by what they see, hear, and sense that our words and emotions have the power to hurt—and to heal.

With their sharply tuned senses and their ability to perceive the most subtle signals, dogs and cats are intimately involved with everything around them. They react to things that we are barely aware of, from the sound of the wind or the tone of our voices to the composition of the light that surrounds them. Some holistic veterinarians believe that these and thousands of other things emit a kind of vibrational energy, which, if properly directed, can be used to heal the body as well as the mind.

In the last few decades, an increasing number of veterinarians have begun using "energy therapies" derived from nature's invisible but potent healing potential. They have found that they can use such things as music, light, color, crystals, and even thoughts to treat a variety of problems, from pain and emotional stress to problems with the immune system, says Teresa Fulp, D.V.M., a holistic veterinarian in private practice in Springfield, Virginia.

These therapies are still in their infancy, however, so veterinarians aren't entirely sure how they work. But research suggests that they *do* work, in some cases better than medications and other conventional treatments. Researchers have found, for example, that listening to music for as little as 15 minutes may bolster the immune system. Lowering stress has also been shown to strengthen immunity, which is why you can make dogs and cats stronger simply by acting—or even thinking—calmly around them, says Deborah C. Mallu, D.V.M., a holistic veterinarian in private practice in Sedona, Arizona.

The wonderful thing about energy healing is that you don't have to be a veterinarian to use these techniques. Everyone can learn how to use music or crystal therapy. In fact, keeping your pet healthy is sometimes as simple as talking to her when she needs reassurance or switching on the radio when she is feeling stressed.

Since these therapies are still quite new, not all holistic veterinarians practice them. In some communities, in fact, the only place you will find animal communicators or color or crystal healers will be on the bulletin boards in health food stores. Some of these practitioners will be veterinarians, but others will not. It will probably be another 10 years or longer before energy healing becomes widely available. In the meantime, you can start using the healing energy from your own mind and body to keep your pets healthy.

## Healing with Thoughts

When you have a backache or your head throbs, you are able to tell your doctor how rotten you feel. This is important because much of your doctor's diagnosis is based on your "history," or what you tell him. Dogs and cats don't have the advantage of speech, but understanding what they are feeling is just as important for their health. The problem is that many people, including veterinarians, don't know how to "listen."

Dogs and cats understand a lot more than we give them credit for—not only the words we use but also the pitch, intonation, and emotions in our voices. Their uncanny attention to detail makes them seem like mind readers, and it explains why they always seem to be hiding when we are ready to give them baths. "We share a consciousness with our pets," says Dr. Mallu. "We are not separate, but are interconnected on an energetic level."

Veterinarians have noticed, for example, that pets often get depressed or sick or refuse to eat when there is a lot of emotional turmoil in their families. This is because pets and people inhabit the same fields of energy, says Dr. Mallu. When you are feeling poorly, those feelings will spill over to some degree to your pet.

Positive feelings also spill over, which is why it may be possible to heal physical and emotional pet problems by changing negative thoughts to ones that are more upbeat, says Kathleen Carson, D.V.M., a holistic veterinarian in private practice in Hermosa Beach, California.

This isn't the same thing as telepathy, Dr. Fulp adds. Your pet doesn't literally read your thoughts any more than you will hear little dog and cat voices in your head. But people do mentally communicate with their pets in subtle ways. Holistic veterinarians call this animal communication, but you will recognize it as plain old intuition.

You have probably had a vague feeling at one time or another that something isn't quite right with your pet, and then come home from work or gotten up in the morning to discover a soiled rug that proved you were right. By trusting more in your intuition, it may be possible to get a jump on your pet's health problems. And once you start communicating positive messages with your thoughts, you will find that your pet will feel better and heal more quickly, no matter what is causing the underlying problem, says Dr. Fulp.

## Developing Your Inner Ear

Some people have such a strong natural gift for animal communication that dogs and cats may as well shout messages in their ears. But for most of us, it takes practice, and faith, to develop a clear sense of what our pets are trying to tell us, says Dr. Carson.

Dogs and cats communicate in dozens of ways—with their tails, their facial expressions, the way they stand or sit, even with the light in their eyes. The more attentive you are, the more quickly you will learn how to read this silent language to understand what your pet is thinking and feeling. "You will develop a connectedness with your pet that you can't put into words, but it will just start happening," says Dr. Mallu. "Then one day you will hear her tell you something. Maybe you will wake up knowing that she doesn't feel well, and then you will discover that you were right."

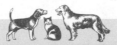

# Healing with Color and Crystals

When you deck out your dog with a bright red sweater or put a jeweled collar on your cat, you are doing more than making a fashion statement. You may be focusing nature's energy in such a way that it can result in powerful healing.

Many holistic veterinarians have begun treating pets with crystals and light therapy, which they believe collect and transmit energy from the world around them. This energy consists of vibrations, which penetrate deep into the body. When properly directed, the vibrations can rebalance the body's natural energy and help restore pets to physical and emotional health, says Lauren Chattigré, D.V.M., a holistic veterinarian in private practice in Boring, Oregon.

Scientists have long been aware that light has healing properties. When light travels into the eyes, for example, it signals the pineal gland to produce melatonin, a hormone that controls rest and relaxation, says Kathleen Carson, D.V.M., a holistic veterinarian in private practice in Hermosa Beach, California. Different colors of light have different effects, she adds. Farmers sometimes bathe their animals in blue light, which makes them calmer and easier to handle. Pink light, by contrast, appears to make animals more aggressive.

Crystals act a little bit differently, says Dr. Chattigré. Like little generators, they store and focus energy from nature and pass it into the body. "You will actually feel a little zing from the resonance when you hold the right stone," she says.

There are many types of crystal and light therapy, and every pet will have different needs, says Dr. Chattigré. To start out, you will need to see a holistic veterinarian who specializes in these forms of healing. Once you know what your pet needs, you can buy the appropriate crystals in gem and crystal shops and from specialty catalogs. Light therapy is even easier to use because you can buy colored lightbulbs in hardware stores.

Most people have trouble trusting their intuition, Dr. Mallu adds. Don't. Even if the images that form in your mind seem really weird, make a note of them. Write them down or tell someone. Once you start keeping track, you will be amazed how often your intuition turns out to be right.

Dr. Mallu recommends setting aside 10 to 15 minutes every few days when you can simply relax without distractions. Ideally, your pet will be in the same room, but you can practice even when she is off doing her own thing. All you have to do is let your mind wander and consciously be receptive to what your pet is thinking and feeling or what she wants to tell you. You won't get a flood of messages all at once, she says, but over time you will find that you are much more aware of what your pet is feeling. And when there is something wrong, you will know it at the same time she does and will be prepared to take action.

Animal communication goes both ways, of course, so you will want to be sure that your pet understands what you are saying to her. One of the best ways to do this is to mentally visualize what you are trying to communicate. Dogs and cats don't completely understand human speech, but pets and people see exactly the same things. These mental pictures can provide common ground between you and your pets.

## Healing with Love

With every stroke and kind word, we tell our pets we love them— and their purrs and tail-wags leave no doubt that they are returning our affection. But the love we have for our pets goes beyond making us (and them) happy. There is some evidence that love can heal the body as well as the emotions.

Every living thing is flooded with a type of energy, or life force, that comes from nature, says Dr. Fulp. This energy is responsible for nourishing the body as well as the mind, just as the oxygen we breathe nourishes cells throughout the body. In order for this energy to work, however, it must flow freely into and throughout the body. That doesn't always happen because emotions such as fear or depression can cause blockages that prevent the energy from getting in. This can result in a variety of problems, from aggression or destructive behavior to heart disease, she says.

Veterinarians who specialize in energy healing believe it is possible to use your own life force to clear these blockages from your pet's body, allowing healing energy to pour in. Energy healers often transmit energy by a laying on of hands. Physical contact isn't always necessary, however, because you can use the power of your mind to affect the energy field, called the aura, that surrounds living things. This is called off-the-body healing, and it seems to work even when the healer and the pet are miles apart, says Dr. Fulp.

Energy healing may sound like wishful thinking, and in fact, nobody understands exactly how it works. Scientists are trying to develop tools or techniques that will explain what happens when life-force energy is exchanged and healing takes place. In the meantime, you can still practice energy healing. There are many testimonials—not only from pet owners but also veterinarians and former skeptics—that suggest it may be effective.

One of Dr. Fulp's colleagues, a mainstream veterinarian, consulted her about a tortoiseshell cat that belonged to a staff member. "Sissy had been paralyzed for three days, and they couldn't figure out what was wrong," she says. So Dr. Fulp rolled up her sleeves and went to work. Surrounded by six skeptical staff members, she stroked the palms of her hands just above Sissy's body, using them like metal detectors to find the problem area. When her palms passed over Sissy's neck she felt a tingle similar to static electricity, indicating that's where the energy was blocked. So she focused her life-force energy into the blockage. "Even though I wasn't physically touching her, Sissy and I both felt a kind of snap, and we flinched," says Dr. Fulp. Sissy jumped up and walked away, and everyone cried. "I suspect the energy broke up a blood clot, but there is no way to know for sure," she says.

You don't have to worry about something going wrong when you use energy healing. "Trust yourself," says Dr. Mallu. "Healing energy is pure love. It can't do harm, and it will only help. Here is how to begin.

**Get grounded to contain the energy.** "If you aren't grounded during the healing, your energy just bounces around like a Ping-Pong ball," says Dr. Mallu. Grounding connects you to the earth and directs life-force energy just as a leash helps direct your pet's bouncing energy. You don't have to stand in a certain place, she adds. All you have to do is stand in a relaxed position with your back straight and say out loud, "I want to be grounded." Concentrating on your energy gives it direction and purpose, she explains.

**Ask your pet what's wrong.** Don't worry about clearing your thoughts or getting into a meditative state, says Dr. Mallu. When you suspect something is wrong, just ask—and listen to the answer. It may be as subtle as a vague impression about a certain part of the body or as distinctive as a voice telling you that she swallowed a bee or hates your new work schedule. Once you know what the problem is, you will be in a much better position to begin solving it.

## ALTERNATIVE

# 🐾SUCCESS

## HEALED WITH ENERGY

Annee was less than a year old when her owner, Meredith Hart of Mosier, Oregon, noticed a problem with her affectionate calico cat. It started when Annee began licking her fanny for long periods of time. Then Annee began to shake and shiver when she slept. "Her whole body jerked and trembled every time she lay down," says Meredith. Annee lost her appetite, too, and soon she was down to about eight pounds and was refusing to eat at all.

Lauren Chattigré, D.V.M., a holistic veterinarian in private practice in Boring, Oregon, found Annee to be thin but otherwise fairly normal. She offered Meredith conventional testing, but Meredith wanted to try a noninvasive approach first. Dr. Chattigré decided to use intuitive methods to find "blockages" in Annee's energetic field. "Her mental and physical bodies were fighting each other instead of working together," she says. She suspected the problem might be related to a rough recovery from anesthesia, which had occurred when Annee was spayed.

In the meantime, Dr. Chattigré treated Annee with Reiki, an energetic healing modality; flower essences; and blue light. Within a day, Annee's twitching and licking had been reduced. And a week later, she was symptom-free.

**Open your heart to healing.** Consciously ask that your emotional blocks, worries, and concerns be let go. If you don't do this, your own blockages will interfere with the healing. It is also important to ask that your heart be opened to help with your pet's healing. This sets the "intent" in place, which is like priming a pump to get the energy flowing, says Dr. Mallu.

**Heal with your hands.** The palms of your hands are the pipeline that feeds healing energy into the problem area, says Dr. Mallu. For instance, you will place your hands on your pet's shoulders to ease stiff joints or over her lower back above her kidneys to help with kidney problems. The energy may not flow evenly from each hand, so Dr. Mallu suggests that you balance the energy by using both hands, putting your dominant hand (that's your right hand if you are right-handed) over the problem spot and the other hand on the opposite side of the body. You can touch your pet or hold your hands just above her body.

Even though energy healing works best when it is done under the supervision of a holistic veterinarian, it is effective even when you don't know exactly what is wrong with your pet, says Dr. Mallu. "The unity consciousness means that your hands are energetically connected to your pet, so trust that your hands know where to go."

**Send love into the hurt.** The key to energy healing is to flood the problem area with love, says Dr. Mallu. Try to imagine a healing light that pours from you into your pet. "You melt and soften problems with energy, and that energy is love," she explains.

## Healing with Sounds

Rambunctious kittens settle down when Mom-cat purrs them to sleep, and fretful puppies get quiet when you put a ticking clock in their beds to remind them of their mother's heartbeat. Every pet owner knows that certain sounds calm their pets, while others make them upset. It makes sense because sound is vibration, and vibration is transmitted through the skin to all parts of the body.

Holistic veterinarians have found that sounds influence the body's natural rhythms. Some sounds speed up these rhythms and cause an increase in energy; other sounds slow them down, says Mary Lee Nitschke, Ph.D., professor of psychology at Linfield College in Portland, Oregon, and an animal behaviorist in Beaverton.

Research has shown that sound causes physical changes in the body. Music with a rhythm of about 60 beats a minute, for example, slows electrical activity in the brain, causing pets to feel more relaxed and peaceful, says Dr. Nitschke. It also slows breathing and the heartbeat and helps the body's metabolism work more efficiently. Studies have also shown that listening to music releases endorphins, natural painkillers that are produced by the brain, and reduces the levels of stress hormones in the body.

Sound therapy is still pretty new, although some of its applications have been around for a while. For instance, veterinarians and doctors use a form of sound called ultrasound to take pictures of the inside of the body. Doctors have also used sound waves to break up kidney stones. More recently, doctors as well as veterinarians have begun using sound therapy to treat a wide range of emotional problems, says Donna M. Starita, D.V.M., a holistic veterinarian in private practice in Boring, Oregon.

Some holistic veterinarians suspect that sound therapy will someday be as powerful and widely used as acupuncture, homeopathy, or other modern therapies. More research needs to be done, but sound therapy, which often includes the use of music, clearly has potential, says Dr. Starita. "I use music to communicate with the body at an electromagnetic level to bring it into balance," she adds. In other words, music may be able to retrain the body's cells, such as those in the heart or lungs, to operate at a normal, healthy rhythm.

Some holistic veterinarians have begun using pure tones—a single sound frequency generated by a tuning fork—to heal a variety of illnesses. The advantage of this type of sound is that it can be directed through the skin to problem areas in the body. "For instance, it is very effective at reducing inflammation and bringing energy into an unbalanced area, like an inflamed disk in the back," says Dr. Starita. Experts in sound therapy use a variety of tuning forks—there are 12 different tones in Western music—to get specific results, she explains.

A simpler way to get the benefits of sound therapy is to use music. Dogs and cats that are stressed or upset will often calm down when they listen to soft music with a slow, steady rhythm, says Dr. Nitschke. There is even some evidence that this type of music helps pets with arthritis relax their muscles and improve their range of motion.

Many pets seem to enjoy Mozart or other classical composers. Soft jazz and New Age music can also be very soothing. So are sounds from nature, says Dr. Mallu, who has installed a water fountain in her examining room because the sound of running water helps pets stay calm.

Of course, some pets don't need soothing music—quite the opposite. Dogs and cats that are tired and lethargic will often benefit from louder music with more of a driving beat. This will temporarily raise their blood pressure and, in many cases, their spirits as well.

# CHAPTER 8

# Exercising for Total Health

Puppies and kittens bounce off the walls as if they had springs on the bottoms of their feet. Their high energy may drive you nuts at times, but it is a natural leftover from life on the wild side, when it prepared furry babies for survival as adults. Pets evolved to race and pounce their way through life.

Today, of course, many dogs and cats happily spend their leisure time snoozing on the sofa or lounging on windowsills. But before they were domesticated, they had to work for a living. Unless they stayed in great shape, dogs and cats went hungry. It was the only way they could capture mice, birds, rabbits, and other prey. This day-to-day business of feeding themselves kept their muscles toned, their bellies trim, and their bones, hearts, and digestive tracts strong.

Nothing changed at first when dogs and cats became a part of the human family. They continued to work, but as partners with their owners. Dogs worked as hunters, trackers, herders, guardians, and shepherds. Cats continued to perform rodent patrol, keeping down the marauding mice that threatened grain stores. And since most owners lived in rural areas, dogs and cats usually had access to the outdoors with unlimited fields to roam in. They stayed in pretty good shape.

## Slower Times

Fast-forward to modern life. People began moving from farms to suburbs and cities, and dogs and cats came with them. Within a few decades, most dogs and cats were spending their days in living rooms, backyards, or city parks, often at the end of a leash. The only exercise they got was when their owners had time to take them out—and most people were too busy to be thinking about exercise. So pets spent their days lounging around. According to holistic veterinarians, that is when their health went downhill. Dogs and cats began to have problems they'd rarely had before, like weight gain, constipation, and arthritis, says Ihor Basko, D.V.M., a holistic veterinarian in private practice in Honolulu and Kilauea, Hawaii.

About one in three dogs and cats in this country are overweight because they don't get enough exercise. They are prone to joint problems—without exercise, the joints don't stay lubricated. They have behavior problems since pets without outlets for their energy are more likely to become aggressive, frustrated, or destructive, says Wayne Hunthausen, D.V.M., a veterinary behaviorist in Westwood, Kansas, and author of the *Handbook of Behaviour Problems in Dogs and Cats*. Veterinarians have become accustomed to hearing stories about dogs chewing through linoleum or pulling the stuffing out of sofas or cats who spend their days shredding the living-room drapes. In just the last 10 to 20 years, behavior problems have become so common that many veterinarians expect most pets to develop them at some time in their lives, he says.

## Back to Basics

Holistic veterinarians and their mainstream counterparts now believe that regular exercise is among the most important tools for keeping pets healthy, both physically and emotionally, says Dr. Basko. Dogs and cats that exercise regularly live up to 30 percent longer than those who don't. They have stronger lungs and hearts, and they have more energy. Regular exercise can even reverse health problems. In one study, dogs with congestive heart failure exercised for two hours a day. Four weeks later, their hearts were significantly healthier when compared with dogs who didn't move their furry tails. Veterinarians have even found that exercise may play a role in healing nerve damage, allowing some pets with paralysis to walk again.

Exercise also gives the digestive system a kick in the pants. It allows food to be digested more completely, which means that there is less waste in the body to put a strain on the kidneys, says Kathleen Carson, D.V.M., a holistic veterinarian in private practice in Hermosa Beach, California. It also keeps the intestines toned so that stools move along more efficiently, which prevents constipation.

On an emotional level for pets, exercise reduces boredom, frustration, and aggression. It stimulates the mind so that dogs and cats stay interested in life, says Mary Lee Nitschke, Ph.D., professor of psychology at Linfield College in Portland, Oregon, and an animal behaviorist in Beaverton.

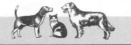

## Puppy Precautions

Puppies have energy levels that can leave their owners gasping for air. It seems logical that vigorous exercise would be the perfect way to cool their exuberance a bit. But what works for adult pets isn't so good for puppies. Even though they will run around as much as you will let them, too much exercise can injure their growth plates (the areas near joints that generate new bone) and interfere with their normal growth.

Dogs mature at different rates, so there are different guidelines for every breed. As a rule, small breeds under 25 pounds can handle vigorous exercise once they reach 8 months. Dogs 45 to 90 pounds shouldn't be taking long walks or runs until they are about 12 months old, and giant breeds should take it easy until they are 18 months old.

Dogs and cats don't have to turn into furry athletes to get the benefits of exercise, Dr. Hunthausen adds. For most pets, a romp in the backyard, a walk around the block, or running up and down the stairs does the trick. "You need to wear them out," he says. "And hopefully, your pet will get tired before you do."

Dogs and cats should exercise 20 to 40 minutes twice a day, says Dr. Basko. But it doesn't have to be the same routine every day. In fact, it shouldn't be because pets enjoy doing new things just as much as people do. You could go for a walk in the morning, then play in the backyard in the evening. Or jog one day and swim the next. It really doesn't matter what you do as long as you get their feet moving, he says.

*(continued on page 86)*

# Walking in Style

Just as dogs come in all sizes and temperaments—from the powerhouse Akita to the slow-moving basset hound—there are many styles of walking gear. Using the right equipment not only keeps pets safe and under control but also makes walks easier and more pleasant. Here are a few of the options.

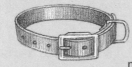

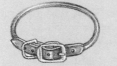

**Buckle collars.** These are great all-purpose collars that fasten with a buckle or snap. Round buckle collars are fine for smaller dogs, but large breeds need the wide, flat collars. Buckle collars aren't recommended for cats because they tend to slip off or put too much pressure on their delicate necks.

**Slip collars.** Also called choke collars, these tighten when you pull the leash and loosen when you release the tension. They are good for training but shouldn't be worn all the time. To prevent slip collars from drawing too tight, arrange them in a P shape before putting them on.

**Harnesses.** These are usually used for cats or dogs who are prone to getting neck injuries. An H-harness is fine for dogs. Cats can wiggle out of them, however, so they need a different style called a figure-eight harness.

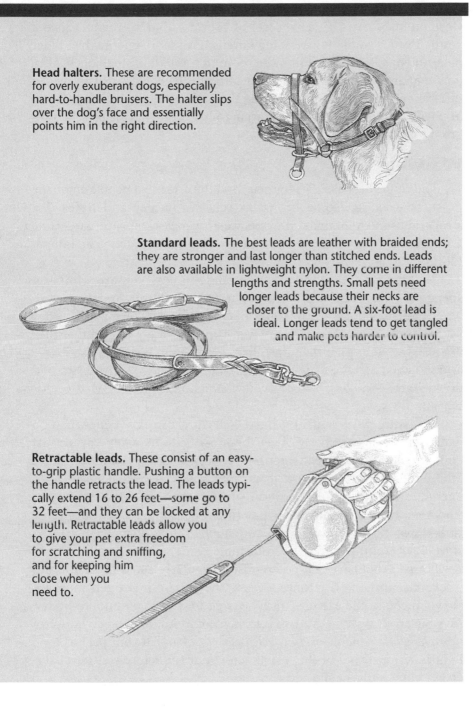

**Head halters.** These are recommended for overly exuberant dogs, especially hard-to-handle bruisers. The halter slips over the dog's face and essentially points him in the right direction.

**Standard leads.** The best leads are leather with braided ends; they are stronger and last longer than stitched ends. Leads are also available in lightweight nylon. They come in different lengths and strengths. Small pets need longer leads because their necks are closer to the ground. A six-foot lead is ideal. Longer leads tend to get tangled and make pets harder to control.

**Retractable leads.** These consist of an easy-to-grip plastic handle. Pushing a button on the handle retracts the lead. The leads typically extend 16 to 26 feet—some go to 32 feet—and they can be locked at any length. Retractable leads allow you to give your pet extra freedom for scratching and sniffing, and for keeping him close when you need to.

Of course, every pet is different, and you wouldn't give an elderly German shepherd the same level of exercise that you would give a young Border collie. Puppies and kittens have more energy than older pets, and big dogs need a bit more room to romp than small ones. Also, pets that are out of shape or have health problems like arthritis need a different exercise plan than those in the pink of health, says Dr. Basko. You will want to ask your veterinarian to help you plan an exercise program that's right for your pet.

## Walking

The single best exercise for pets, and the one most people enjoy the most, is walking. Going for walks releases energy and flexes and strengthens the joints. And it works well for pets of all ages, says Anne Lampru, D.V.M., a holistic veterinarian in private practice in Tampa, Florida.

Walking isn't ideal for cats, of course, unless you are willing to spend time training them to accept a harness and lead. And it is not always the best choice for big dogs like Great Danes or mastiffs. They love to walk, but unless they are well-trained, you may find that they are walking you rather than the other way around. But for most dogs—and for cats, as long as you are walking around the yard or up and down stairs—walking is about your best choice. Here is what veterinarians advise.

**Get your pet breathing hard.** A leisurely walk is better than no walk at all, but your pet will get the most benefits when you go fast enough and long enough to get him breathing hard. For most pets, a 20-minute walk twice a day is about right, says Dr. Basko. Of course, an energetic dog needs to cover more ground than an older, slower pet. And pets that are out of shape may find a 20-minute walk—or even a walk down the driveway—a little too much at first. So you will want to start slowly until your pet is comfortable going farther and faster.

For pets that haven't been exercising regularly, start with 5 minutes of exercise three to five times a week, then, as your pet gets more fit, slowly increase the exercise until he is getting 20 to 60 minutes a day, says Susan G. Wynn, D.V.M., a veterinarian in Atlanta and co-editor of *Complementary and Alternative Veterinary Medicine*. If your pet has been ill or is seriously out of shape, talk with your vet before you start exercising him regularly, she adds.

Dogs are often more interested in smelling—and wetting—the roses than just walking past them, so you may have to struggle a bit to keep your pet moving. You will know that you are moving fast enough when his breathing rate speeds up and stays elevated for most of the walk. Panting won't hurt him, but be prepared to slow down if he struggles to get his breath, is slowing down, or simply sits down and refuses to move. Let him rest for a few minutes before moving on, says Dr. Nitschke.

Small dogs can often get by with shorter walks than large ones can, simply because their short legs have to move pretty fast to keep up with your normal stride. So don't be surprised when a dog such as a toy poodle is ready to go home sooner than a golden retriever, says Dr. Nitschke.

**Work around his schedule.** No one wants to exercise after a big meal, dogs and cats included. It is best to take dogs and cats for walks before meals, says Dr. Nitschke. And once you get outside, be prepared to stop a few times while he makes his pit stops. Most pets will take care of their business in the first few minutes, and you can walk pretty steadily after that.

**Plan for the weather.** Dogs and cats can't take off their coats the way you can, and temperatures that feel comfortable to you may be uncomfortably warm for them. When the humidity or temperature is high, walk more slowly than usual and be prepared to go home early if he seems to be dragging. Pets will do their best to please you, which means they will keep pushing themselves even when they are overheating.

You need to be especially cautious if you have a bulldog or another breed with a short, pushed-in face. They don't breathe as efficiently as other dogs and have a higher risk of getting heatstroke, says Dr. Hunthausen.

Where you walk also makes a difference. Concrete sidewalks can get hot even on relatively mild days. Your pet's foot pads provide a lot of protection, but they aren't proof against scorching heat, says Dr. Carson.

Winter causes its own problems, Dr. Carson adds. Air that is colder than about 20°F is hard on the lungs. In addition, your pet's paw pads won't protect him from constant moisture, road salt, or sharp shards of ice.

Many winter walkers invest in a stout pair of booties for their pets, available in pet supply stores. They are very effective at protecting the paws, but most dogs don't like wearing them; they are often more trouble than they are worth, says Dr. Nitschke. Sweaters, however, are another story. Short-haired pets like Chihuahuas are especially vulnerable to winter's chill and will enjoy having an extra layer of comfort, she adds.

**Vary the routine.** Dogs and cats love new sights, smells, and sounds, and they will get bored if you walk the same route every day. Walking in different directions and neighborhoods or even in different parts of a park will help keep them interested. In fact, you will get more exercise bang for your buck when you change routes because pets get more enthusiastic when they are going someplace new, says Dr. Nitschke.

## Swimming

Walking is the most convenient exercise, but for pets that like water, swimming is hard to beat. It works almost every muscle in the body, and the buoyancy of the water reduces stress on the legs and back. Pets that are overweight or have arthritis or previous injuries can often swim with no discomfort at all, says Donn W. Griffith, D.V.M., a holistic veterinarian in private practice in Dublin, Ohio.

Of course, some pets take to the water more readily than others. A Labrador retriever may dive in and refuse to climb out, while cats will do just about anything to stay high and dry. Big dogs need quite a bit of water to swim comfortably, so it may be hard to find a good place to take them, adds Kathy Kern, a registered veterinary technician and owner of Animal Fitness Center at Almaden Valley Animal Hospital in San Jose, California. Small pets, on the other hand, may be able to do laps in your bathtub.

Since many dogs (and even some cats) take naturally to water, you don't have to worry about giving them swimming lessons. You do have to make sure, however, that they are comfortable as well as safe.

**Stick to warm-water swimming.** Even though cold-climate breeds like Labradors don't object to frigid water, the cold causes muscles to tighten and contract, which can lead to injuries if you aren't careful, Kern says. Ponds, swimming pools, and even the ocean are fine as long as the outside temperature is warm, she adds. For small pets who are swimming in the tub, the water should be between 85° and 90°F.

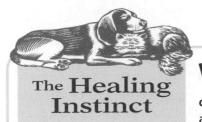

## The Healing Instinct

Whether they are swiping your socks, tumbling on the floor, or chasing a ball around the house, dogs and cats love games. Their high jinks may look like silly fun, but it is one of their strategies for staying healthy.

Pets experience stress just like people do. A change in your schedule, workers in the house, or a neighbor's dog visiting the yard can put their tails in a twist. Too much stress can weaken the immune system and cause a host of emotional and physical problems, says Michael W. Fox, B.V.M. (bachelor of veterinary medicine, a British equivalent of D.V.M.), Ph.D., a veterinary consultant in Washington, D.C., and author of *The Healing Touch*.

When stress levels rise, dogs and cats instinctively try to blow off steam—and their favorite way to do it is with vigorous play. A few minutes' running around stimulates their minds, defuses frustration, and helps keep them emotionally and physically fit, Dr. Fox explains.

**Give some support.** Pets that don't swim well or are recovering from health problems may need a little help staying afloat, Kern says. She recommends gently holding the base of the tail while your pet paddles away from you. He won't make any progress, but he won't know this, and swimming in place is excellent exercise, she says. It also ensures that he won't bash into the sides of the tub or pool.

**Limit his exertion.** Swimming is vigorous exercise, and pets that aren't used to it will get sore if you let them go too long. Kern recommends letting your pet swim for 5 to 10 minutes two days in a row. This will loosen up stiffness and get his muscles in shape. As time goes by, you can let him swim for longer periods. For most pets, though, 10 to 20 minutes is plenty, she says.

**Rinse him well.** Chlorine, ocean salt, and other things in water can irritate the skin. And pond scum will perfume your house for days at a time. It is worth hosing your dog off right after his swim. Dry him well, and dab excess water from inside the ears, which will help prevent infections, Dr. Hunthausen says.

## Fun and Games

Dogs and cats love to play, and left to their own devices, they will invent entertaining games of their own, like shredding the potted plants or strewing linens down the hall. That is why every exercise plan should include plenty of planned playtime. It is especially important for cats since play is often the main way they exercise, says Dr. Griffith. As with any form of exercise, games should be fast-paced and vigorous enough to get your pet's heart and lungs working for about 20 minutes at a stretch.

You can find all kinds of toys at pet supply stores or through catalogs, but it is just as easy—and cheaper—to make your own. You may not even need any toys at all. Cats, for example, often love chasing the covers when you are making the bed. You can make a real game out of it if you want to. And dogs—especially terriers—really dig digging. The next time your dog shows an interest in helping you garden, hide a few treats in his personal patch of ground and watch the dirt fly. He will get a great workout, and all you have to do is sit back and smile.

Every dog and cat enjoys different kinds of games, and what excites one pet will leave another yawning, but here are some common favorites.

***Catch.*** Almost all dogs—and even some cats, especially Siamese— love chasing things, although they are not always interested in bringing them back, says Dr. Griffith. It is pretty hard to go wrong tossing a tennis ball, a ball of string, or a catnip mouse. Just be sure that whatever you are throwing is too big for your pet to swallow and that it doesn't have sharp edges or splinters.

***Herding games.*** Some dog breeds, like corgis and Border collies, are bred for herding. One way to keep them entertained—and to distract them when they are trying to "herd" the cat—is to get a toy called a boomer ball. This is a large rubber ball that dogs can bump, bite, and bully all over the yard.

***Keep-away.*** Cats and some terriers love games of chase and capture, in which they tackle a moving object, hold onto it for a moment, then tear after it when it gets away. Pet supply stores sell fishing pole–style toys, in which you cast a furry lure across your pet's line of sight. But it is just as easy to put a feather or a piece of fabric on the end of a string and toss it around, says Dr. Lampru. Just be sure to let him catch it periodically, which will keep him from getting frustrated, she adds. In addition, cats have a hard time detecting objects that are coming straight toward them, so always draw the string and lure across his line of sight.

*Hide-and-seek.* It doesn't work for cats, but dogs adore a good treasure hunt, with food being the treasure. Take some of your dog's favorite treats and stash them around the house—under a book, leaning against a table leg, or under a corner of the carpet. Lead him to one treat so he gets the idea, then relax while his nose goes to work. Some dogs will search for food by the hour, says Dr. Hunthausen. You can play a variation of this game by getting your dog a toy such as the Buster Cube or Goody Ship. These toys have hidden compartments that you fill with food. The food only comes out a little at a time, so dogs have to nose, nudge, and shake them around to get their reward.

*King of the mountain.* A fun way to get your cat moving is to take advantage of his natural inclination to climb to high places. Put his favorite toy or a tasty tidbit in a high place—on top of a bookcase or, for out-of-shape cats, midway up the stairs—so that he will have to jump or climb to get it.

# CHAPTER 9

# Old-Fashioned Care

Dogs and cats have more exuberance than common sense. Their full-speed-ahead enthusiasm makes them a lot of fun, but it also leaves them hobbling with cuts or bruises when they have run without looking or throwing up after they have gobbled pilfered snacks. Which is why most owners, sooner or later, discover the value of old-fashioned care.

Some pet problems always require a trip to the vet, but the majority can be handled at home, says Michelle Tilghman, D.V.M., a holistic veterinarian in private practice in Stone Mountain, Georgia. In fact, many old-fashioned home treatments are the same ones that veterinarians use, and for good reason: They work.

Consider ice. Nothing complicated or high-tech about it, but it is still one of the best remedies for relieving pain and reducing swelling and inflammation. Vinegar is another one. Vets recommend and use it all the time for treating skin problems, although they usually call it acetic acid, just to be fancy. Even remedies as simple as herbal teas and cool-water rinses can work as well as or better than modern medications.

This isn't to say that there isn't a place for the latest drugs and sophisticated procedures. Dogs and cats are living longer, healthier lives thanks to advances in veterinary medicine. The problem is that over the years there has been a gradual shift toward using only the newest and shiniest and most impressive treatments. This makes sense for life-threatening or complicated illnesses and conditions, but it isn't always the best approach for common complaints.

Despite the many benefits of modern medicine, it leaves a lot to be desired, says Dr. Tilghman. A pill may stop your pet's cough, but it won't necessarily cure the underlying problem that caused the cough in the first place. And drugs sometimes bring side effects along with their benefits, causing additional problems.

There is really nothing "old-fashioned" about old-fashioned care because some of the simplest remedies are also the most effective, says Dr. Tilghman. That is why many veterinarians, especially those specializing in holistic care, continue to recommend and use traditional home remedies.

## Simple Power

One reason veterinarians feel comfortable recommending old-fashioned treatments is that research has shown that they work. In fact, many traditional remedies contain ingredients that are identical or similar to those used in modern drugs and treatments. Warm milk, for example, calms pets down and helps them sleep because it contains the amino acid tryptophan, which is converted in the brain to serotonin, a chemical that tells the body when to rest, says Mary Lee Nitschke, Ph.D., professor of psychology at Linfield College in Portland, Oregon, and an animal behaviorist in Beaverton.

One of the best-known (and best-loved) traditional remedies is chicken soup. Experts used to chuckle when their patients swore it had healing powers. But evidence suggests that chicken soup slows the action of neutrophils, cells that cause inflammation when they rush to an infection. It also clears congestion, stimulates the appetite, and, when you add garlic, controls infection by killing viruses and bacteria.

One of the best things about old-fashioned care is that you don't have to be a veterinarian to help your pet. You probably won't even have to drive to the drugstore because many old-fashioned treatments use ingredients that you already have at home. Suppose, for example, your dog has a hot spot. This is a painful skin infection that can spread within hours. You could rush to your vet or the pet supply store to get a commercial hot-spot remedy. Or you could moisten a tea bag and

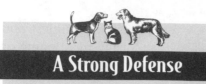

## A Strong Defense

Your pet's immune system is designed to recognize and destroy most germs that it comes into contact with. Sometimes, however, the immune system doesn't work as well as it should, which gives the germs a dangerous advantage.

Researchers have spent decades and billions of dollars in the search for germ-killing drugs and treatments. But one of the most powerful germ-fighters is also one of the oldest—and it is something that you have at home: common household bleach.

Unlike antiseptics, which are applied to the skin, disinfectants such as bleach are used to clean floors, litter boxes, and other places where germs thrive. When your pet has been ill with ringworm, for example, treating the environment is just as important as treating the disease because it is the only way to stop him from getting reinfected, says Robert Kennis, D.V.M., a veterinary dermatologist at Texas A&M University College of Veterinary Medicine in College Station.

There are many disinfectants, but veterinarians like bleach because it is inexpensive and works against almost every kind of germ. They recommend diluting 1 part bleach in 10 parts water and using the solution to wash bedding and food and water bowls and to wipe down hard surfaces where your pet spends his time.

apply it to the spot. Tea contains tannic acid, a natural astringent that dries hot spots and helps them heal, says Lowell Ackerman, D.V.M., a veterinary dermatologist in Mesa, Arizona, and author of the *Guide to Skin and Haircoat Problems in Dogs*.

For some illnesses, of course, old-fashioned care isn't going to work. But since you are taking care of your pet yourself, you will know very soon whether or not you need to call your veterinarian. Some holistic vets are happy to give information over the telephone as long as your pet is one of their regular patients. This means that you get the best of both worlds: the natural effectiveness and safety of home care and advice from an expert when you need it most, telling you what to do next, says Deborah C. Mallu, D.V.M, a holistic veterinarian in private practice in Sedona, Arizona.

Dogs and cats usually recover more quickly when they are treated at home with old-fashioned care, says Dr. Mallu. The close bond that you share with your pets reassures them and helps them recover more quickly. This also eliminates stressful trips to the vet, which can slow recovery. Even when dogs and cats are hospitalized, veterinarians usually ask that owners spend as much time with them as possible. The love and energy from owners help them recover better than any drug, she says.

## How to Use Old-Fashioned Care

Home remedies are very safe compared to drugs, but there are limits to what you can do at home, says Pat Zook, D.V.M., a holistic veterinarian in private practice in Stone Mountain, Georgia. A little Kaopectate may ease diarrhea after your dog has raided the trash, but won't do a bit of good if he has a more serious problem like salmonella or parvovirus. "Most of the time, pets can fight off a mild infection or injury. But if they are totally overwhelmed, your pet is going to need more extensive treatments that only your vet can give," she says. As a rule, it is a good idea to call your vet when your pet doesn't get better— or starts getting worse—within a day or two or when the problem goes away and then comes back, says Dr. Zook.

Even when your pet is being treated by your vet, there is still a place for home remedies, Dr. Zook adds. For most conditions that dogs and cats get, like diarrhea, itching, or cut paw pads, they need a little support as much as they need medical treatment. Keeping your pet comfortable and relieving the symptoms take some of the burden off the body, allowing it to direct more of its energy to healing itself. Nutrition is especially important because pets that are sick tend to lose their appetites, which means that they don't get all the nutrients they need to keep the immune system strong.

Veterinarians sometimes use drugs like diazepam (Valium) to stimulate the appetite, but this is hardly ever necessary, says Dr. Zook. A simpler, safer strategy is to brew up some chicken or beef broth. Pets can't resist it, and even a drizzle of the broth will provide essential vitamins and minerals.

Something as simple as hand-feeding will often encourage pets to eat, adds Alice Wolf, D.V.M., professor of medicine at Texas A&M University College of Veterinary Medicine in College Station.

Old-fashioned care tends to work best for digestive complaints, some skin problems, and minor skin infections—conditions that come on suddenly or within a few days. When you know what to do, most of these problems will clear up almost as quickly as they appeared, says Dr. Zook.

## Treating Digestive Problems

Living with dogs and cats is like having a baby in the house. It seems that no matter what they eat and drink, they will invariably have bouts of diarrhea and vomiting. This is partly because pets eat a lot of things they shouldn't. Nibbling garbage from the trash can or chomping an old dead mouse will cause the body to react in predictable and unpleasant ways. Some digestive problems are serious, but most of the time you can clear them up and help your pet feel better with simple home remedies. You will find more information on using these remedies throughout the book, but here is a quick look.

*Yogurt.* Pets love the taste, and it is one of the best medicines that you can find for stopping diarrhea and helping the digestive tract work more efficiently. Live-culture yogurt contains beneficial bacteria that aid in digestion and help keep harmful intestinal bacteria in check, explains Roger L. DeHaan, D.V.M., a holistic veterinarian in private practice in Frazee, Minnesota.

*Petroleum jelly.* It is not as tasty as yogurt, but petroleum jelly is a very versatile remedy. It lubricates the intestines, which is especially helpful for hair balls. In fact, it works better than some commercial hair-ball remedies, which often contain artificial flavors and preservatives, says James R. Richards, D.V.M., director of the Cornell Feline Health Center at Cornell University in Ithaca, New York.

*Kaopectate.* A medicine-cabinet staple, Kaopectate contains a mineral found in clay called attapulgite, coats the digestive tract, and absorbs toxins that cause diarrhea. It is not just a home remedy, adds H. Ellen Whiteley, D.V.M., a veterinary consultant in Guadalupita, New Mexico, and consultant for *The Country Vet's Home Remedies for Cats*. Most veterinarians use it, too.

*Fiber.* This is one of nature's most powerful remedies. Found in generous amounts in products such as Metamucil and in grains, bran, fresh vegetables, and canned pumpkin, dietary fiber is a superb digestive aid that can relieve constipation and diarrhea, says Dr. Whiteley.

## Treating Skin Problems

The skin shields dogs and cats from the elements. It regulates temperature and protects against viruses, bacteria, and environmental toxins. It takes quite a beating, and it is a testimony to its toughness that serious skin problems don't occur more often. It is far from invulnerable, however. Minor skin problems are fairly common, says Dr. Ackerman. Cuts, scrapes, and other irritations occur from time to time. And some dogs and cats suffer from itching a lot more than people do.

Most skin problems are easy to treat at home, says Dr. Ackerman. In fact, many old-fashioned remedies, such as the following, work as well as or better than their medicinal counterparts.

*Oatmeal.* An important ingredient in some commercial shampoos and conditioners, oatmeal is an excellent remedy for itching caused by dry skin, allergies, and insect bites and stings, says Carolyn Blakey, D.V.M., a holistic veterinarian in private practice in Richmond, Indiana. You can make your own skin-soother by filling a cotton sock with breakfast oatmeal and running water through it. Or you can use colloidal oatmeal (like Aveeno), which has been ground to a powder so that it dissolves in water.

*Oil.* Oils used for cooking, like safflower and olive, are easily absorbed by the skin and are good for treating small areas of dryness and irritation. Many vets recommend using oil to relieve chapped noses or cracked paw pads, says Joanne Stefanatos, D.V.M., a holistic veterinarian in private practice in Las Vegas. Hand creams that contains lanolin, a natural oil that comes from sheep's wool, are also good moisturizers.

*Ammonia.* It doesn't smell pretty, but it is one of the best remedies for insect bites and stings. A number of commercial products, like After Bite, use ammonia as the active ingredient.

*Heating pads and cold packs.* When you are looking for a safe alternative for aspirin (which can be toxic for cats) and other drugs, you can't do better than applying hot or cold. Veterinarians often recommend using cold to relieve the pain of bruises and pulled muscles. Heat is one of the best ways to ease long-term problems like painful joints. Hot and cold treatments can be as fancy as using commercially made packs or as simple as filling a washcloth with ice or applying a hot-water bottle.

*Water.* This ubiquitous wet stuff is so common that it is hard to think of it as medicine, but it is one of the best remedies for itchy skin, says Allen M. Schoen, D.V.M., director of the Veterinary Institute for

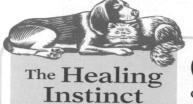

## The Healing Instinct

One of the most potent of nature's remedies, and certainly the most common, is water. Dogs and cats know instinctively that water makes them feel good. Veterinarians have found, for example, that dogs that have been bitten by ants or stung by bees will often lie in a puddle of water or plaster their bellies against wet grass. In the wild, wolves and moose know instinctively that the quickest way to get away from fleas or flies is to stand neck-deep in the nearest water, and some dogs do the same thing.

So don't be surprised when your pet suddenly makes a run for the nearest mud puddle or pool of water. He is not trying to make a mess. He is just trying to make himself feel better.

---

Therapeutic Alternatives in Sherman, Connecticut, and author of *Love, Miracles, and Animal Healing*. A cool-water rinse or bath moisturizes the skin and soothes the nerve endings.

## Stopping Infections

One area in which old-fashioned care excels is stopping infections. Veterinarians often use creams or oral medications to kill infection-causing germs, but medications are mainly used only after pets are sick. Holistic veterinarians feel that it makes more sense to strengthen the immune system by giving pets a wholesome, all-natural diet, for example, so that it is better able to resist germs before they multiply. Even when dogs and cats do get infections or when they have a high risk of getting one such as after an injury, you can usually protect them with traditional home care. For example, here are some home remedies for skin infections.

*Soap and water.* Simple soaps kill most germs, and the suds and flushing action will wash the rest away. You don't even need to use an antibacterial soap. In fact, you may not want to because these soaps are often too harsh, says Steven A. Melman, V.M.D., a veterinarian with practices in Potomac, Maryland, and Palm Springs, California, and author of *Skin Diseases of Dogs and Cats*.

*Saline solution.* The same stuff that you use to clean contact lenses, and that vets use during surgery, is perfect for flushing the eyes and ears and for rinsing wounds. Saline doesn't sting like plain water because its composition is similar to the body's natural fluids.

*Vinegar.* It contains a mild acid that inhibits the growth of yeast and other organisms that cause infection as well as those that cause dandruff or an oily coat, says Anne Lampru, D.V.M., a holistic veterinarian in private practice in Tampa, Florida. Vinegar also works as an ear cleaner and rinse. Many commercial ear cleansers contain vinegar.

*Hydrogen peroxide.* This old-fashioned remedy can be a helpful antiseptic for dental care, says Ihor Basko, D.V.M., a holistic veterinarian in private practice in Honolulu and Kilauea, Hawaii. Wetting a toothbrush with two or three drops of hydrogen peroxide and dipping it in baking soda makes a very effective toothpaste, he says.

*Isopropyl alcohol.* This is an antiseptic that kills germs quickly. It is really too harsh to apply to cuts or scrapes, says Dr. Lampru. But when your pet has been sick and can't tolerate any more problems, you can use alcohol, along with soap and hot water, to sterilize food bowls, kennel floors, and other things that your pet comes in contact with.

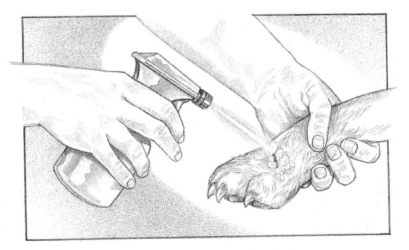

To disinfect cuts and scrapes, spritz the area forcefully with clean water to remove surface debris. Follow this by spraying the area with a solution made from six ounces of aloe vera juice and eight ounces of saline solution or distilled water. The aloe vera juice will help the wound heal.

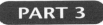

**PART 3**

# Common Health and Behavior Problems

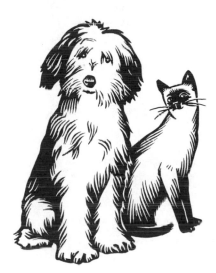

# ACNE

## The Signs

- Your pet has pimples, blackheads, or crusty sores on the chin or lower lip.
- His chin is swollen or inflamed.

## The Cause

Dogs and cats don't worry about their complexions, but acne can plague them just the same. When pimples or blackheads get infected, they can make the skin itchy and sore, says Steven A. Melman, V.M.D., a veterinarian with practices in Potomac, Maryland, and Palm Springs, California, and author of *Skin Diseases of Dogs and Cats*.

Some pets have a genetic tendency to develop acne. Dogs often get it during their "teenage" years, while for cats it can be a lifelong problem, explains Dr. Melman. You don't need harsh chemicals or medications to control acne in pets, he adds. In most cases, you can control or eliminate the problem with a few gentle—and natural—home remedies.

## The Solutions FOR DOGS & CATS

**Stop the infection.** Pimples occur when bacteria get trapped under the skin. The herb calendula (*Calendula officinalis*), available as a tincture or made into a tea, will soothe the skin

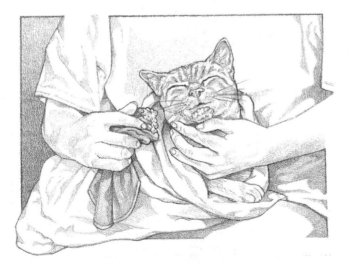

Wrap your pet securely in a towel, leaving his head unwrapped and making sure that the towel is loose enough for him to breathe. Moisten his chin with a washcloth dipped in warm water. Apply a drop of pet shampoo to the washcloth and work up a lather. Then rinse the cloth, wring it out, and wipe off all the suds and soapy residue, repeating until the soap is completely rinsed.

while also stopping infection, says Michelle Tilghman, D.V.M., a holistic veterinarian in private practice in Stone Mountain, Georgia. Soak a cotton ball or gauze pad in the tincture (dilute the tincture with an equal amount of water) or tea (made by soaking a tablespoon of dried herb in a cup of hot filtered water)—squeeze out the excess, and apply it to the sore spots for about five minutes. Used for a compress, calendula can be applied every day and will help acne heal more quickly, she explains.

**BEST BET!** **Apply a little warmth.** A warm-water compress will help open blocked pores and increase circulation to flush out infection, says Dr. Melman. He recommends soaking a cloth with warm water and holding it on the affected area until the cloth turns cool. You can repeat this every day until the acne clears up, he says.

**BEST BET!** **Keep him clean.** Washing your pet's face every day with an antibacterial pet wash or hypo-allergenic shampoo will help open blocked pores and allow pimples to heal more quickly, says Alexander Werner, V.M.D., a veterinary dermatologist in private practice in Studio City, California. Daily washing is especially important for flat-faced breeds like Persian cats and bulldogs. These pets often get a lot of food in their facial folds, and these tasty leftovers provide a perfect breeding ground for bacteria, he explains.

**Treat it from the inside out.** The flower essence crab apple is often recommended for stopping infections, including those in the skin, says Teresa Fulp, D.V.M., a holistic veterinarian in private practice in Springfield, Virginia. She recommends giving pets with acne four drops of crab apple flower essence four times a day. You can drip the medicine directly in your pet's mouth, she says.

**Give them a tonic.** Herbal tonics can help remove toxins from the body and strengthen the immune system, both of which can help relieve acne and other skin problems, says Nancy

## Meet the Experts

**Teresa Fulp, D.V.M.,** is a holistic veterinarian in private practice in Springfield, Virginia.

**Steven A. Melman, V.M.D.,** is a veterinarian with practices in Potomac, Maryland, and Palm Springs, California, and the author of *Skin Diseases of Dogs and Cats*.

**Nancy Scanlan, D.V.M.,** is a holistic veterinarian in private practice in Sherman Oaks, California. She is certified in acupuncture and chiropractic.

**Michelle Tilghman, D.V.M.,** is a holistic veterinarian in private practice in Stone Mountain, Georgia. She is certified in acupuncture.

**Alexander Werner, V.M.D.,** is a veterinary dermatologist in private practice in Studio City, California.

Scanlan, D.V.M., a holistic veterinarian in private practice in Sherman Oaks, California. "I like a tonic called Hokamix, which helps decrease inflammation and builds the body up," she says. Pets like the flavor, so you can mix the tonic in their food, following the directions on the label, she adds.

## The Solutions  *FOR CATS*

**Do a dish switch.** Some cats are allergic to plastic and will break out in acne when their faces touch their food or water bowls, says Dr. Melman. It is a good idea to use glass or ceramic dishes and wash them every day.

# AGGRESSION

## The Signs
- Your pet is staring you down.
- He stands in your way and doesn't move when you approach.
- He is growling at you.
- He plays too rough, and sometimes playfulness turns into anger.
- He chases people or threatens to bite.

## The Cause

Dogs bark at strangers, and cats resent animals that trespass on their turf. This type of behavior is normal and shouldn't cause problems in the family. But when dogs and cats are turning their aggression—and their teeth and claws—toward people and other pets, you have to act quickly because a touch of aggression can quickly become dangerous.

Pets sometimes get aggressive when they perceive themselves as "top dog" over the humans in their lives. And any pet, even a shrinking-violet type, can get aggressive when he is scared, in pain, or under stress.

It's not always easy to tell what is causing dogs and cats to act up—and act out. Even if you don't know what is causing the aggression, however, there are ways to stop it. For dogs, this has traditionally meant starting a training program or taking a refresher course with a professional trainer or behaviorist. For dogs and cats, veterinarians sometimes recommend sedatives or mood-altering drugs as a way of getting bad behavior under control.

## Call the VET

Dogs and cats with dominant personalities will sometimes use aggression to get their way, and with their sharp claws and strong jaws, they can do considerable damage in a very short time. That's why aggression, especially in dogs, is such a serious problem.

Don't wait until you have actually been bitten to get some help, says Wayne Hunthausen, D.V.M., a veterinary behaviorist in Westwood, Kansas, and author of the *Handbook of Behaviour Problems in Dogs and Cats*. "A dog that's growling at a family member warrants immediate attention. Go to your veterinarian for help or get a referral to somebody that works with behavior problems," he advises.

---

Even if your pet does need professional help, there are natural ways to take the edge off his anger and make him happier and more secure.

## The Solutions FOR DOGS & CATS

**Use scent to restore their sense.** Pets can get so wound up because of anxiety or other strong emotions that they lose all common sense. Treating them with aromatherapy may help reset their brains. "Essential oil of bergamot especially helps very wild or fractious animals," says Donna M. Starita, D.V.M., a holistic veterinarian in private practice in Boring, Oregon. She recommends putting three drops of the oil on a bandanna and tying it around your pet's neck. The scent will stay active for four to six hours. You can repeat the treatment once a day until the aggression starts to fade.

**Balance his emotions.** A mixture of flower remedies called Bach Rescue Remedy soothes pets very quickly and helps calm negative emotions, says Joanne Stefanatos, D.V.M., a holistic veterinarian in private practice in Las Vegas. "Drip two to four drops directly on your pet's gums two to four times a day or before a stressful event, or three times a day while traveling," she suggests. Or you can squirt a dropperful of the remedy on his food.

**Adjust his attitude with magnets.** Aggressive behavior can sometimes be eliminated by using a magnet to alter the brain's electromagnetic field, says Dr. Stefanatos. Hold the "north pole" of the magnet against your pet's forehead for about 20 minutes, once a day while you are watching TV or reading, for example, she advises. You can get healing mag-

ALTERNATIVE SUCCESS

# A SUCCESSFUL ADJUSTMENT

One cool evening, H. T. Spunkenheimer sneaked under the hood of a car for a warm nap—and was rudely awakened when the engine started. "H. T. recovered, but he lost a toe and needed some surgery," says Albert J. Simpson, D.V.M., a holistic veterinarian in private practice in Oregon City, Oregon. "The trauma and the terrible scare turned old H. T. into a very mean cat."

His aggression got so bad, in fact, that Dr. Simpson and his staff dreaded the times when H. T. was due to visit. "He was nearly impossible to treat," he says, "so we finally decided to try to figure out what was going on."

They discovered that one of H. T.'s vertebrae was out of alignment, and he had a trigger point—a painful knot in a muscle—in his left hip. The muscle had tightened after the accident and was throwing off his posture. H. T. hurt, and the pain was making him uncommonly cranky.

Dr. Simpson treated the trigger point with acupuncture and gave H. T. a chiropractic adjustment for his bum back. And that's all it took. "Now he's fine when he comes in," he says. "We pet him, and everything's cool."

H. T. still gets stiff and sore occasionally, Dr. Simpson adds, and when he does, his bad mood comes back. So he gets another treatment and turns into a pussycat again.

nets from holistic veterinarians and some pet supply catalogs.

**Touch away aggression.** Linda Tellington-Jones, an animal trainer and consultant in Santa Fe, New Mexico, and author of *Tellington Touch: A Breakthrough Technique to Train and Care for Your Favorite Animal*, has developed a technique called TTouch, a type of massage that affects the limbic system, the part of the brain that controls the emotions.

Dogs and cats that are acting aggressively may get calmer and more relaxed if you trace circles with your fingertips on their ears, mouth, and tail for a few minutes each day, says Tellington-Jones. Most pets enjoy the touches, but those that are aggressive may struggle or bite, so be prepared to back off if it doesn't seem to be working.

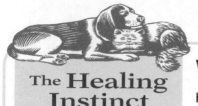

## The Healing Instinct

When cats walked in the wild, confrontations—which consisted of a lot of hissing, tail-puffing, and posturing—occurred all the time. The fur rarely flew, however, because one of the cats would usually turn tail and run, says John C. Wright, Ph.D., a certified applied animal behaviorist and professor of psychology at Mercer University in Macon, Georgia, and author of *The Dog Who Would Be King*. But indoor cats can't get away from each other, so aggression may be inevitable, he explains.

Fortunately, cats have developed a very effective way to cool their hot tempers and calm down after a fight: They groom themselves. Behaviorists refer to this as displacement grooming, and it lowers body temperature and reduces stress, Dr. Wright explains.

**BEST BET!** **Heal with your heart.** Angry, aggressive pets are often insecure pets. You can help them feel better about themselves by giving them some of your healthy life force, says Deborah C. Mallu, D.V.M., a holistic veterinarian in private practice in Sedona, Arizona. Begin by focusing your own energy, which you can do by saying out loud, "I am rooted like a tree." Discard all your worries for a moment and let your mind and body fill with love. Then move your hands over your pet where it feels right, stroking from the head toward the tail, she says. Dogs and cats have enormous powers of intuition, and they will sense and be affected by the strength of your emotions.

**BEST BET!** **Ease his mind.** Dogs and cats can sense when you are upset, and their concern may come out as aggressive behavior. It is important to be honest with your pet so that he knows what you are going through, says Kathleen Carson, D.V.M., a holistic veterinarian in private practice in Hermosa Beach, California. "Say out loud, 'I'm upset, but it's not your fault,'" she says. "Just talk things out."

**BEST BET!** **Help them blow off steam.** Some pets get aggressive because they have too much energy and not enough to do—much as children will pick on each other during long trips in the car. "Pets weren't designed to sit around. They were designed to hunt and run and play," says Pat Zook, D.V.M., a holistic veterinarian in private practice in Stone Mountain, Georgia. You can often curb early signs of aggression simply by wearing out your pet, she explains. Go for longer walks—or, better yet, jogs, as long as your dog is fit enough. Get your cat running with a game of chase-the-string. Run in circles. Throw a ball. Go swimming. As long as you get your pet moving for at least 20 minutes a few times a day (some breeds, like Border collies, need more exercise), he will be sufficiently tired and won't feel like causing trouble.

"Play therapy is also a great way to distract one pet from bullying another pet," adds John C. Wright, Ph.D., a certified applied animal behaviorist and professor of psychology at Mercer University in Macon, Georgia, and author of *The Dog Who Would Be King.*

**BEST BET!** **Avoid aggressive games.** With dogs especially, people like to wrestle or play tug-of-war and other rough games. There is nothing wrong with these games most of the time, but some pets have trouble distinguishing appropriate play from inappropriate aggression. "Don't encourage behaviors that you don't want to see in another context," says Wayne Hunthausen, D.V.M., a veterinary behaviorist in Westwood, Kansas, and author of the *Handbook of Behaviour Problems in Dogs and Cats.*

**Show them the kindness of strangers.** Since aggression is often caused by fear, it is important to socialize young pets by encouraging them to explore the world. The more they encounter when they are young—such as noisy streets, loud people, and other pets—the less likely they will be to develop aggression later on.

If your pet is naturally shy, encourage his adventurous spirit by giving him something to eat whenever he does something novel and exciting. "If they get a little tidbit every time they meet somebody, they will learn to look forward to meeting people," explains Dr. Hunthausen.

**Get them used to attention.** A key to preventing adult aggression is to handle young pets every day. This process, called habituation, is nothing more than touching your pet all over, head to tail. If you get him used to human contact when he is young, he will be more friendly later on—and less likely to object to getting groomed or having his tail or ears touched.

"You should have little mini-handling sessions throughout the day," says Dr. Hunthausen. Do them when your pet is calm, he adds. If you suspect that he is getting restless, stop the handling *before* he asks you to stop. "If you stop only when your puppy or kitten bites the brush or wiggles away, you have taught him that he can be aggressive to get what he wants," he explains.

**Block the view.** Cats and dogs often act aggressively toward strange animals that trespass on their property. And when they can't get through the window or door to confront the interloper, they may turn their aggression toward other pets in the family, says Dr. Wright. One of the simplest solutions is to make it harder for your pet to see outside by drawing the blinds when other pets are in the

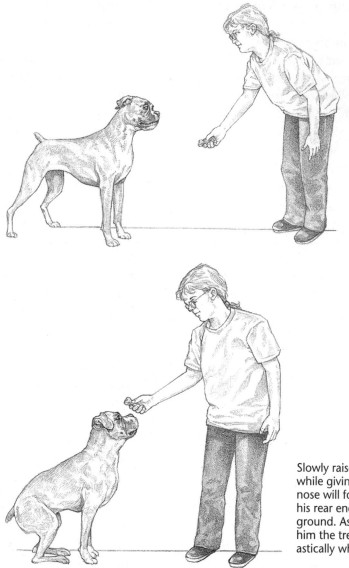

Teaching your dog basic obedience is a great way to curtail aggression. Most dogs can learn the "sit" command in a few lessons. Start by holding a dog treat just in front of his nose to get his attention.

Slowly raise the treat over his head while giving the command. His nose will follow the food, causing his rear end to drop to the ground. As soon as he sits, give him the treat and tell him enthusiastically what a smart dog he is.

neighborhood, for example, or by moving the furniture in such a way that your pet can't get a clear view of the street or yard.

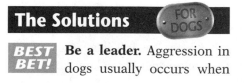

**The Solutions** FOR DOGS

**BEST BET!** **Be a leader.** Aggression in dogs usually occurs when they get the idea that they are more important than other family members, says Dr. Hunthausen. Whether you have a puppy or an older dog, it is essential to take command. You can do this by training your dog to earn attention, food, lap time, or anything else he wants. Make him sit before you let him outside. Have him heel or lie down before you hand over a treat. If you do this consistently, your dog will quickly learn that he is working for you, making him more subordinate and less prone to aggression.

If you haven't taken your dog to obedience school or aren't sure how to train your puppy, a good place to start is with the "sit" command, says Dr. Hunthausen. All you have to do is hold a tasty tidbit in front of his nose, then raise it over his head. "As his nose goes up to follow the food, the rear end goes down to ground," he says. "When that happens, say 'sit' and give him the treat."

**Interrupt the aggression.** Unless you stop it fast, aggression invariably gets worse, says Dr. Hunthausen. So it is important to interrupt every form of aggression, no matter how reasonable it seems. When your dog is barking at the mail carrier, for example, interrupt your dog right away by giving him a command and rewarding him when he complies. This will remind him that you are in charge. In addition, the reward will put him in a good mood—and it is hard for dogs to be aggressive when they are feeling good.

## Meet the Experts

**Kathleen Carson, D.V.M.,** is a holistic veterinarian in private practice in Hermosa Beach, California.

**Wayne Hunthausen, D.V.M.,** is a veterinary behaviorist in Westwood, Kansas, and the author of the *Handbook of Behaviour Problems in Dogs and Cats*.

**Deborah C. Mallu, D.V.M.,** is a holistic veterinarian in private practice in Sedona, Arizona. She is certified in acupuncture.

**Albert J. Simpson, D.V.M.,** is a holistic veterinarian in private practice in Oregon City, Oregon. He is certified in acupuncture and chiropractic.

**Donna M. Starita, D.V.M.,** is a holistic veterinarian in private practice in Boring, Oregon

**Joanne Stefanatos, D.V.M.,** is a holistic veterinarian in private practice in Las Vegas. She is certified in acupuncture and chiropractic.

**Linda Tellington-Jones** is an animal trainer and consultant in Santa Fe, New Mexico, and the author of *Tellington Touch: A Breakthrough Technique to Train and Care for Your Favorite Animal*.

**John C. Wright, Ph.D.,** is a certified applied animal behaviorist and professor of psychology at Mercer University in Macon, Georgia, and the author of *The Dog Who Would Be King*.

**Pat Zook, D.V.M.,** is a holistic veterinarian in private practice in Stone Mountain, Georgia. She is certified in acupuncture.

# AGING

## The Signs

- Your pet sleeps more and plays less than she used to.
- Her muzzle and the tips of her ears have turned gray or white.
- She moves slowly and carefully or has trouble getting up.
- She doesn't always hear you when you approach.

## The Cause

We don't like to think about our pets getting old, but it is an issue that every pet owner must face. Pets typically live only a fraction of the amount of time that we do, so they age faster and need help earlier, says Albert J. Simpson, D.V.M., a holistic veterinarian in private practice in Oregon City, Oregon.

Old age isn't a disease, but it weakens many parts of the body—from the joints and muscles to the immune system—making troublesome problems much more likely to occur. "Older pets tend to get sick more easily, and it takes them longer to get well," says W. Jean Dodds, D.V.M., adjunct professor of clinical sciences at the University of Pennsylvania School of Veterinary Medicine in Philadelphia and owner of Hemopet, a national nonprofit animal blood bank in Irvine, California.

For a long time, veterinarians focused mainly on treating the symptoms of age-related illnesses, such as using aspirin to ease arthritis. But holistic veterinarians feel that there is a better approach. Rather than treating symptoms, they look for ways to strengthen the entire body so that the pet is much less likely to get sick in the first place. "The goal is to prevent problems and not wait for trouble to develop," says Dr. Dodds.

## The Solutions FOR DOGS & CATS

**BEST BET!** **Feed them naturally.** Veterinarians have found that the chemical additives and preservatives in many commercial foods as well as the low ratio of proteins to carbohydrates in them may speed up the aging process by causing the body to produce more waste products. The extra work involved in getting rid of the wastes can strain the kidneys, liver, and other organs, says Dr. Dodds.

Natural foods are easy to digest and produce fewer wastes than commercial foods, says Nancy Scanlan, D.V.M., a holistic veterinarian in private practice in Sherman Oaks, California.

ALTERNATIVE

SUCCESS

## YOUNG AGAIN

As a hard-core canine athlete, Serling competed in nearly every dog sport, from retriever trials to flyball. But by his 12th birthday, the 80-pound Newfoundland-Labrador mix had started to slow down. "We really had to cut back on his exercise and walks when he developed arthritis," says his owner, Cheryl Smith of Port Angeles, Washington. "And then he was diagnosed with early kidney disease," she adds.

After watching Serling get more depressed from giving up his active lifestyle, Cheryl talked to her veterinarian, who recommended giving Serling homeopathic Detoxification to help his kidneys, along with a nutritional supplement called glucosamine to help his arthritic joints.

After about three months, Cheryl saw an amazing sight. "We were out walking, and Serling started running up steep hills," she says. "I was afraid he'd fall over, roll down the hill, and die, but he obviously felt better."

So much so that Cheryl started Serling on an active exercise program again, which included 1½-mile walks and swims in the pond near her house. Serling has regained much of his former energy, and both his kidneys and his joints are in much better shape. "He runs my life," Cheryl says. "But at his age, he deserves to run my life!"

You can choose from a number of high-quality, all-natural foods, such as Innova, Solid Gold, and Wysong, which are available in some pet supply stores and through mail order, or you can make your pet's meals at home. Holistic veterinarians advise giving dogs a diet consisting of one-third meat, one-third raw vegetables, and one-third cooked carbohydrates, such as rice or potatoes.

For cats, a natural-food diet should consist of one-half meat, one-quarter raw vegetables, and one-quarter cooked carbohydrates. For more on natural-food diets, see page 61.

**Decrease the servings.** Older pets burn two to four times fewer calories than youthful ones. They also exercise less, so they tend to get a little tubby. The extra weight puts additional strain on muscles and joints. You have to feed them less to keep them trim and healthy, says Dr. Scanlan.

Every pet needs different amounts of food, she adds. A good way to check is with the rib test: You should be able to feel, but not see, your pet's ribs. In cats, take a look at their bellies—when there is too much sway, they need to eat a little less. "Just feed them less of the same food," says Dr. Scanlan. Start by decreasing the amount by about one-quarter. If your pet seems hungry on this amount of food, mix in a little rice, which is filling but lower in calories than her usual food.

**Give a digestive aid.** In nature, dogs and cats swallowed helpful digestive enzymes when they ate the internal organs of their prey. Commercial and homemade diets lack these enzymes, which means that your pets are unable to unlock the full benefits of their food. Some holistic veterinarians recommend giving older pets digestive enzymes, such as F-Biotic for cats and C-Biotic for dogs, following the directions on the label.

**Protect their joints.** The cartilage in the joints is extremely tough, but it doesn't last forever. Over time, it begins to break down, causing pain and stiffness. Holistic veterinarians have found that dietary supplements containing glucosamine or a combination of glucosamine and chondroitin sulfate, like Cosequin, can help heal damaged cartilage and keep it strong in the future.

You can give pets 10 milligrams of Cosequin per pound of body weight twice a day. The combination of glucosamine and chondroitin sulfate shouldn't be given to pets with liver disease or clotting disorders, says Susan G. Wynn, D.V.M., a veterinarian in Atlanta and co-editor of *Complementary and Alternative Medicine*.

**Keep them limber.** Flexing your pet's back will help relieve general stiffness and keep internal organs healthier, says Randy Caviness, D.V.M., clinical instructor of small animal acupuncture at Tufts University School of Veterinary Medicine in North Grafton, Massachusetts, and a holistic veterinarian in Concord.

This technique, called motion palpation, also helps keep nerve connections healthy, adds Michael W. Fox, B.V.M. (bachelor of veterinary medicine, a British equivalent of D.V.M.), Ph.D., a veterinary consultant in Washington, D.C., and author of *The Healing Touch*.

**BEST BET!** **Give them a massage.** Older pets often tire easily, in part because their circulation isn't as efficient as it used to be. Massaging pets helps stimulate blood flow, which nourishes tissues and washes away pain-causing lactic acid crystals that collect in tired muscles, says Michelle Rivera, a certified massage therapist, a veterinary dental technician, and co-owner of the Healing Oasis Veterinary Hospital in Sturtevant, Wisconsin.

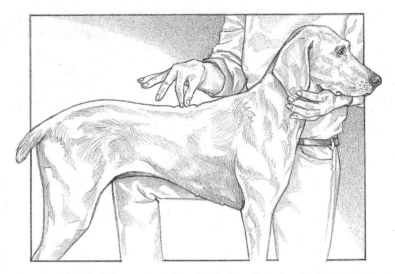

Place the thumb and index finger of one hand together. Find the dip between the vertebrae on either side of your pet's backbone. This indentation feels like the area between your knuckles. Gently press straight down with your thumb and index finger for one to two seconds, then release. (If your pet is sensitive to this type of touch, press with the flat of your hand.) Starting at the shoulders, do the press/release technique between each vertebra in turn, using just enough pressure to slightly move the spine. Continue the entire length of your pet's back and stop at the hips.

The best massage technique for older pets, called effleurage, involves using long, firm strokes over your pet's entire body. It keeps the muscles toned and can help prevent stiffness, says Dr. Fox. Massaging your pets daily also allows you to detect problems, such as lumps beneath the skin that you might otherwise miss, he adds.

**BEST BET!** **Get them moving.** Regular exercise is important for pets of all ages, and it is especially beneficial for older dogs and cats. It helps keep joints working smoothly because it literally pumps in lubricating fluids. It also strengthens the immune system and causes the body to release endorphins, natural chemicals that help relieve pain, says Dr. Dodds. Vets recommend giving pets as much exercise as they can comfortably handle. Try to get them moving by taking them on regular walks or just by playing in the house for at least 20 minutes, twice a day.

**Give them extra strokes.** "Many 20-year-old cats and dogs I see have spent a lifetime being handled and petted—sitting on the owner's lap, spending time with them, staying connected," says Dr. Fox. Petted and loved pets live longer, not only because they are emotionally happy but also because touch keeps the body healthy.

Gentle petting and massaging can increase circulation to muscles and decrease spasms, adds Dr. Scanlan.

**Provide extra comfort.** "Older pets appreciate a soft place to rest," says Dr. Simpson. You can buy pet beds—everything from rubber mats to thickly padded foam pillows—at pet supply stores, but you don't really need anything fancier than an old blanket on the floor, he says.

**Keep her warm.** "Pets really appreciate having a warm light nearby," says Dr. Simpson. When using heat, however, be sure it doesn't burn the skin. Keep heat lamps several feet away from your pet's bed, says Dr. Simpson, and give your pet space to move away from the heat if she gets overheated. You can buy a heat lamp (brooder) bulb at most hardware stores or feed stores.

**Raise your voice.** As dogs and cats age, the tiny bones inside the ears that amplify sound tend to lose their mobility and become less sensitive, which is why your dog or cat may appear to be ignoring you or will sometimes get startled when you come up and touch her from behind. Talking more loudly will often help, says Dr. Dodds. It is also a good idea to lightly stamp your foot when you are trying to get your pet's attention but you are not in her line of sight.

**BEST BET!** **Give them a boost.** It is normal for dogs and cats to become a little less agile with the

## Meet the Experts

**Randy Caviness, D.V.M.,** is a clinical instructor of small animal acupuncture at Tufts University School of Veterinary Medicine in North Grafton, Massachusetts, and a holistic veterinarian in Concord. He is certified in acupuncture and chiropractic.

**W. Jean Dodds, D.V.M.,** is an adjunct professor of clinical sciences at the University of Pennsylvania School of Veterinary Medicine in Philadelphia and the owner of Hemopet, a national nonprofit animal blood bank in Irvine, California.

**Michael W. Fox, B.V.M., Ph.D.,** is a veterinary consultant in Washington, D.C., and the author of *The Healing Touch*.

**Michelle Rivera** is a certified massage therapist, a veterinary dental technician, and co-owner of the Healing Oasis Veterinary Hospital in Sturtevant, Wisconsin.

**Nancy Scanlan, D.V.M.,** is a holistic veterinarian in private practice in Sherman Oaks, California. She is certified in acupuncture and chiropractic.

**Albert J. Simpson, D.V.M.,** is a holistic veterinarian in private practice in Oregon City, Oregon. He is certified in acupuncture and chiropractic.

**Susan G. Wynn, D.V.M.,** is a veterinarian in Atlanta and co-editor of *Complementary and Alternative Medicine*.

passing years. If your pet is accustomed to a favorite place—a window perch, for example, or a chair in the living room—you may want to put a low stool or platform underneath so that they can help themselves up, says Dr. Simpson. This not only helps them get comfortable, but it also provides a great emotional boost since older pets may get depressed when they can't do the things that they used to.

## The Solutions FOR DOGS

**Take her swimming.** Swimming is one of the best exercises for dogs because the water supports their weight and prevents punishing strain on muscles and joints, says Dr. Fox. Swimming is great for cats, too—if they like the water. Most don't, of course, so water sports are really limited to dogs.

# ALLERGIES

## The Signs

- Your pet is licking or biting his feet.
- He is rubbing his face on the floor or against furniture.
- There is a rash on his belly.
- His nose is runny and his eyes are red.
- He keeps getting ear infections.

## The Cause

Cats and dogs can be allergic to many of the same things as humans, like pollen and mold. They can also be sensitive to fleas, yard chemicals, or even grass. But unlike humans, who usually sniffle and sneeze when they have allergies, pets get extremely itchy. This is because histamine, the natural chemical that triggers allergic symptoms, is more abundant in pets' skin than in their nasal passages.

The traditional approach to allergies, apart from keeping your pets away from whatever bothers them, is to give antihistamines or to use medicated shampoos to control itchy flare-ups. But holistic veterinarians take a slightly different approach. Rather than focusing only on the allergy-causing substance, they try to figure out why the immune system is making "mistakes" and attacking harmless things like pollen in the first place.

"Allergies mean that the immune system is being thrown off by things in the environment," says Greig Howie, D.V.M., a holistic veterinarian in private practice in Dover, Delaware. Food additives, chemicals in the air and water, and even vaccinations may cause the immune system to react to the wrong things, says Dr. Howie. That is why holistic veterinarians favor more of a whole-body approach—one that controls the symptoms and helps the immune system stay on track.

## The Solutions FOR DOGS & CATS

**BEST BET!** **Try a simple diet.** One of the best ways to calm allergies and hay fever is to give your pet a natural diet, one that doesn't contain the artificial additives found in many commercial foods, says Karen Komisar, D.V.M., a holistic veterinarian in private practice in Lynn, Massachusetts. "A natural diet often helps quiet the immune system."

The best meals for pets with allergies are those that are homemade, adds Deborah C. Mallu, D.V.M., a holistic veterinarian in private practice in Sedona, Arizona. She recommends giving dogs meals that are one-third meat (preferably raw or lightly steamed), one-third cooked grains, and one-third finely chopped vegetables. Cats need more protein than dogs, she adds. Their meals should be 60 percent meat, 20 percent cooked grains, and 20 percent cooked vegetables.

When you don't have the time or inclination to cook from scratch, look for all-natural pet foods that don't contain chemical additives or preserva-

tives, says Dr. Mallu. You can get natural foods from holistic veterinarians and from some pet supply or health food stores.

**Calm the skin with calendula.** Calendula (*Calendula officinalis*) ointment is an herbal preparation that quickly relieves itching caused by allergies, says Adriana Sagrera, D.V.M., a holistic veterinarian in private practice in New Orleans. She recommends applying a thin coat of the ointment two or three times a day to the areas your pet is scratching.

**Strengthen the immune system with echinacea.** Echinacea (*Echinacea purpurea* or *Echinacea angustifolia*) is a healing herb that helps the immune system work more effectively, and it is often recommended for pets with allergies, says Sandra Priest, D.V.M., a veterinarian in private practice in Knoxville, Tennessee. She recommends adding two to four drops of echinacea extract to an ounce of spring water and putting a dropperful in your pet's mouth once a day or every other day. Echinacea works best when it is given before allergies actually start—in the early spring, for example, before pollens fill the air.

**Put vitamins to work.** Vitamins C and E have been shown to help the body fight the inflammation that accompanies allergic reactions. You can give cats or dogs under 15 pounds 250 milligrams of vitamin C (preferably in the form of sodium ascorbate) a day during allergy season. Pets 15 pounds

## Call the VET

Most pets with hay fever or allergies will be a little uncomfortable during flare-ups, but they won't have serious problems. In some cases, however, they get so itchy that they scratch themselves raw, causing sores or infections, says Karen Komisar, D.V.M., a holistic veterinarian in private practice in Lynn, Massachusetts.

When the itchiness isn't going away, or your pet has other symptoms like an eye discharge or sores or a bad odor on the skin, you will need to see your vet. He may recommend allergy tests to find what, exactly, your pet is allergic to. And in some cases, he may give your pet medications until gentler, more natural remedies have time to work.

and over need more, usually between 500 and 1,000 milligrams a day, says Cheryl Schwartz, D.V.M., a holistic veterinarian in San Francisco and author of *Four Paws, Five Directions: A Guide to Chinese Medicine for Cats and Dogs*. "If you give them too much, they will get diarrhea. When that happens, you will want to lower the dose until the diarrhea goes away."

Vitamin E is also good for the skin, Dr. Schwartz adds. She recommends 50 international units (IU) for cats and dogs weighing less than 10 pounds. Give 200 IU to pets weighing from 10 to 40 pounds and 400 IU for dogs over 40 pounds. It should be given once a day during allergy season. To prevent stomach upset, it is best to give vitamin E (as well as vitamin C) with food, she adds.

Vitamin E increases blood pressure, adds Dr. Schwartz, so don't give it to pets with high blood pressure without first checking with your vet.

**Provide some essential fats.** Another way to fight skin inflammation is with essential fatty acids, found in flaxseed oil and fish oil. "In order to get a balanced anti-inflammatory effect, look for a supplement that has both omega-3 and omega-6 fatty acids," advises Dr. Priest. You can buy fatty-acid supplements made specifically for pets. Just follow the directions on the label.

**Shower them with flowers.** Holistic veterinarians often use flower essences to soothe itchy pets. A good combination of essences is agrimony, beech, cherry plum, crab apple, olive, and walnut, says Wanda Vockeroth, D.V.M., a holistic veterinarian in private practice in Calgary, Alberta, Canada. To prepare the mixture, put two or three drops of each essence in a one-ounce dropper bottle filled with spring or purified water. Give your pet a dropperful of the mixture twice a day. "You can also put it in a spray bottle and spritz the itchy spots or dab some on a cloth and wipe it on," she adds.

**Change their water.** Chemicals in drinking water can make the immune system act a little haywire, says Anne Lampru, D.V.M., a holistic veterinarian in private practice in Tampa, Florida. "Give them distilled water for six to eight weeks, which will help them slowly detoxify," she says. "Then put them on good filtered water."

**Wash them with oatmeal.** You can give itchy pets quick relief by washing them with an oatmeal shampoo, available in pet supply stores, says Dr. Komisar. Or, if they will put up with it, you can add some colloidal oatmeal (like Aveeno) to their bathwater and give them a soothing soak for 10 to 15 minutes.

**Ease their eyes with eyebright.** Pets with allergies may get weepy, itchy eyes, much the way people do. When they do, you may want to rinse the eyes with an herbal eyewash. Dr. Priest recommends boiling a cup of pure water and adding two to four drops of eyebright (*Euphrasia officinalis*) extract. Boil the solution for another minute, then let it cool entirely. Draw some solution into a dropper and rinse your pet's eyes once a day.

There are many conditions besides allergies that can cause red eyes,

---

## Meet the Experts

**Greig Howie, D.V.M.,** is a holistic veterinarian in private practice in Dover, Delaware. He is certified in acupuncture and homeopathy.

**Karen Komisar, D.V.M.,** is a holistic veterinarian in private practice in Lynn, Massachusetts. She is certified in homeopathy.

**Anne Lampru, D.V.M.,** is a holistic veterinarian in private practice in Tampa, Florida. She is certified in acupuncture and homeopathy.

**Deborah C. Mallu, D.V.M.,** is a holistic veterinarian in private practice in Sedona, Arizona. She is certified in acupuncture.

**Sandra Priest, D.V.M.,** is a holistic veterinarian in private practice in Knoxville, Tennessee. She is certified in chiropractic.

**Adriana Sagrera, D.V.M.,** is a holistic veterinarian in private practice in New Orleans.

**Cheryl Schwartz, D.V.M.,** is a holistic veterinarian in San Francisco and the author of *Four Paws, Five Directions: A Guide to Chinese Medicine for Cats and Dogs*. She is certified in acupuncture.

**Wanda Vockeroth, D.V.M.,** is a holistic veterinarian in private practice in Calgary, Alberta, Canada. She is certified in acupuncture.

---

Dr. Priest adds. So if the redness doesn't go away after two days—or you are not sure that allergies are responsible—you should ask your vet to take a look. Pets that squint or paw at their eyes may be in pain, and you will want to call your vet right away.

**Use soothing pressure.** Your pet's body has a number of acupressure points that help control the immune system, says Dr. Schwartz. For dogs and cats with allergies, she recommends pressing one or more of these points for 30 seconds to a minute several times a day. The best points for allergies are as follows:

🐾 LI4, located in the web of the dewclaw, on the inside of the front legs, just below the uppermost pad or in this area if the dewclaw is removed.

🐾 LI11, located on the outside of the front leg where the elbow bends.

🐾 GB20, located at the base of the skull about halfway between the spine and the bottom of the ear on both sides of the head.

**Vaccinate with care.** Many holistic veterinarians believe that giving pets a lot of vaccines may compromise the immune system, causing it to overreact to ordinary substances. It is worth asking your veterinarian if vaccines may be contributing to the problem and whether it is a good idea for your pet to get fewer vaccines or to get vaccinated less often.

# Anal-Sac Problems

## The Signs
- Your pet is scooting across the floor.
- He is licking his bottom more than usual.
- The anal area is swollen or inflamed, or there is a discharge.

## The Cause

Dogs and cats have an amazing sense of smell, which is why they spend so much time with their noses to the ground. What they are sniffing for, in most cases, are traces of other pets. Whenever they have a bowel movement, dogs and cats release small amounts of fluid from the anal sacs—two storage areas on either side of the anus. The smell of the fluid is unique to each pet. It is one way of saying, "I was here."

The anal sacs normally empty and refill every day. When stools aren't firm enough, however, they don't exert enough pressure to empty the sacs. This causes fluid to accumulate, making the anal area itchy and sore,

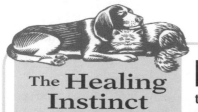

## The Healing Instinct

**D**ogs and cats with blocked anal sacs will sometimes scoot across the floor on their bottoms. It looks as though they are giving themselves a little scratch—and in many cases, they probably are. But the scooting may serve another purpose as well. It is nature's way of putting extra pressure on the sacs, says Susan G. Wynn, D.V.M., a veterinarian in Atlanta and co-editor of *Complementary and Alternative Veterinary Medicine*. This can help the sacs empty, relieving the pressure and making pets feel better, she explains.

says Jeffrey Feinman, V.M.D., a holistic veterinarian in private practice in Fairfield County in Connecticut.

Vets aren't sure why, but small dogs tend to have more anal-sac problems than larger breeds. Cats will occasionally have blocked anal sacs, but it is generally more of a problem in dogs.

The traditional treatment is to unblock the sacs by manually pressing out the fluid. It is an easy procedure—vets can do it in just a few seconds—but the problem often comes back. That is why holistic veterinarians favor more of a whole-body—and hands-off—approach. "When the anal sacs act up, it is kind of like an oil light going on in a car," says Junia Borden Childs, D.V.M., a holistic veterinarian in private practice in Ojai, California. It is a sign that something is wrong somewhere in the body. Treating the problem by emptying the sacs, she ex-

plains, "is like taking out the oil light. It doesn't solve the problem."

## The Solutions FOR DOGS & CATS

**Put water to work.** One of the most effective ways to relieve discomfort and help the anal sacs drain is to soak your pet's bottom in a mixture of warm water and Epsom salts (about one cup of salts in two gallons of water) for about 10 minutes, says Dr. Childs. Doing this once or twice a day for a few days will help liquefy the fluid in the sacs so that it flows more easily. The salts can be drying, however, so it is a good idea to apply a little petroleum jelly or mineral oil after the bath, she adds.

**Apply a warm compress.** Many pets won't sit for a sitz. An easy alternative is to soak a washcloth in the Epsom salts–water mixture and hold it to your pet's rear for about 10 minutes, twice a day. "A lot of times this will open the sacs," says Dr. Childs. You can also try placing your palm over your pet's bottom and gently rocking it back and forth, without squeezing. The slight pressure will often help the sacs drain, she explains.

**Try a new diet.** Switching pets to a higher-quality food—one that has at least two meat sources among the first three ingredients—or giving them homemade food may help prevent blocked anal sacs from coming back, says Susan G. Wynn, D.V.M., a veterinarian in Atlanta and co-editor of *Complementary and Alternative Veterinary Medicine*.

**Give your pet extra fiber.** Even if you decide not to switch foods, you can improve your pet's diet by giving him fresh vegetables, which are high in dietary fiber. Fiber absorbs tremendous amounts of water in the intestine, which causes stools to get larger. Larger stools put more pressure on the anal sacs, helping them empty normally, says Dr. Wynn. She recommends giving cats and dogs under 15 pounds about one-eighth cup of minced vegetables such as broccoli or carrots each day. Pets weighing 15 to 50 pounds can have between one-fourth cup and one-half cup. Dogs over 50 pounds can have as much as two cups of vegetables each day.

Cats are fussier than dogs about

## Call the VET

Many pets will have anal-sac problems at least once in their lives, and some pets have them all the time. The problems usually aren't serious and will clear up within a few days. But the anal area isn't the cleanest environment, and blocked anal sacs sometimes get infected. This can cause inflammation, impaction, or a painful abscess, says Susan G. Wynn, D.V.M., a veterinarian in Atlanta and co-editor of *Complementary and Alternative Veterinary Medicine*. Infections can be dangerous, so it is important to call your vet when your dog or cat is suddenly scooting a lot more than usual or the anal area looks red or swollen. Your vet may need to clean out the sacs thoroughly and possibly install a temporary "drain." Your pet may need oral antibiotics as well.

what they eat, she adds. If your cat turns up his whiskers at the minced vegetables, you can run them through a blender—adding a little water or chicken broth—and mix them with his food.

**BEST BET!** **Get those paws moving.** Regular exercise strengthens the rectal and abdominal muscles so that they put more pressure on the anal sacs. As long as they are healthy, dogs and cats should get at least 20 minutes of exercise twice a day.

**Soothe them with Silica.** Silica is a homeopathic remedy that can help the anal sacs empty normally, says Allen M. Schoen, D.V.M., director of the Veterinary Institute for Therapeutic Alternatives in Sherman, Connecticut, and author of *Love, Miracles, and Animal Healing*. He recommends giving two or three drops or three to five pellets of Silica 6C twice a day for three days. For some pets, this is all you will need to do to relieve the discomfort.

## The Solutions FOR DOGS

**Relieve his allergies.** Vets aren't sure why, but anal-sac problems in dogs may be related to allergies. If your dog is scratching a lot and licking his feet and he has anal-sac problems, there is a good chance that the problems are related, says Dr. Wynn. The best "cure" for allergies is to help your dog avoid whatever he is allergic to.

### Meet the Experts

**Junia Borden Childs, D.V.M.,** is a holistic veterinarian in private practice in Ojai, California.

**Jeffrey Feinman, V.M.D.,** is a holistic veterinarian in private practice in Fairfield County in Connecticut.

**Allen M. Schoen, D.V.M.,** is the director of the Veterinary Institute for Therapeutic Alternatives in Sherman, Connecticut, and the author of *Love, Miracles, and Animal Healing*. He is certified in acupuncture and chiropractic.

**Susan G. Wynn, D.V.M.,** is a veterinarian in Atlanta and co-editor of *Complementary and Alternative Veterinary Medicine*.

That's not always easy to do, of course, especially if he is allergic to something like common pollen.

An alternative is to give him dog supplements containing omega-3 fatty acids, such as fish oil or flaxseed oil, which can help reduce itching and inflammation. Vets usually recommend giving dogs under 15 pounds 250 to 500 milligrams of fatty acids twice a day, says Dr. Wynn. Dogs between 15 and 50 pounds can have 1,000 milligrams one or two times a day. Dogs 50 pounds and over can take between 1,000 and 2,000 milligrams twice daily. Every pet reacts differently to supplements, however, so ask your vet for the correct dose.

# ANEMIA

## The Signs
- Your pet's gums are pale or white.
- The insides of her eyelids are pale instead of pink.
- She seems weak and tired.
- Her breathing is labored, and her pulse is fast.

## The Cause

Anything that causes blood loss—from fleas to wounds to internal diseases—can cause anemia, a condition in which dogs and cats don't have enough red blood cells to deliver all the oxygen their bodies need. Without enough oxygen, pets get tired and weak.

Anemia by itself isn't always dangerous—at least not at first. But because it is always a symptom of another, more serious problem, it is a warning sign that your pet needs immediate veterinary attention, says Michael W. Lemmon, D.V.M., a holistic veterinarian in Renton, Washington, and past president of the American Holistic Veterinary Medical Association.

The idea—both in conventional and alternative medicine—is to restore your pet's energy by treating whatever is causing blood loss and to encourage the growth of new red blood cells. Here are a few ways to naturally strengthen your pet's body, spirit, and energy.

## The Solutions FOR DOGS & CATS

**BEST BET!** **Put meat on the menu.** The proteins in turkey, lamb, beef, chicken, or other raw meats will help dogs and cats create more red blood cells, enhancing the body's ability to transport oxygen, says Dr. Lemmon. Be sure to buy high-quality organic or free-range meats because they are less likely to contain dangerous organisms like salmonella, he adds.

Or, to help eliminate possible organisms, you can lightly steam the meat before adding it to your pet's food, says Alan M. Schoen, D.V.M., director of the Veterinary Institute for Therapeutic Alternatives in Sherman, Connecticut, and author of *Love, Miracles, and Animal Healing*. Check with your vet on the amount of meat that is appropriate for your anemic pet.

**Serve a hearty stew.** Another way to "strengthen" the blood is to give your pet some chicken-and-vegetable soup or stew. Boil the chicken in water until it is tender, remove the bones, then add some vegetables like beets, spinach, and carrots to the broth, Dr. Lemmon suggests. Don't use onions, however, which can be dangerous for cats.

**Buoy the blood with the B vitamins.** Bone marrow produces oxygen-carrying red blood cells. You can strengthen your pet's bone marrow by supplementing her diet with a B-vitamin elixir, says Jan Facinelli, D.V.M., a holistic veterinarian in private practice in Denver. Every pet needs different amounts of B vitamins, she adds, so ask your vet for the correct dose.

**Add some vitamin C.** This powerful nutrient helps the body soak up blood-building iron from the intestinal tract, says Junia Borden Childs, D.V.M., a holistic veterinarian in private practice in Ojai, California. Twice a day, give pets weighing less than 15 pounds 250 milligrams of vitamin C, she advises. Pets that weigh 15 pounds or more can take up to 1,000 milligrams of vitamin C a day.

Vitamin C occasionally causes diarrhea, she adds, so be prepared to cut back the amount until you find a dose that her stomach will tolerate.

**Offer liquid liver.** A raw-liver extract like Livaplex can help relieve anemia because it contains large amounts of nutrients like iron and B-complex vitamins, which are essential for healthy blood, Dr. Lemmon says.

You can buy liver extracts from vets or health food stores. He recommends giving cats one-quarter to a whole capsule of Livaplex once a day. Dogs can take between one-half capsule and four capsules a day, depending on their size and overall health. Your vet will help you choose the proper dose. Don't give liver extracts without checking with your vet because they can be dangerous for dogs that have a liver disorder called copper-related hepatitis.

**Give her some greens.** Chlorophyll, a pigment found in plants, can help the body produce healthier blood, Dr. Lemmon says. Fresh, juiced, or powdered barley grass and wheat grass contain highly concentrated forms of chlorophyll. Pets usually don't mind the taste, especially when you mix the greens in their food, he says. You can give one-quarter teaspoon to pets that weigh less than 15 pounds. Larger pets can have one to two teaspoons.

Other supplements containing chlorophyll include algae- and spirulina-based chlorophyll-complex powder. Give pets weighing up to 15 pounds one-eighth to one-quarter teaspoon of the supplement once a day. Pets weighing more than 15 pounds can take up to two teaspoons a day.

**Put herbs to work.** A natural way to ease anemia is with nettle (*Urtica dioica*), red clover (*Trifolium pratense*), and burdock root (*Arctium lappa*)—

## Call the VET

Anemia is sneaky because the main cause—losing blood—isn't always obvious. It is up to you to notice the subtle signs: a sudden lack of energy, a distended abdomen, or gums that have gone from bubble-gum pink to pale or even white. If signs do appear, you need to call your vet immediately, says Jan Facinelli, D.V.M, a holistic veterinarian in private practice in Denver.

One easy test is to check your pet's stool every day, she adds. Since anemia may be caused by internal bleeding due to ulcers, for example, or more serious conditions such as cancer, stools that are much darker than usual or are black and tarry-looking are a serious warning sign, and you should call your vet right away.

herbs that are bursting with nutrients and minerals, especially iron, says herbalist Gregory L. Tilford, co-owner of Animals' Apawthecary in Conner, Montana, and author of *Edible and Medicinal Plants of the West*. These herbs have the added advantage of strengthening the liver, which plays a role in producing blood cells and cleansing the blood, he explains. The herbs can be mixed together or given separately. Once a day, give dogs a level tablespoon of the dried herbs for every 30 pounds of weight, he suggests. Add approximately one-half teaspoon to a cat's food each day.

You can buy dried herbs at most health food stores. If you are using fresh burdock root, however, just grate some onto your pet's food, he adds. Pets under 15 pounds can have about

a teaspoon of burdock root a day. Larger pets can take up to two table spoons, says Susan G. Wynn, D.V.M., a veterinarian in Atlanta and co-editor of *Complementary and Alternative Veterinary Medicine*. Pets don't love the taste of burdock, so be prepared to adjust the amount, depending on how much your pet will eat.

**Try a homeopathic remedy.** "Phosphorus is a remedy for many types of bleeding," says Dr. Facinelli. "It's one of the first homeopathic remedies to think of when you are treating anemia caused by blood loss."

She recommends giving dogs and cats three pellets of Phosphorus 30C three times a day for about three days. Crushing the pellets and putting them in a teaspoon of milk will make them easier to take, she adds.

**ALTERNATIVE**

## ❧ SUCCESS

# A NATURAL VICTORY

Dogs and cats are living longer than ever because of steady advances in veterinary medicine. But sometimes modern "miracle drugs" cause additional problems.

That's what happened with Annie, an Old English sheepdog with autoimmune hemolytic anemia, a serious condition in which the immune system "accidentally" destroys red blood cells. "She was on conventional drugs, including prednisone, and she was dying," says Jan Facinelli, D.V.M., a holistic veterinarian in private practice in Denver. "The drugs were basically killing her, and she was not responding to them."

Dr. Facinelli tried a different approach. She gave injections of vitamin $B_{12}$ into selected acupuncture points to stimulate the bone marrow to produce red blood cells. She also treated Annie with homeopathic Phosphorus.

The results, Dr. Facinelli recalls, were stunning. "The next day, Annie was able to walk on her own," she says. "She was still weak, but the spark was back in her eyes. We weaned her off the conventional drugs as quickly as possible, and she has done fine. She really turned around."

Other homeopathic remedies are also recommended for anemia, depending on your pet's other symptoms. For example:

❧ Arsenicum album 6X may be helpful for anemic dogs and cats that are also weak, restless, or chilled, says Dr. Lemmon. Pets that weigh less than 15 pounds can take one or two pellets. Larger pets can take three to five pellets two or three times a day for up to two weeks.

❧ Sulfur 6X is often recommended when pets with anemia also have fleas or skin problems, he says. Give two to four pellets to pets weighing 15 pounds or more. Smaller pets can take one pellet two or three times a day for up to two weeks.

**Cleanse them with flower essences.** Since pets with anemia are often exhausted as well as stressed, holistic veterinarians feel that it is important to help them relax and gain strength. One of the best ways to do this is with the flower essences olive and star-of-Bethlehem, says Dr. Childs. "If the anemia is due to blood loss from fleas or worms, I would add crab apple for physical and emotional cleansing," she says.

She recommends putting 4 drops of each essence in a one-ounce amber glass bottle filled with spring water. Shake it well before using, and give your pet 4 drops four times a day. You can put the drops directly on her gums or nose, or rub them into the tips of her ears, she says. Or you can put 10 drops in her water twice a day until she is feeling better.

**Press for healing.** Acupressure can help relieve fatigue that is caused by anemia, and it can also strengthen the immune system, says Dr. Lemmon. He recommends pressing the following points for half a minute twice a day.

The ST36 point, located on the outside of each back leg just below the knee where the bone meets the muscle, can be used to increase your pet's energy.

The GV14 point, located where the neck meets the shoulder blades, will help strengthen the immune system.

**Try a healing touch.** Another way to help your pet relax is with a hands-

on therapy called TTouch. Starting anywhere on her body, massage the skin in small, clockwise circles, beginning at the six o'clock position, says Dr. Lemmon. Complete a full circle, plus a little more. Then move on to another spot. You can keep doing this as long as your pet seems comfortable and is enjoying it, he says.

## Meet the Experts

**Junia Borden Childs, D.V.M.,** is a holistic veterinarian in private practice in Ojai, California.

**Jan Facinelli, D.V.M.,** is a holistic veterinarian in private practice in Denver. She is certified in acupuncture and homeopathy.

**Michael W. Lemmon, D.V.M.,** is a holistic veterinarian in Renton, Washington, and past president of the American Holistic Veterinary Medical Association.

**Allen M. Schoen, D.V.M.,** is the director of the Veterinary Institute for Therapeutic Alternatives in Sherman, Connecticut, and the author of *Love, Miracles, and Animal Healing.* He is certified in acupuncture and chiropractic.

**Gregory L. Tilford** is an herbalist and co-owner of Animals' Apawthecary in Conner, Montana, and the author of *Edible and Medicinal Plants of the West.*

# APPETITE LOSS

## The Signs

- Your pet is suddenly eating less than usual or is losing weight.

## The Cause

It is not uncommon for dogs and cats to go through cycles in which they eat less than usual. A temporary loss of appetite is a natural response to such things as stress, decrease in exercise, or even changes in the weather. Pets that suddenly stop eating or are losing weight, however, need to be seen by a vet because they could have internal problems such as parasites, an infection, or even cancer, says Junia Borden Childs, D.V.M., a holistic veterinarian in private practice in Ojai, California.

You should call your vet if your cat hasn't eaten in 24 hours or if your dog hasn't eaten in 48 hours. Most changes in appetite aren't serious, however. For example, cats will sometimes eat less when they have an upper respiratory infection that temporarily reduces their ability to smell their food. Both dogs and cats may lose their appetites when they are feeling stress such as when another pet in the family is pushing them

around. Restoring a lost appetite usually isn't difficult as long as you approach things from a pet's point of view. Here are a few tips you may want to try.

## The Solutions FOR DOGS & CATS

**Do a food swap.** Some pets will stop eating for a day or two simply because they are ready for a change in food. There is nothing wrong with switching them to a new one for a while, says Susan G. Wynn, D.V.M., a veterinarian in Atlanta and co-editor of *Complementary and Alternative Veterinary Medicine*. If they eat the new food with gusto, you can be pretty sure that they are healthy and are enjoying the change in the menu. Let them eat the new food for a few days, then ease them back into their old diets, she says.

**Create a comfort zone.** Dogs and cats are very adaptable and usually adjust easily to noise and commotion in the family. But some pets are more sensitive than others, and when life is tumultuous, such as when you have weekend guests, they may stop eating. You may want to try moving their food to a quieter place, like inside a pantry. This will allow them to regain their

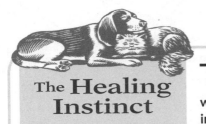

## The **Healing Instinct**

There is nothing like devouring a load of greasy fries or what you suspect is a week-old hamburger to send your appetite into a free fall. Your body doesn't respond well to unwholesome foods, and going without food for a while gives it time to recover.

What works for people is equally effective for pets. Dogs and cats understand instinctively that a temporary fast allows the body to recover from such things as fever or infections, or even from midnight raids on the trash. "It's not uncommon for pets to stop eating after they have eaten something they shouldn't, like a dead mouse," says Junia Borden Childs, D.V.M., a holistic veterinarian in private practice in Ojai, California. Temporarily going without food allows the body to devote less energy to digestion and more to healing itself.

sense of calm and eat in peace, says Pam Johnson Bennett, a feline behavior consultant in Nashville and author of *Twisted Whiskers*.

**Stimulate the appetite with aromatherapy.** The scent of two essential oils, rose and vetiver, acts very quickly to reawaken flagging appetites, says Thomas Van Cise, D.V.M., a holistic veterinarian in private practice in Norco, California. He recommends putting a few drops of either of these oils on a bandanna and tying it around your pet's neck until he starts eating again. The drops are highly concentrated, so don't put them on the fur or skin, he adds. Most pets don't mind wearing a bandanna, but some won't put up with it. An alternative is to put one or two drops of oil on your pet's bedding, he advises.

**Get them eating with homeopathy.** Two homeopathic remedies, Lycopodium and Nux vomica, are very helpful for pets who have lost their appetites, Dr. Van Cise says. He recommends giving cats two pellets of either remedy, using a potency of 6C or 12X, twice a day for no more than 24 hours. Dogs can take three pellets twice a day for no longer than two days.

**BEST BET!** **Serve it warm.** Dogs and cats love foods with strong smells—the smellier the better. One of the best ways to get them eating again is to warm their food, which releases more of the pungent aroma. Dr. Van Cise recommends putting the food in a bowl and slightly heating it in a shallow pan of water on the stove.

**Punch up the flavor with garlic.** Dogs love garlic, and mixing a little fresh garlic in their food may be all it takes to coax their noses into their bowls, says Dr. Van Cise. He recommends giving dogs weighing over 15 pounds one-quarter teaspoon of garlic a day, either chopped fine or pressed into their food. Smaller dogs can have one-eighth teaspoon a day.

Cats enjoy garlic, too, but they can't have too much because it can cause a type of anemia. You can give them up to one-eighth teaspoon a day for two weeks at a time.

**Use acupressure to restore eating energy.** There are two important acupressure points that control the flow of energy to the stomach and intestines: ST36, located in a depression on the outside of the back legs just below the knees, and BL20, located on either side of the spine in the hollow between the last two ribs. Pressing

these points for about 60 seconds once a day will help correct energy imbalances that may be causing your pet's appetite to flag, says Dr. Van Cise.

---

## Meet the Experts

**Pam Johnson Bennett** is a feline behavior consultant in Nashville and the author of *Twisted Whiskers* and *Psycho Kitty*.

**Junia Borden Childs, D.V.M.,** is a holistic veterinarian in private practice in Ojai, California.

**Thomas Van Cise, D.V.M.,** is a holistic veterinarian in private practice in Norco, California. He is certified in acupuncture.

**Susan G. Wynn, D.V.M.,** is a veterinarian in Atlanta and co-editor of *Complementary and Alternative Veterinary Medicine*.

---

# ARTHRITIS

## The Signs
- Your pet is having trouble getting up or climbing stairs.
- He moves stiffly, especially when he first wakes up.

## The Cause

Dogs and cats are designed for movement. Their joints are wrapped in strong muscles and held together with flexible ligaments and tendons. The ends of bones within the joints are coated with cartilage, a protective, plasticlike substance that enables the bones to slide smoothly back and forth. In addition, the natural movement of the joints causes the body to pump in lubricating fluid that keeps them operating smoothly.

As with other parts of the body, however, joints may deteriorate with age. When cartilage gets thinner or wears away entirely, bones grind instead of glide. This often causes painful friction and inflammation, a condition known as wear-and-tear arthritis, or osteoarthritis. "The body tries to fix the problem by growing extra bone around the joints," says Randy Caviness, D.V.M., clinical instructor of small animal acupuncture at Tufts University School of Veterinary Medicine in North Grafton, Massachusetts, and a holistic veterinarian in Concord. The extra bone doesn't really help, though. If anything, it makes the joints more painful, making it harder for pets to move. When they move less, muscles shrink and lose their strength, which makes the joint problems even worse.

Many dogs and cats get only a touch of arthritis and never experience anything worse than a little morning stiffness. Other pets, big dogs especially, may be seriously affected. Drugs like aspirin, cortisone, and carprofen (Rimadyl) are the conventional answers for treating arthritis, and in certain cases, surgery may be needed to repair damaged joints. But even though arthritis always needs a veterinarian's care, there are many natural remedies that can relieve pain without the side effects of medications. More important, it is often possible to protect cartilage and strengthen the joints so that a touch of arthritis doesn't get a lot worse. Here is what holistic veterinarians advise.

## The Solutions FOR DOGS & CATS

**BEST BET!** **Strengthen the cushion.** Veterinarians have found that two dietary supplements, glucosamine sulfate and chondroitin sulfate, which are available in health food stores, can help repair damaged cartilage and increase lubrication in the joint, reducing pain and stiffness, says Nancy Scanlan, D.V.M, a holistic veterinarian in private practice in Sherman Oaks, California.

A good supplement is Cosequin. Available from veterinarians, it contains both ingredients, says Susan G. Wynn, D.V.M., a veterinarian in Atlanta and co-editor of *Complementary and Alternative Veterinary Medicine.* You can give pets 10 milligrams of Cosequin per pound of body weight twice a day. Don't give Cosequin to pets with liver problems or clotting disorders.

Supplements containing green-lipped mussels, like Glyco-Flex, are also helpful because they contain glucosamine-like compounds, says Dr. Scanlan. "Green-lipped mussel supplements smell like dead fish, so pets think they are a wonderful treat," she says. You can buy these supplements from vets and some pet supply catalogs. Follow the dosage directions on the label.

**Give Mobility.** Specialists in traditional Chinese medicine have found

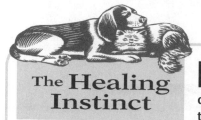

**D**ogs and cats have their priorities straight. Not only do they spend their days contentedly snoozing, but they also take the time to stretch when they wake up. "Pet yoga" is nature's way of keeping their joints limber and helping prevent painful problems such as arthritis.

After resting, pets launch into a fairly vigorous stretching routine, explains Albert J. Simpson, D.V.M., a holistic veterinarian in private practice in Oregon City, Oregon. First, they arch their backs. Then they bow their backs, putting their heads down and their tails in the air. They finish up by taking a few steps forward while stretching each hind leg behind them.

While dogs do a little bit of stretching, cats do a lot more—and it pays off. "Cats don't get a lot of joint problems," says Dr. Simpson. "They can arch their backs and contort themselves in ways that would pinch a dog's back."

that an herbal combination called Mobility 2 can help pets with arthritis move more easily, says Dr. Scanlan. Available in tablet form from veterinarians, the usual dose is one-half tablet twice a day for cats and dogs weighing less than 15 pounds and one to two tablets twice a day for larger pets.

**Flex the spine.** You can use a touch technique called motion palpation to limber up the back and relieve general stiffness and discomfort, says Albert J. Simpson, D.V.M., a holistic veterinarian in private practice in Oregon City, Oregon. Beginning at the shoulders and working backward to the hips, simultaneously press with your thumb and forefinger in the depressions on either side of the spine between each vertebra. Press for two to three seconds, release, then move to

the next spot, he advises. You can repeat the massage once a day until your pet is feeling better, he says.

**Rub away the pain.** Dogs and cats with arthritis often don't move a lot because it hurts when they do. A daily massage will get blood flowing into the muscles and quickly relax painful tightness, says Patricia Whalen-Shaw, a registered massage therapist and owner of Optissage, an animal massage school in Circleville, Ohio.

She recommends starting with a technique called effleurage, in which you use slow, firm strokes, beginning at the head and working back to the tail. After your pet is feeling warm and relaxed, hold your fingertips together and rub firm circles into the muscles. Concentrate on the muscles on either side of the spine, around the hips, and on the shoulders—wherever your pet seems to be hurting, Whalen-Shaw says. You can continue the massage for 15 minutes to an hour, once a day.

**Give daily vitamins.** Veterinarians have found that giving dogs and cats vitamin C and E supplements every day can reduce inflammation in the joints and protect the cartilage. Dr. Simpson recommends giving cats and dogs weighing less than 15 pounds about 10 international units (IU) of vitamin E a day. Pets 15 to 50 pounds can take 20 IU, and larger dogs can take 30 IU. For vitamin C, give about one-quarter teaspoon of 1,000-milligram vitamin C powder to dogs over 50 pounds, one-eighth teaspoon of 500-milligram powder to dogs 15 to 50 pounds, and just a sprinkling (about 250 milligrams) of 500-milligram powder to smaller pets. Vitamin C can cause diarrhea, so you may have to reduce the dose until you find an amount your pet will tolerate. Dr. Simpson recommends using ester vitamin C because it is less likely to cause diarrhea. "Just sprinkle it once a day on their food," he says.

**Press the "aspirin" point.** "One of the best acupressure points for arthritis pain is BL60, which is located on the outside of the rear ankle," says Dr. Simpson. When your pet seems to be hurting, press this point for about 60 seconds, once or twice a day, he suggests. For very small dogs and all cats, your fingertip may be too big to hit the spot exactly. It is fine to use the eraser end of a pencil as long as you press gently, he advises.

**Help the hips.** Arthritis often affects the hips, especially in big dogs, says Dr. Caviness. To relieve pain and stiffness quickly, he recommends pressing all around the head of the femur, the end of the thighbone where it fits into the pelvis. This will hit three important acupressure points—BL54, GB29, and GB30—that can help relieve hip pain, he says. You can repeat this two or three times a day, or as often as needed to help your pet feel better.

**BEST BET!** **Keep them moving.** Dogs and cats don't like to move when arthritis is flaring, but it is worth pushing them a little. Flexing the joints pumps in synovial fluid, which lubricates and nourishes tissues within the joints, says Dr. Simpson. Even gentle exercise may be uncomfortable at first, but the joints and muscles will quickly relax and loosen, he explains. It is a good idea to begin with about five minutes of gentle exercise twice a day, working up to 20 minutes twice a day as soon as your pet can handle it.

## The Solutions FOR DOGS

**Stop the swelling.** "An herb called boswellia (*Boswellia serrata*) naturally fights joint inflammation, and it is the number one arthritis product used in India," says Dr.

Simpson. Veterinarians usually recommend giving 150 to 200 milligrams twice a day. Every dog is different, however, so be sure to ask your vet for the correct dose.

**Lead them to water.** Swimming is one of the best exercises for arthritis because the water supports the body and takes the strain off tender joints. Some dogs take to water naturally, but others need a little coaxing. Once you get them in, they will often stick around as they discover that the water helps soothe their pain, says Kathy Kern, a registered veterinary technician and owner of Animal Fitness Center at Almaden Valley Animal Hospital in San Jose, California.

Dogs are natural swimmers, but it is important to stay nearby to bail them out if they need some help, she says. While large dogs need three to four feet of water for swimming, smaller pets can make do in a shallow pool or even a bathtub. "I recommend 88° to 92°F water for the best results," Kern says. Let your dog swim for about 10 minutes at first. You want him to be breathing hard when he is done, but not gasping. After he is done, towel him dry and finish up with a blow-dryer, set on low and held at least six inches from the fur. He will appreciate the extra warmth, she says.

**Add some spice to his life.** The scent of essential oil of ginger (*Zingiber officinale*) can help relieve in-

---

## Meet the Experts

**Randy Caviness, D.V.M.,** is a clinical instructor of small animal acupuncture at Tufts University School of Veterinary Medicine in North Grafton, Massachusetts, and a holistic veterinarian in Concord. He is certified in acupuncture and chiropractic.

**Teresa Fulp, D.V.M.,** is a holistic veterinarian in private practice in Springfield, Virginia.

**Kathy Kern** is a registered veterinary technician and owner of Animal Fitness Center at Almaden Valley Animal Hospital in San Jose, California.

**Nancy Scanlan, D.V.M.,** is a holistic veterinarian in private practice in Sherman Oaks, California. She is certified in acupuncture and chiropractic.

**Albert J. Simpson, D.V.M.,** is a holistic veterinarian in private practice in Oregon City, Oregon. He is certified in acupuncture and chiropractic.

**Patricia Whalen-Shaw** is a registered massage therapist and the owner of Optissage, an animal massage school in Circleville, Ohio.

---

flammation in the joints, says Teresa Fulp, D.V.M., a holistic veterinarian in private practice in Springfield, Virginia. Dilute the oil half-and-half with peanut oil, then massage it on the inside tip of your dog's ear, she advises.

# ASTHMA

## The Signs

- Your cat has coughing fits throughout the day.
- He crouches with his neck extended.
- There is a whistling sound when he breathes.
- He is taking rapid, shallow breaths or breathing with his mouth open.
- He tires easily, especially after exercise.

## The Cause

If you have ever watched your cat tearing around and noticed his easy breathing, you know how efficient his lungs can be. But for cats with asthma (dogs don't get it), the airways in their lungs get inflamed and narrow. During asthma flare-ups, these cats can hardly draw a good breath.

Veterinarians aren't sure what causes asthma, although it appears to be an inherited condition. The attacks may be triggered by such things as pollen, chemical fumes, or emotional stress, says Jeanne Olson, D.V.M., a holistic veterinarian in private practice in North Pole, Alaska. Once an attack is underway, pets begin to panic, making it even harder for them to breathe.

Asthma is always serious, and the conventional approach is to treat the actual attacks by giving medications such as steroids. While medications are often necessary for emergencies, holistic veterinarians feel that it is just as important to treat the underlying problems that are causing the attacks in the first place, says Dr. Olson. Here is what they advise.

## The Solutions

**FOR CATS**

**Soothe the emotions.** Life's little upsets—anything from moving to a new home to having houseguests—may trigger attacks in pets with asthma. One way to keep them calm is with a flower essence called Bach Rescue Remedy, says Arthur Young, D.V.M., a holistic veterinarian in private practice in Stuart, Florida. "Put three or four drops in his mouth." If your pet doesn't like taking medications, you can put the drops on his earflap. "Just flip the ear over to expose the leathery skin, put on the drops, and wipe the area with your finger real quick," he says. You can give Rescue Remedy every

## ✸✸ SUCCESS

### BREATHING EASY

It doesn't happen often, but sometimes the vaccines used to keep pets healthy make them sick. That's what happened with Isis, a five-year-old Egyptian Mau cat who developed severe asthma after getting her annual shots.

"She had to be hospitalized and then was sent home with a lot of medications," says Christina Chambreau, D.V.M., a holistic veterinarian in Sparks, Maryland, and education chairperson for the Academy of Veterinary Homeopathy. "A year and a half later, she still couldn't come off the medication without having severe respiratory problems."

That's when Isis's owner asked Dr. Chambreau to step in. "We put her on a raw-food diet and gave her a homeopathic remedy called Thuja to help counteract the negative effects of the vaccines," she says. "Within three months, she was off all of the drugs, and she was happy, healthy, and playing like she had before her asthma attacks began."

15 minutes until your pet is calm again.

**Stop the sadness.** "Any kind of grieving or sadness will make a lung problem worse," says Cheryl Schwartz, D.V.M., a holistic veterinarian in San Francisco and author of *Four Paws, Five Directions: A Guide to Chinese Medicine for Cats and Dogs.* "It's not unusual for animals to get asthma attacks after a loss in the family, for example."

One way to lift your pet's spirits is with a flower essence called star-of-Bethlehem, which you can give for two weeks to a month. "Put three drops in his water bowl," Dr. Schwartz advises. "Every time you change the water, put the drops in again."

**BEST BET!** **Treat the environment.** Cats can be very sensitive to chemical fumes from such things as room deodorizers, fabric softeners, and insecticides. Cigarette smoke will also trigger asthma attacks in some pets, says Allen M. Schoen, D.V.M., director of the Veterinary Institute for Therapeutic Alternatives in Sherman,

Connecticut, and author of *Love, Miracles, and Animal Healing*. Pets with asthma will breathe a lot easier if you avoid chemical products and use natural alternatives instead, he says. If you smoke, it is best to do it outside. Using an air filter in your home will help remove airborne particles that can irritate the lungs, he adds.

**BEST BET!** **Take advantage of antioxidants.** Holistic veterinarians often recommend giving cats daily supplements of vitamins C and E. These nutrients help the body resist environmental toxins that can trigger asthma attacks, says Dr. Olson. Cats can take 200 milligrams of vitamin C a day. "I prefer ester C, not the ascorbic acid that people take," she adds.

Vitamin C in large doses can cause diarrhea, so you may have to reduce the dose by one-quarter or one-half, says Susan G. Wynn, D.V.M., a veterinarian in Atlanta and co-editor of *Complementary and Alternative Veterinary Medicine*.

For vitamin E, Dr. Wynn recommends giving cats 50 to 100 international units (IU) a day. "I poke the capsule with a pin and squirt it on the

## Call the VET

Asthma isn't like bacterial bronchitis or pneumonia, which can be cured with medications. "It's a progressive disease, not something that happens once and goes away," says Jeanne Olson, D.V.M., a holistic veterinarian in private practice in North Pole, Alaska. Even though pets with asthma always need to be under a veterinarian's care, most people learn to prevent their pets' attacks and treat occasional flare-ups at home.

The danger with asthma is that even a minor attack can become serious with very little warning. One of the most serious symptoms is a blue color to the gums or tongue. Called cyanosis, this means that the body's cells are dangerously low in oxygen. Cyanosis is always an emergency, says Dr. Olson. In fact, any time your pet's breathing is labored, or he is coughing and having trouble breathing, you need to call your vet right away.

## Meet the Experts

**Christina Chambreau, D.V.M.,** is a holistic veterinarian in Sparks, Maryland, and education chairperson for the Academy of Veterinary Homeopathy.

**Anitra Frazier** is an animal behavior consultant in New York City and the author of *The New Natural Cat* and *It's a Cat's Life*.

**Jeanne Olson, D.V.M.,** is a holistic veterinarian in private practice in North Pole, Alaska.

**Allen M. Schoen, D.V.M.,** is director of the Veterinary Institute for Therapeutic Alternatives in Sherman, Connecticut, and the author of *Love, Miracles, and Animal Healing.* He is certified in acupuncture and chiropractic.

**Cheryl Schwartz, D.V.M.,** is a holistic veterinarian in San Francisco and the author of *Four Paws, Five Directions: A Guide to Chinese Medicine for Cats and Dogs*. She is certified in acupuncture.

**Susan G. Wynn, D.V.M.,** is a veterinarian in Atlanta and co-editor of *Complementary and Alternative Veterinary Medicine*.

**Arthur Young, D.V.M.,** is a holistic veterinarian in private practice in Stuart, Florida. He is certified in homeopathy.

food," she says. Or you can mix it in a food treat.

**Rub the lungs into action.** There is an area between the shoulder blades that has "association points" for the lungs. During an asthma attack, "use the balls of your fingers and rub forward and backward, in the head-to-tail direction," says Dr. Schwartz. "It's very helpful in quieting down an attack."

**Create a refuge.** Cats can get very upset by changes in their routines, and any kind of stress can trigger asthma attacks. To keep cats calm during trying times, it is important to give them a snug retreat, says Anitra Frazier, an animal behavior consultant in New York City and author of *The New Natural Cat*. She recommends turning a sturdy cardboard box on its side and putting it in a warm, secluded place. Put a soft towel or an old sweatshirt in the box to make it more cozy. "Cats love this, and it keeps them calm," she says.

**Check his weight.** Cats that are obese have less space for their lungs to move, says Dr. Wynn. If your cat is overweight, talk to your vet about putting him on a weight-loss plan. Your cat will be healthier overall, and his asthma will be a little less of a problem.

**Use soothing words.** "Communication is very important in keeping stress down," Frazier says. Rather than speaking in negatives, such as saying, "No one is going to hurt you," she recommends being very positive. "Tell your pet, 'You're safe; everything is fine,'" she advises.

# Back Problems

## The Signs

- Your pet hunches her shoulders, neck, or back.
- She has trouble moving.
- She cries when you pet her or pick her up.
- She limps, or her hind legs wobble when she walks.

## The Cause

Dogs and cats don't walk upright the way we do, so their backs do a lot less bending and twisting. But even small problems like a pulled muscle or a spot of arthritis can cause a lot of pain and stiffness. Back pain is particularly common in long-bodied dogs, such as dachshunds, because their stretched-out shapes provide relatively little support for the spine, leaving them prone to injuries like herniated disks.

Traditional treatments for back problems include drugs, weeks of confinement and rest, and sometimes surgery. Except in the most serious cases, natural remedies like gentle exercise (or reducing exercise), acupressure, and dietary supplements will relieve the pain and, in some cases, slow the progression of the underlying problem as well, says Susan G. Wynn, D.V.M., a veterinarian in Atlanta and co-editor of *Complementary and Alternative Veterinary Medicine*.

## The Solutions  FOR DOGS & CATS

**Put pressure to work.** The body has a natural—but painful—method for dealing with back problems: Muscles in the area suddenly tighten and go into spasms. Spasms help stabilize the back and give it a chance to heal. The problem with spasms is that they don't always go away when the problem does. Spasms can persist for weeks, months, or even years, causing excruciating pain and stiffness.

When your pet is suddenly stiff and sore, feel the muscles along either side of the spine. If you discover a hard little muscle "knot"—the telltale sign of a spasm—press directly on the spot with your thumb or finger, says Dr. Wynn. Maintain the pressure for 10 seconds to two minutes. "You may be able to feel the knot suddenly relax," she says. Then move farther along the spine, pressing muscle spasms as you go. Muscle spasms are tender, and your pet won't like the pressure, but it is one way to stop the pain.

**Magnetize the pain.** The BL60 acupressure point (located on the outside of the back leg in the depression at the base of the Achilles tendon midway between the tendon and the ankle-bone) has been called the aspirin point because it is well-known for controlling pain, says Randy Caviness, D.V.M., clinical instructor of small animal acupuncture at Tufts University School of Veterinary Medicine in North Grafton, Massachusetts, and a holistic veterinarian in Concord. You can stimulate the point with direct pressure or by using a magnet. "The magnet stimulates the point in a very gentle but prolonged way," he says. "It's great for a pet with long-term pain."

You can get healing magnets from holistic veterinarians. Some have a self-stick adhesive on the back, he explains, so that you can stick them on the skin and leave them in place for up to a week. Or you can wrap it in place with a piece of gauze or first-aid tape.

**Ease it with ice.** One reason back problems are so painful is that they are often accompanied by inflammation, which puts pressure on nearby muscles and nerves. To relieve temporary pain and inflammation, apply cold to the area. You can freeze water

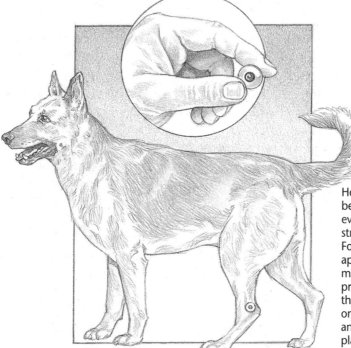

Holistic veterinarians have begun using magnets for everything from reducing stress to relieving pain. For pets with back pain, apply an adhesive-backed magnet to the BL60 acupressure point (also called the aspirin point), located on the outside of the ankle, and leave it in place for up to a week.

## Call the VET

**B**ack problems are worrisome because the body's main communication pathways, the spinal cord and adjoining nerves, run through and exit from the spine. Anything that presses on one of the spinal nerves—a misaligned vertebra, for example, or a slipped disk—can prevent it from carrying messages to and from the brain and spinal cord.

Any back problem is potentially serious. Symptoms of a bad back include a wobbly walk or difficulty getting up. Don't take chances if the symptoms came on suddenly. Serious back problems that cause paralysis of the hind legs are an emergency, and you need to get your pet to the vet right away.

in a paper cup, then peel away the paper to use the "ice stick" on areas that feel hot to the touch, says Dr. Caviness. Apply the cold for 15 to 20 minutes, or until your pet makes it clear she has had enough. Repeat the treatment two or three times a day for a few days until the inflammation goes away, he advises. You will know that your pet is feeling better when she is less sensitive to touch and moves more easily.

**Add a little heat.** When your pet has long-term back pain that isn't accompanied by swelling, you may want to apply warmth to the area. This loosens muscles, relieving painful stiffness, says Dr. Caviness. He recommends wrapping a hot-water bottle in a towel and holding it on your pet's

back for about 20 minutes, three times a day, for two to three days.

**Protect the joints.** A dietary supplement called glucosamine, available in health food stores, can help heal connective tissues between the vertebrae, says Albert J. Simpson, D.V.M., a holistic veterinarian in private practice in Oregon City, Oregon. He recommends giving cats 3 to 4 milligrams of glucosamine per pound of body weight once a day. Dogs under 15 pounds can take 5 milligrams per pound, and larger dogs can take up to 15 milligrams per pound, he says.

Some veterinarians recommend giving Cosequin, a combination of glucosamine and another supplement called chondroitin sulfate, which can help repair damaged cartilage. You can give pets 10 milligrams of it per pound of body weight twice daily, says Dr. Wynn. Glucosamine is safe, but when combined with chondroitin, it may cause bleeding problems. Cosequin is available only through your veterinarian and should not be used in pets that have liver problems or clotting disorders.

**Walk it off.** Veterinarians have traditionally recommended that dogs and cats with back problems be kept virtually immobile until they start feeling better. Holistic veterinarians feel that it is better to keep them moving, at least in a gentle way. For pets with chronic back problems, gentle, sustained exercise can help muscles stabilize the spine, Dr. Wynn says. (For pets with neck problems, use a harness instead of a collar when taking walks.) But keep in mind that pushing too hard before an injury is healed will slow recovery rather than speed it along.

Start with five minutes of gentle walking three to five times a week, says Dr. Wynn. As your pet gets better, gradually increase the duration of the walks from 20 to 60 minutes a day. Be sure to check with your vet before starting an exercise program, she adds. It may not be good for pets with serious injuries.

**Watch her weight.** Pets that are overweight are more likely to have back problems because of the extra pressure on the spine. Helping over-

## Meet the Experts

**Randy Caviness, D.V.M.,** is a clinical instructor of small animal acupuncture at Tufts University School of Veterinary Medicine in North Grafton, Massachusetts, and a holistic veterinarian in Concord. He is certified in acupuncture and chiropractic.

**Kathy Kern** is a registered veterinary technician and the owner of Animal Fitness Center at Almaden Valley Hospital in San Jose, California.

**Nancy Scanlan, D.V.M.,** is a holistic veterinarian in private practice in Sherman Oaks, California. She is certified in acupuncture and chiropractic.

**Albert J. Simpson, D.V.M.,** is a holistic veterinarian in private practice in Oregon City, Oregon. He is certified in acupuncture and chiropractic.

**Susan G. Wynn, D.V.M.,** is a veterinarian in Atlanta and co-editor of *Complementary and Alternative Veterinary Medicine*.

weight pets lose a few pounds can relieve or even eliminate some back problems, says Nancy Scanlan, D.V.M., a holistic veterinarian in private practice in Sherman Oaks, California. To check your pet's weight, feel her sides. If you can feel the ribs, but they aren't clearly visible, she is probably in good shape. If she seems a little heavy, cut back on her food a bit or ask your vet to recommend a safe weight-loss plan.

## The Solutions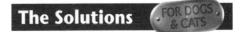

**Head for the water.** Swimming is almost the perfect exercise for dogs with back problems because the water supports your pet's weight and reduces stress on the spine. It also gets the joints moving, which loosens tight muscles and eases pain and stiffness, says Kathy Kern, a registered veterinary technician and owner of Animal Fitness Center at Almaden Valley Animal Hospital in San Jose, California.

# BAD BREATH

## The Signs
- Your pet's breath has recently taken a turn for the worse.
- His breath smells like ammonia or urine, or it is unusually sweet.

## The Cause

Things that humans consider unspeakably smelly, like last week's garbage, are ambrosia for dogs and cats. They will eat—and try to digest—just about anything that has a strong flavor and a stronger smell. So it is not surprising that they occasionally have bouts of smelly breath—as well as indigestion, which can make their breath even worse.

Even though occasional bad breath is normal, foul odors that don't go away usually mean that something is wrong, either in the mouth itself or somewhere else in the body, says Kimberly Henneman, D.V.M., a holistic veterinarian in private practice in Utah. Brushing your pet's teeth won't hurt and may, in fact, solve the problem, but holistic veterinarians usually take a broader view. "The mouth is like a gateway into the body, and bad breath can signal disease or a more serious chronic condition," she says.

In most cases, you can improve your pet's breath with a combination of basic hygiene and changes in his diet, along with a variety of all-natural remedies that attack the problem from the inside out. Here are a few tips you may want to try.

## The Solutions

**Give them some leafy greens.** Fresh alfalfa and parsley are filled with vitamins, minerals, and other compounds such as chlorophyll that can aid digestion and sweeten the breath at the same time, says Dr. Henneman. You can buy fresh parsley at any supermarket, although you will probably have to go a health food store to purchase alfalfa sprouts. Whichever herb you choose, finely chop it and sprinkle one-half to one teaspoon on your pet's food every day.

You can also use dried herbs, says Dr. Henneman. When using dried herbs, soak one tablespoon in a cup of hot filtered water to make an herbal tea. Once it cools to room temperature, strain the tea and add it to your pet's food, she suggests. Pets under 15 pounds can take one-half to one teaspoon of the tea. Give one teaspoon to one tablespoon to pets weighing 15 to 50 pounds and one to three tablespoons to larger dogs.

**BEST BET!** **Remove the plaque.** Just like humans, dogs and cats have problems with plaque—an invisible, bacteria-filled film that accumulates on the teeth and is one of the leading causes of bad breath. Brushing your pet's teeth will help remove plaque before it hardens in place. Brushing twice a day is ideal, says Anthony Shipp, D.V.M., a veterinarian in private practice in Beverly Hills, California. Twice a week, however, is okay.

You can buy toothbrushes made especially for dogs and cats, but an easier solution is to rub the outer surfaces of their teeth with a small piece of gauze coated with a dab of pet toothpaste. Pet toothpastes come in a variety of flavors, like poultry, beef, or malt, which make brushing more enticing to pets. Look for a toothpaste with all-natural ingredients like Doctors Foster and Smith All Natural Toothpaste, which is available in the Doctors Foster and Smith catalog. Don't use human toothpastes because they may contain ingredients that can cause stomach upset in pets, says Wendy Beers, D.V.M., a veterinarian in private practice in Albany, California. This is especially important if your pet is currently being treated with homeopathy. Peppermint as well as other common ingredients in human toothpastes can make homeopathic remedies ineffective.

**BEST BET!** **Improve their diets.** Another way to fight plaque is to make a few changes in your pet's diet. Animals on excellent diets tend to get a lot less tooth plaque, says Dr. Henneman. She recommends feeding pets a homemade diet made up of raw meat, vegetables, and grains. For more on homemade diets, see page 61.

**Give them dry food.** Dogs and cats love the aroma and taste of moist foods, but these foods don't always love them back. Moist foods stick to the teeth, which encourages foul-smelling bacteria to proliferate. "Switching to dry food may help to

## Call the VET

Nearly every pet gets bad breath now and then, and it usually goes away within a few days. While a little stinky breath isn't cause for alarm, there are a few serious conditions that can cause distinct mouth odors, says Albert S. Dorn, D.V.M., professor of surgery at the University of Tennessee College of Veterinary Medicine in Knoxville. Call your vet if you notice one of the following.

- An ammonia- or urine-like smell. This is a dead giveaway for kidney problems.

- A rotten smell. This is usually a sign of intestinal problems or gum or tooth disease.

- A sweet, almost sugary smell. This often signals diabetes. Pets with diabetes will also be drinking a lot of water and losing weight.

improve mouth odor," says Lisa Freeman, D.V.M., Ph.D., assistant professor and clinical nutritionist at Tufts University School of Veterinary Medicine in North Grafton, Massachusetts. Cats may need both wet and dry food because they don't always drink a lot of water and can use the extra fluids they get from moist foods.

**Take advantage of nature's toothbrush.** Raw carrots are great for the teeth because they act like natural tooth scrapers, says Cheryl Schwartz, D.V.M., a holistic veterinarian in San Francisco and author of *Four Paws, Five Directions: A Guide to Chinese Medicine for Cats and Dogs*. If your pet is reluctant to eat carrots, try freezing them first. Most dogs and cats enjoy

crunching ice cubes and other cold treats, and freezing the carrots will make them more tempting.

**Settle the stomach.** Since bad breath is often caused by indigestion, you may want to give your pet some ginger (*Zingiber officinale*), which helps calm an upset stomach, says Susan G. Wynn, D.V.M., a veterinarian in Atlanta and co-editor of *Complementary and Alternative Medicine*. She recommends adding one tablespoon of fresh sliced ginger to a cup of hot filtered water and letting the tea cool. Strain the tea and give pets under 15 pounds one-half to one teaspoon of the tea, using a dropper or needleless syringe, she says. Give one teaspoon to one tablespoon to pets weighing 15 to

50 pounds and one to three table-spoons to larger dogs.

Another way to quell indigestion is with homeopathy. Dr. Henneman recommends giving dogs and cats one to two pellets of Nux vomica 30X or any 3 potency of Arsenicum. You can repeat the treatment once in a few hours if your pet is feeling better and his breath seems to be improving. If the problem continues despite this treatment, check with your vet.

**Rub him the right way.** Massaging your pet's belly, using a technique that is similar to Lamaze, will often help ease the cramping that can cause bad breath, Dr. Henneman says. Starting on the flank near the hip, use your fingertips to make gentle, sweeping circles, moving down the side of the flank and onto the abdomen. Once you have reached his tummy, massage your way onto the chest and then back toward the groin. "Most pets love it, but it must be done softly," she says. "It should be relaxing to your pet, but not painful."

**Care for the gums.** Dogs and cats often get smelly breath when they have a gum infection. An effective way to help the gums heal is to give them a supplement called coenzyme $Q_{10}$, says Ihor Basko, D.V.M., a holistic veterinarian in private practice in Honolulu and Kilauea, Hawaii. He recommends giving pets weighing up to 20 pounds 10 milligrams of coenzyme $Q_{10}$ a day. Pets 21 to 50 pounds

## Meet the Experts

**Ihor Basko, D.V.M.,** is a holistic veterinarian in private practice in Honolulu and Kilauea, Hawaii, and the creator of the video *The Healing Touch for Your Dogs*. He is certified in acupuncture.

**Wendy Beers, D.V.M.,** is a veterinarian in private practice in Albany, California.

**Albert S. Dorn, D.V.M.,** is a professor of surgery at the University of Tennessee College of Veterinary Medicine in Knoxville.

**Lisa Freeman, D.V.M., Ph.D.,** is an assistant professor and clinical nutritionist at the Tufts University School of Veterinary Medicine in North Grafton, Massachusetts.

**Kimberly Henneman, D.V.M.,** is a holistic veterinarian in private practice in Utah. She is certified in acupuncture and chiropractic.

**Cheryl Schwartz, D.V.M.,** is a holistic veterinarian in San Francisco and the author of *Four Paws, Five Directions: A Guide to Chinese Medicine for Cats and Dogs*. She is certified in acupuncture.

**Anthony Shipp, D.V.M.,** is a veterinarian in private practice in Beverly Hills, California. He specializes in dentistry.

**Susan G. Wynn, D.V.M.,** is a veterinarian in Atlanta and co-editor of *Complementary and Alternative Medicine*.

can take up to 30 milligrams once a day, and larger dogs can take 30 milligrams twice a day.

**Shed some light on the problem.** Breath that is suddenly pungent may be caused by something that is stuck in the mouth. Place one hand over the muzzle and gently open the lower jaw with your other hand. Pets may bite when they are in pain, so you will want to be cautious. You can use a flashlight to take a look inside. If you see something stuck between the teeth or under the gum, you will need to have it removed by the vet.

# BARKING

## The Signs

- Your dog barks for long periods of time.
- He barks even when nothing is going on.

## The Cause

It's natural for dogs to bark. It's one of their ways of communicating and letting you (and other dogs) know that something exciting is going on. But when your dog is barking for hours and is driving you, your neighbors, and everyone who comes within a block of your house crazy, it can be a real problem.

Incessant barking is often caused by emotional problems, says Robin Cannizzaro, D.V.M., a holistic veterinarian in private practice in St. Petersburg, Florida. "It can stem from nervous excitability, excess energy, fear, or a need for attention," she explains.

It is possible to train dogs to bark less often, but it is equally important to deal with the underlying emotions that are causing the barking in the first place, says Dr. Cannizzaro. Here are some natural—and gentle—ways to turn down the volume.

## The Solutions

**Try a distraction.** Dogs usually bark in response to something they see or hear. One way to keep them quiet is to put their noses to work. "Get a very strong smelling essential oil, such as lavender or citrus, and spritz some in the air when they are barking," says Deborah C. Mallu, D.V.M., a holistic veterinarian in private practice in Sedona, Arizona. Use a spray bottle and dilute five

**ALTERNATIVE**

# 🐾SUCCESS

## RELIEF FROM FEAR

Dancer, a two-year-old Great Dane, was calm and quiet as long as people were around. When he was left alone, however, he would go slightly berserk, barking and tearing up rugs, furniture, and anything else that he could get his teeth around. It was his way of coping with the fear and anxiety he felt when he was by himself.

His owners, besieged by angry neighbors and faced with mounting repair bills, finally took him to Pat Bradley, D.V.M., a holistic veterinarian in private practice in Conway, Arkansas. After an examination and a lot of questions, she decided to treat Dancer with the homeopathic remedy Pulsatilla.

"It worked beautifully, and today he is much calmer," she says. "He still gets a bit anxious when he is left alone, but he doesn't go into the frantic barking and destructiveness anymore."

drops of the oil in a cup of water. Shake the mixture very well before using. You don't need to spray it in his face, she adds. Just putting a new smell in the air will help, distracting him from his noise-making. Avoid spraying essential oils near your dog's eyes.

**Try a "bark alarm."** Veterinarians sometimes recommend shock collars as training tools to stop barking. A gentler option is to use a citronella collar. "You put this collar on the dog, and when he barks, he gets a little spray of citronella," says Karen Komisar, D.V.M., a holistic veteri-narian in private practice in Lynn, Massachusetts. Dogs dislike the smell of citronella and will soon learn that barking can have odoriferous conse-quences, she explains.

**Soothe their emotions.** Dogs often bark because they are afraid or nervous or simply want some atten-tion, Dr. Cannizzaro says. You can turn down the volume by giving them flower essences, which will help keep their emotions calm. The essence mimulus will quiet barking caused by fear, for example. Agrimony or cherry plum will calm anxiety, and impatiens is good for nervous irritability. You can give dogs

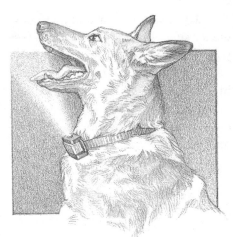

One way to teach your dog not to bark is to use a citronella collar. Unlike shock collars, which deliver an electrical jolt when dogs bark, these release a mist of citronella, along with a "psst" sound. Once your dog makes the connection between his barking and the unpleasant smell and strange sound, he will think twice about sounding off. Citronella collars are available in pet supply stores and catalogs.

several drops a day of a flower essence by putting the drops either in their water or directly in their mouths.

**Tell him what you think.** Dogs don't mean any harm when they bark, and they will often quiet down when they understand how you feel about it, says Dr. Mallu. "Tell your dog exactly what you think," she advises. "He will pick up on what you're trying to say on some level, whether it's the intonation of your voice, the mental picture you send him, or your body language."

**Move the furniture.** Dogs get ex-

cited by things they see outside the house—trucks going by, for example, or a neighbor watering his lawn. You may want to try moving the furniture a bit in order to block the view by putting a couch in front of a low window or simply pulling the blinds, says Dr. Mallu. Don't cut off all outside views, she adds, just the ones where the view seems to be causing a lot of excitement.

**Return to school.** Barking dogs often need reminders that their jobs

## Meet the Experts

**Pat Bradley, D.V.M.,** is a holistic veterinarian in private practice in Conway, Arkansas. She is certified in homeopathy.

**Robin Cannizzaro, D.V.M.,** is a holistic veterinarian in private practice in St. Petersburg, Florida. She is certified in acupuncture and homeopathy.

**Christina Chambreau, D.V.M.,** is a holistic veterinarian in Sparks, Maryland, and education chairperson for the Academy of Veterinary Homeopathy.

**Karen Komisar, D.V.M.,** is a holistic veterinarian in private practice in Lynn, Massachusetts. She is certified in homeopathy.

**Deborah C. Mallu, D.V.M.,** is a holistic veterinarian in private practice in Sedona, Arizona. She is certified in acupuncture.

are to please the human members of the family, says Christina Chambreau, D.V.M., a holistic veterinarian in Sparks, Maryland, and education chairperson for the Academy of Veterinary Homeopathy. "He needs to know who is in charge and that you are unhappy with what he is doing,"

she says. You don't have to go to obedience school, but you do need to give your dog lessons by telling him, "No!" when he starts barking or by putting him in a room by himself for a minute or two. "You need to think of a consequence that will work for your particular pet," she says.

# BEGGING

## The Signs
- Your pet won't get out of the kitchen.
- She stares at you or whines when you are eating.
- She swipes food when you are not looking.

## The Cause

Pets love people food, and if you share your dinner even once, they will get optimistic and start asking for more—again and again. Dogs can be incorrigible beggers, although cats do their share of mooching, too.

Whether begging is caused by your past generosity or your pet's freewheeling tastebuds, the only solution is to help her understand that your food isn't automatically her food—and to keep reminding her until she gives up and lets you eat in peace. Here are

some simple remedies that you may want to try.

## The Solutions · FOR DOGS & CATS

**Try a raw-meat diet.** Dogs and cats will occasionally turn to begging when they aren't getting all the nutrients they need from their regular food, which can make them feel hungry all the time, says Adriana Sagrera, D.V.M., a holistic veterinarian in private practice in New Orleans. "When I put pets on a raw-meat diet, they tend to beg less because they are getting all the proteins and enzymes they need," she explains. For more information on raw diets, see page 67.

**Help digestion.** Even healthy pets given high-quality foods aren't always able to absorb all the nutrients in their food, says Pat Bradley, D.V.M., a holistic veterinarian in private prac-

## Call the VET

Dogs and cats usually mooch for the same reason children do: There is something tasty around that they like better than what they already have. But some pets may have health problems such as diabetes or hyperthyroidism that can make them ravenously hungry even when they have cleaned out their bowls, says Pat Bradley, D.V.M., a holistic veterinarian in private practice in Conway, Arkansas.

If the begging is a recent thing, or if your pet is losing weight or her fur is looking dry and dull, she may not be getting essential vitamins and minerals, and you should call your vet right away.

---

tice in Conway, Arkansas. This can make them hungry all the time and less likely to mind their manners. Holistic veterinarians often recommend giving pets digestive enzymes formulated specifically for pets, which make it easier for them to get all the vitamins and minerals their bodies need. Follow the dosage directions on the label.

**BEST BET!** **Give her some quiet time.** Rather than scolding your pet for begging at the dinner table, try putting her in a room by herself until you are done eating, says Robin Cannizzaro, D.V.M., a holistic veterinarian in private practice in St. Petersburg, Florida. The idea isn't to punish her, but to help her understand that your dinner hour and hers don't necessarily coincide. Giving her a bone to chew or a toy to play with will keep her happily occupied. You may want to play some soothing music as well, which will help keep her mind off her stomach, she adds.

**Move the snack tray.** There is nothing wrong with giving pets tasty tidbits from the table as long as you do it in a different location from where you eat, says Anitra Frazier, an animal behavior consultant in New York City and author of *The New Natural Cat*. Pets who learn that they will get something special after you are done eating will be less likely to beg at the table. "Keep a little plate on the table and use it for things you want your pet to have later," she suggests. "Then, after you have eaten, say something like, 'Come on, it's leftover time!' and feed her, using the same plate in the same place, but not near the table."

**BEST BET!** **Be consistent.** In every family, there is bound to be a softie who will slip the dog or cat snacks while you are the one laying down the law. It is important that everyone in the family buy into the anti-begging program. Otherwise, your pet will get mixed signals and will keep asking for more, says Deborah C. Mallu, D.V.M., a holistic veterinarian in private practice in Sedona, Arizona.

**Feed her more often.** Some dogs and cats get hunger pangs when they are fed only once a day, and their appetites can lead them into temptation. You may want to feed your pet the same amount of food but divide it into several servings throughout the day. This will help keep her satisfied and less likely to beg, says Dr. Mallu.

## The Solutions  FOR CATS

**Feed her first.** Feeding your cat before the family sits down at the

table is often all it takes to get a little peace. "Cats will usually go off to wash and preen once they have had enough to eat," Dr. Mallu explains.

# BLADDER-CONTROL PROBLEMS

## The Signs
- Your pet dribbles urine when she sleeps.
- Her bedding or back legs are damp.
- She has started having accidents in the house.

## The Cause
Dogs have been our best friends for thousands of years, but they never would have been invited across the threshold if they weren't naturally clean. They have an instinctive need to keep their "nests" tidy, which is why they are reluctant to urinate in areas

where they play or sleep. But despite their best intentions, even well-trained dogs may lose control occasionally or for prolonged periods of time.

Spayed female dogs are the ones most likely to have problems with bladder control because they produce so little estrogen, a hormone that gives tension to the urinary sphincter (the muscle that controls urination), says George Carley, D.V.M., a holistic veterinarian in private practice in Tulsa, Oklahoma. Urinary tract infections, which are readily treated with antibiotics, can also cause a loss of control. In addition, older pets, both males and females, sometimes forget their training or lose control. Cats almost never have bladder control problems; they mainly occur in dogs, he adds.

Conventional veterinarians sometimes control problems by giving dogs a form of synthetic estrogen called diethylstilbestrol or an over-the-counter "diet" medication that strengthens and tightens the urinary sphincter. Nature has provided many sources of estrogen, however, so it isn't always necessary to resort to drugs, says Dr. Carley. It is possible to use home remedies to help your dog produce more estrogen naturally. Here are a few things you may want to try.

## The Solutions FOR DOGS

**Restore control with acupressure.** There are several acupressure points that control the bladder as well as the adrenal glands. Pressing these points may strengthen the urinary sphincter and help the body produce more estrogen, says Joanne Stefanatos, D.V.M., a holistic veterinarian in private practice in Las Vegas. The acupressure points for bladder control include the following.

- BL67, located on the outside edge of the outside toe on each rear foot.

- BL1, located on the inside corner of each eye.

- SP6, located on the inside rear leg above the hock (the ankle).

- SP10, located just above the bend on the rear knee.

Put pressure on each of these points for about 60 seconds, two or three times a day, recommends Dr. Stefanatos. Once your dog regains control, repeat the treatments once or twice a week.

**Rebalance the body.** Some holistic veterinarians treat bladder-control problems with a homeopathic combination called, appropriately enough, Urinary Incontinence. It contains healing amounts of Gelsemium, Alumina, Plantago, Causticum, and Cantharis, and it helps change your dog's hormonal balance so that the bladder and urinary sphincter work more efficiently. Dr. Stefanatos recom-

## ALTERNATIVE

# ☙ SUCCESS

## NATURAL CONTROL

Judith wasn't happy when Jill, her poodle companion of 14 years, began dribbling urine in the house, but she wasn't about to let a damp carpet get in the way of their wonderful relationship. So she took Jill to a conventional veterinarian, who prescribed synthetic estrogen to be given every day.

Judith faithfully gave the medication for three months. Jill's control did improve, but the medicine was making her sick. She wouldn't eat, she was bloated, and generally didn't feel very well. "Jill had all the signs of estrogen overdose when I saw her," says George Carley, D.V.M., a holistic veterinarian in private practice in Tulsa, Oklahoma.

Dr. Carley stopped the estrogen and started treating Jill with digestive enzymes and herbal supplements, along with a procedure called aquapuncture, in which dilute substances, including vitamin $B_{12}$, are injected near acupuncture points.

The treatments worked, and within just a few weeks Jill was both dry and healthy, and she quickly regained her usual energy, says Dr. Carley.

mends giving half a dropperful of the remedy twice a day until things start to improve.

**Replace estrogen with glandular supplements.** Dogs with bladder-control problems may improve when given supplements containing extracts from the ovaries and adrenal, thyroid, and pituitary glands. Called raw-gland concentrates or multiple-glandular dietary supplements, these products help the body produce more natural estrogen, says Dr. Carley.

Holistic veterinarians sometimes use a product called Symplex F, available from veterinarians only, which contains all the necessary extracts. Or you can use a glandular supplement designed for humans, such as Solaray, available in health food stores, says Anne Lampru, D.V.M., a holistic veterinarian in private practice in Tampa, Florida. She recommends giving dogs weighing under 15 pounds one-quarter of the human dose. Dogs 15 to 50 pounds can take one-third of the human dose, and larger dogs can take one-half of the human dose. Most dogs will need to take the supplements for the rest of their lives, she adds.

**Strengthen the nerves with massage.** Back and spinal disk injuries sometimes put pressure on the nerves that control urination, resulting in incontinence, says Susan G. Wynn, a veterinarian in Atlanta and co-author of *Complementary and Alternative Veterinary Medicine*. You can use a technique called motion palpation to flex the spine and reduce pressure on the nerves.

Motion palpation is easy to do. Hold your thumb and index finger together and find the dip between the vertebra on either side of your pet's backbone. Gently press straight down for one to two seconds, then release. (Some pets are sensitive to the pressure, and you may want to press with the flat of your hand.) Starting at the shoulders and going to the hips, press between each vertebra, using just enough pressure to slightly move the spine. Because motion palpation helps keep the spine flexible, it can be used to help prevent as well as treat incontinence, says Dr. Wynn.

**Keep the mind sharp.** Older dogs sometimes lose control because they forget that they are supposed to wait until they get outside. A variety of vitamins, including vitamins A, C, and E, seem to help, says Dr. Wynn. She

recommends using a supplement called Cell-Advance, available from veterinarians, following the directions on the label.

Digestive enzymes such as Pro-zyme and FloraZyme, available in pet supply stores, may also help the intestines absorb nutrients more efficiently, which can play a role in keeping the mind sharp, explains Dr. Carley. Every pet needs different amounts, so follow the directions on the label.

An alternative to store-bought enzymes is to give your pet yogurt containing active cultures with every meal. Pets under 15 pounds can have a few teaspoons, and larger pets can have a few tablespoons.

Egg yolks also act as natural digestion enzymes, says Roger L. De-Haan, D.V.M., a holistic veterinarian in private practice in Frazee, Minnesota. Pets under 50 pounds can have one egg yolk a week, and larger pets can have two, he explains.

# BLADDER STONES

## The Signs
- Your pet is straining to urinate or is urinating more often.
- There is blood in the urine.
- He is urinating in inappropriate places.

## The Cause

Urine leaves the bladder through a tube called the urethra, which isn't much wider than a piece of thread. Urine is mainly water, so it passes through without a hitch—except when pets have bladder stones. Then these jagged accumulations of minerals can scrape the urethra on their way through, causing excruciating pain.

"There are a lot of minerals in the urine, and for reasons that aren't completely understood, the minerals will sometimes crystallize," explains Carvel Tiekert, D.V.M., executive director of the American Holistic Veterinary Medical Association and a holistic veterinarian in Bel Air, Maryland.

Small bladder stones may leave the body without causing discomfort. But when the stones are large, they irritate the lining of bladder, triggering a frequent (and urgent) need to urinate. They can also partially or completely block the flow of urine, forcing pets to strain just to eliminate a feeble stream.

There are two kinds of bladder stones. One kind tends to form in urine that is acidic, and the other may form when urine is alkaline. Each type of stone may require different treatments, so it is important to see your vet to find out which kind your pet has. Surgery is often needed to remove large stones. In many cases, you can use natural remedies to keep them from coming back. Here is what veterinarians advise.

## The Solutions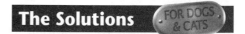

**Put meat on the menu.** Commercial pet foods typically get most of

## Call the VET

Bladder stones are uncomfortable, but they rarely cause life-threatening problems—at least in females. In males, however, the urethra is so narrow that it is easily blocked, even by small stones. This means that large amounts of urine can accumulate, possibly damaging the bladder or kidneys in just a few hours.

Pets with a blocked urethra will strain to urinate, but little or nothing will come out. This condition is painful, so they will probably cry as well, says John M. Simon, D.V.M., a holistic veterinarian in private practice in Royal Oak, Michigan. A blocked urethra is always an emergency, he says, and you will need to get your pet to a vet as quickly as you can.

---

their calories and protein from grains, which make the urine alkaline—an environment that encourages some types of stones to form. "Giving pets more meat tends to acidify the urine and helps dissolve certain types of crystals," says John M. Simon, D.V.M., a holistic veterinarian in private practice in Royal Oak, Michigan.

He recommends giving dogs and cats raw lamb, beef, or venison every day. For dogs, about one-third of the diet should consist of raw meat. For cats, about 40 percent of the diet should consist of meat. Raw meat is more nutritious than cooked or processed meat, says Dr. Simon, but if you are using commercial products, find one with a high percentage of meat and then add some raw meat to it, just to make sure. For more information on raw-meat diets, see page 67.

**Feed him less often.** Frequent feedings can be a problem, says Michele Yasson, D.V.M., a holistic veterinarian in private practice in New York City and Rosendale, New York. "Right after eating, many parts of the body become more alkaline, which can promote the crystallization of stones," she explains.

She recommends feeding pets no more than once or twice a day. This will keep the urine more acidic so that stones are less likely to form.

**BEST BET!** **Provide plenty of water.** Pets that don't drink a lot of water don't urinate very often, which means that bacteria and debris in the bladder aren't flushed out as often as they should be. This can be a problem because pets with bladder infections have a higher risk of developing stones, says Michelle Tilghman, D.V.M., a holistic veterinarian in private practice in Stone Mountain, Georgia. Make sure that your pet's water supply is not only plentiful but also pure since impurities in tap water can irritate the bladder, she says.

Of course, dogs and cats won't drink more water just because you want them to. The easiest way to get more fluids into their bodies is to add water or low-salt broth to their food. "Make the food soupy," Dr. Tiekert advises.

**Give a natural diuretic.** There are a number of herbs, such as corn silk and parsley, that act as natural diuretics and help remove fluids from the body. This can be helpful for pets with bladder stones because the extra urine produced by the kidneys can help flush away debris, says Susan G. Wynn, D.V.M., a veterinarian in Atlanta and co-editor of *Complementary and Alternative Veterinary Medicine*. You can give one corn silk capsule for every 20 pounds of weight, she says. When giving fresh parsley, just add it to your pet's food. Pets under 15 pounds can take one-half to one teaspoon of fresh chopped parsley a day,

| Meet the Experts |
| --- |

**Gerald Buchoff, B.V.Sc.A.H.,** is a holistic veterinarian in private practice in North Bergen, New Jersey. He is certified in chiropractic.

**John M. Simon, D.V.M.,** is a holistic veterinarian in private practice in Royal Oak, Michigan. He is certified in acupuncture and chiropractic.

**Carvel Tiekert, D.V.M.,** is executive director of the American Holistic Veterinary Medical Association and a holistic veterinarian in Bel Air, Maryland. He is certified in acupuncture and chiropractic.

**Michelle Tilghman, D.V.M.,** is a holistic veterinarian in private practice in Stone Mountain, Georgia. She is certified in acupuncture.

**Susan G. Wynn, D.V.M.,** is a veterinarian in Atlanta and co-editor of *Complementary and Alternative Veterinary Medicine*.

**Michele Yasson, D.V.M.,** is a holistic veterinarian in private practice in New York City and Rosendale, New York. She is certified in acupuncture.

she says. Pets 15 to 50 pounds can take one to two teaspoons, and larger pets can have one-half to one tablespoon.

**Give them ascorbic acid.** The most common form of vitamin C is ascorbic acid, which acidifies the urine and helps dissolve and prevent some kinds of stones, says Dr. Yasson. She recommends giving pets under 15 pounds between 250 and 500 milligrams of vitamin C twice a day. Pets 15 to 50 pounds can take 500 milligrams twice a day, and larger dogs can take 1,000 milligrams of vitamin C twice a day. Since vitamin C can cause diarrhea, you may have to cut back the dose until you find an amount that your pet can tolerate.

**Show him the whey.** A mineral supplement called Capra Mineral Whey contains biologically active minerals that help dissolve stones in the bladder, says Dr. Yasson. It usually comes in granule form and is available in some health food stores or from mail-order companies. She recommends giving pets that weigh more than 50 pounds the full human dose once a day. Pets 20 to 50 pounds can take one-half of the human dose, and smaller pets can take one-quarter of the human dose.

## The Solutions

FOR CATS

**Remove the grit with homeopathy.** Cats occasionally develop a condition called feline lower urinary tract disease, in which the urine gets so loaded with minerals that it has a gritty appearance. You can eliminate much of the grit with homeopathic remedies, says Gerald Buchoff, B.V.Sc.A.H. (bachelor of veterinary science and animal husbandry, the Indian equivalent of D.V.M.), a holistic veterinarian in private practice in North Bergen, New Jersey. When the grit is red, the best homeopathic remedy is Lycopodium. When the grit is white, use Sarsaparilla. He recommends giving cats one 30C pellet of either remedy three times a day until the urine looks normal again.

# Bloat

## The Signs

- Your dog's belly is swollen.
- He tries to vomit, but nothing comes up.
- He is drooling heavily.

## The Cause

Humans who eat too much sometimes get a gassy, bloated feeling. It is uncomfortable and sometimes embarrassing, but it is not a serious problem. In dogs, however, bloat (also

# Call the VET

The scary thing about bloat is that it can occur very quickly, sometimes causing the stomach to expand and twist (a condition called volvulus) in an hour or less. That's why it is critical to know the warning signs of bloat before it goes too far.

Dogs with sudden bloat will get a hard, swollen abdomen, which, if you tap it with your finger, will thump like a drum. They will also be uncomfortable and will arch their backs, lick their lips, drool heavily, and try to swallow. They will try to vomit, although nothing will come out. These symptoms mean that your dog is seriously ill, and you need to get him to your veterinarian or an emergency clinic immediately.

called gastric dilation) can be serious or even life-threatening.

Bloat occurs when air and gases accumulate in the stomach, causing it to swell like a balloon. A little bit of gassiness will usually go away on its own. But when bloat comes on suddenly, the stomach may swell so much that it twists within the abdominal cavity, possibly cutting off its supply of blood, explains Maria Chelaru-Williams, D.V.M., a veterinarian in private practice in Boulder, Colorado. Cats rarely get bloat, she adds. It is most common in large, deep-chested dogs like German shepherds and standard poodles.

Although bloat can be serious, the remedies to help prevent it are really quite simple. Here is what veterinarians advise.

## The Solutions FOR DOGS

**Feed him yogurt.** Your dog's digestive tract contains bacteria that help food digest properly. When there aren't enough of these bacteria, bloat-causing gas may accumulate, says Sandra Priest, D.V.M., a holistic veterinarian in private practice in Knoxville, Tennessee. To improve digestion and prevent gas, "I usually suggest giving plain yogurt with no artificial sweeteners," she says. Dogs over 15 pounds can have a teaspoonful of live-culture yogurt once a day, while smaller dogs can have between one-quarter and one-half teaspoon.

**Add some enzymes.** Another way to improve digestion is to give your dog digestive enzymes, available at pet supply stores, once a day, says Dr.

Priest. She recommends following the directions on the label.

**Divide the meals.** Dogs that gobble their food all at once are much more likely to get bloat than those that eat more slowly and more often, says Monique Maniet, D.V.M., a holistic veterinarian in private practice in Bethesda, Maryland. She recommends giving them smaller meals more often. "Try feeding your pet twice a day, and if he is still having problems, increase the frequency to three times a day," she suggests.

**Let him eat in peace.** Dogs will often bolt their food because they are afraid that other pets in the family might get to it first. This type of anxious eating can cause gas, says Cheryl Schwartz, D.V.M., a holistic veterinarian in San Francisco and author of *Four Paws, Five Directions: A Guide to Chinese Medicine for Cats and Dogs.* "Give him his own space to eat in," she suggests.

**Switch to moist food.** Veterinarians often recommend that dogs prone to bloat be given moist or semi-moist food instead of dry kibble. Dry dog food absorbs tremendous amounts of water in the stomach, causing it to suddenly swell, explains Dr. Maniet. An alternative to switching foods is to moisten dry food with water and let it sit for a few minutes before letting your dog eat. This will allow the food to expand before it goes into his stomach.

**BEST BET!** **Start cooking at home.** Research has shown that dogs given a healthful, homemade diet are less likely to bloat, says Susan G. Wynn, D.V.M., a veterinarian in Atlanta and co-editor of *Complementary and Alternative Veterinary Medicine.* You will find a complete guide to homemade diets on page 61.

**Calm the tummy with chamomile.** A healing herb long used for digestive problems, chamomile may

## Meet the Experts

**Maria Chelaru-Williams, D.V.M.,** is a veterinarian in private practice in Boulder, Colorado.

**Monique Maniet, D.V.M.,** is a holistic veterinarian in private practice in Bethesda, Maryland. She is certified in acupuncture.

**Sandra Priest, D.V.M.,** is a holistic veterinarian in private practice in Knoxville, Tennessee. She is certified in chiropractic.

**Adriana Sagrera, D.V.M.,** is a holistic veterinarian in private practice in New Orleans.

**Cheryl Schwartz, D.V.M.,** is a holistic veterinarian in San Francisco and the author of *Four Paws, Five Directions: A Guide to Chinese Medicine for Cats and Dogs.* She is certified in acupuncture.

**Susan G. Wynn, D.V.M.,** is a veterinarian in Atlanta and co-editor of *Complementary and Alternative Veterinary Medicine.*

help prevent bloat, says Dr. Schwartz. "Just make a cup of chamomile tea as you would for yourself, then cool it to room temperature," she suggests. Give dogs under 15 pounds one-half teaspoon of chamomile tea a day. Dogs 15 pounds and over can have one tablespoon a day. You can mix the tea in their food or put it in their mouths before meals with a needleless syringe.

**Work it out.** Food can ferment in sluggish intestines, causing gas to accumulate, says Dr. Priest. "Sometimes the problem is a lack of conditioning," she explains. It is worth taking your dog for a brisk walk at least once a day.

Just be sure to exercise him before—not after—he eats because vigorous exercise after meals may actually cause bloat, adds Dr. Chelaru-Williams. "Wait at least two hours after meals before exercising," she advises.

**Nix it with Nux.** The homeopathic remedy Nux vomica can help reverse buildups of gas right away, says Adriana Sagrera, D.V.M., a holistic veterinarian in private practice in New Orleans. She recommends giving two pellets of a 30C dose every half-hour or two pellets of a 6C dose every 15 minutes when your dog seems to be bloating.

Bloat is always an emergency, however, so you will still need to get your pet to the vet as quickly as possible for treatment.

# Body Odor

## The Signs
- Your pet smells wet even when he is not.
- The odor has been getting worse.
- The odor comes back even after bathing.

## The Cause

Dogs love to roll in manure, dead fish, and other stinky things. For some reason, they relish this canine perfume—a lot more than their owners do. A quick bath is the easiest way to eliminate *eau de dog* when the smell's cause is external. But things get more complicated when the body odor is coming from within.

"The skin is a reflection of the health of the internal organs," says Joanne Stefanatos, D.V.M., a holistic veterinarian in private practice in Las Vegas. If you treat the whole body and make it healthy, your pet's skin will improve naturally. Dogs are

## Call the VET

**S**ome dogs and cats are naturally smellier than others, and a quick bath will usually clear the air. But body odor is occasionally caused by serious problems, like infections, tooth decay, or even kidney disease. "If the odor persists after you have bathed your pet, or it returns in only a day or so, it could point to a bigger problem and you need to see your vet," says Robert Kennis, D.V.M., a veterinary dermatologist at Texas A&M University College of Veterinary Medicine in College Station.

usually smellier than cats, but any pet may occasionally become a little pungent.

Some owners resort to spritzing their pets with cologne or scented powders, but this only masks the odors. The only way to get rid of body odor, according to holistic veterinarians, is to discover and eliminate the underlying cause. It is usually not difficult to do, adds Dr. Stefanatos. Try the following simple tips provided by veterinarians.

## The Solutions FOR DOGS & CATS

**BEST BET!** **Change the diet.** One of the best ways to get rid of body odor is to switch your pet to a natural diet, says Susan G. Wynn, D.V.M., a veterinarian in Atlanta and co-editor of *Complementary and Alternative Veterinary Medicine.* Try one of the high-quality brands like Innova, Wysong,

Flint River Ranch, or PetGuard Premium, she says, which are available in some pet supply stores and through mail order. Or you can switch to a homemade diet. See page 61 for more information on preparing natural foods at home.

**Clean them from the inside out.** Giving your pets barley grass, wheat grass, or chlorophyll can remove toxins from the body that can lead to bad smells, Dr. Stefanatos says. "Each of these will cleanse the gastrointestinal system and help eliminate body odor," she says. For pets under 10 pounds, she recommends giving one-eighth teaspoon of one of these remedies twice a day. Those weighing 10 to 24 pounds can have one-quarter teaspoon, pets 25 to 50 pounds can take one-half teaspoon, and larger pets can take a full teaspoon—all doses given twice a day. The remedies are available in health foods stores and can be mixed in your pet's food.

**Save the skin.** A type of yeast that normally lives on your pet's skin will sometimes multiply, causing infections and sometimes a bad smell, says Steven A. Melman, V.M.D., a veterinarian with practices in Potomac, Maryland, and Palm Springs, California, and author of *Skin Diseases of Dogs and Cats*. Washing your pet with a medicated shampoo, such as MalAcetic, will kill the yeast and help your pet smell sweet again. Ask your vet how often you should use the shampoo.

**Try some supplements.** Giving pets fatty-acid supplements along with their regular food can help eliminate smelly toxins in the body, says Dr. Stefanatos. She recommends a product called Omegaderm Oil, available from vets. Pets under 35 pounds can take a teaspoon of the oil twice a day, mixed into their food, while larger pets can take a tablespoon twice a day. "The multiple veterinary mineral tablet Gerizyme also helps," she says. Gerizyme is also only available through your veterinarian.

**Clean the coat.** Combing and brushing your pet regularly will help remove the thick undercoat, which tends to trap moisture along with bad smells, says Dr. Stefanatos. She recommends "back-combing" your pet, going against the direction of the fur, every day, especially during shed-

ding season. "Wetting the comb with water helps remove loose hair," she adds.

**Schedule a bath day.** Natural oils on your pet's skin will sometimes collect in the fur, turn rancid, and give off bad smells. The odor will usually go away when you give your pet a good sudsing, says Robert Kennis, D.V.M., a veterinary dermatologist at Texas A&M University College of Veterinary Medicine in College Station. Any pet shampoo will work fine, he says. Check with your vet to see how often you should bathe your pet.

To make baths even more effective, give your pet a final rinse with a solution containing two tablespoons

## Meet the Experts

**Robert Kennis, D.V.M.,** is a veterinary dermatologist at Texas A&M University College of Veterinary Medicine in College Station.

**Steven A. Melman, V.M.D.,** is a veterinarian with practices in Potomac, Maryland, and Palm Springs, California, and the author of *Skin Diseases of Dogs and Cats*.

**Joanne Stefanatos, D.V.M.,** is a holistic veterinarian in private practice in Las Vegas. She is certified in acupuncture and chiropractic.

**Susan G. Wynn, D.V.M.,** is a veterinarian in Atlanta and co-editor of *Complementary and Alternative Veterinary Medicine*.

of vinegar in a quart of water, adds Dr. Stefanatos.

**Trim the fur.** Since they don't use toilet paper, dogs and cats will sometimes get smelly deposits around their back ends. This usually occurs in pets with long fur or those that aren't mobile enough to clean themselves properly. Dr. Kennis recommends keeping the hair trimmed short and periodically washing your pet's rear with a cloth and warm water.

# BOREDOM

## The Signs
- Your pet gets destructive when he is alone.
- He begs for attention all the time.

## The Cause

Dogs and cats need interesting hobbies just as much as people do. When they spend a lot of time alone without a lot to do, they become bored—and this can lead to trouble.

"An active pet deprived of stimulation will create activities that make life interesting—like pulling the stuffing out of the couch," says Mary Lee Nitschke, Ph.D., professor of psychology at Linfield College in Portland, Oregon, and an animal behaviorist in Beaverton. Unrolling the toilet paper and knocking things off high shelves are other favorite amusements.

Even when they aren't destroying the house, pets with energy to burn may express their frustration in other ways by digging up the backyard, for example, or running frantically alongside a fence. Some pets turn to food or raiding the trash to pass the time, eventually getting so heavy that their health is endangered.

Not surprisingly, young pets get bored more easily than older ones. When you don't give them something to do, they will come up with something on their own, and you are unlikely to appreciate their idea of fun. Punishing your pet won't help, says Dr. Nitschke. What will help is redirecting his energy to more acceptable activities.

## The Solutions FOR DOGS & CATS

**Keep their noses busy.** Dogs and cats have phenomenal senses of smell, and they can literally wear themselves out sniffing new odors, says Dr. Nitschke. "It takes a 15- to 20-block walk to tire out my giant schnauzer, but if we take an unfamiliar route, he is so busy sniffing that he is ready to crash after only 5 blocks."

The easiest way to stimulate their senses is to give them new places to explore. Walking down a different block or in a different part of the park will open their nsotrils—and their minds—to an exciting new world of smells. Even spending time in the backyard will stimulate their senses. And the more excited they get during their outings, the less likely they are to be bored once they get back home.

**BEST BET!** **Tire them out.** Dogs and cats spend a lot of time sleeping and will happily doze away most of the day as long as you get them tired before you leave. "Sometimes the only good pet is a tired pet," says Dr. Nitschke.

All pets need regular exercise, and those with high energy need even more. Try to walk your dog for at least 20 minutes twice a day. Most cats don't go for walks with their owners, but they need about the same amount of exercise. The time you spend rolling a ball or tossing a stuffed cat toy is time you won't have to spend cleaning up after your pet's shenanigans.

**Calm him with flower essences.** There are dozens of flower essences that holistic veterinarians use to target different emotional problems. For ex-

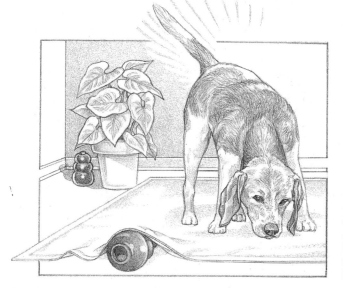

A great way to keep your dog entertained when you are gone is to buy a few Kong toys, stuff the hollow cavities with peanut butter or cheese and seal the openings with a dog biscuit. Then stash the toys around the house. Once his nose alerts him to treasure, he will happily spend hours seeking it out.

ample, the essence wild oat is good for pets that are dissatisfied, frustrated, or bored. Vervain is good for pets that are overly enthusiastic, and impatiens is good for restless and impatient pets, says Jean Hofve, D.V.M., a holistic veterinarian in private practice in Denver. Choose the essence that most closely matches your pet's moods and put two to four drops in his mouth once a day, she advises.

## The Solutions

**Send him on a hunt.** Dogs love to explore, especially when they hope to uncover a tasty treat. To keep your dog busy when you are gone, try hiding dog biscuits around the house, suggests Dr. Nitschke. He will find them all eventually and will have a great time doing it.

**BEST BET!** **Exercise the mind.** Dogs don't play chess or work out math problems, but they do like a challenge. Pet supply stores sell a variety of toys that can be loaded with tasty treats that take some creativity to get out, says Wayne Hunthausen, D.V.M., a veterinary behaviorist in Westwood, Kansas, and author of the *Handbook of Behaviour Problems in Dogs and Cats*. One toy, the Buster Cube, has hidden compartments that contain food. As your dog shoves it around the floor, pieces of food will occasionally fall

---

## Meet the Experts

**Jean Hofve, D.V.M.,** is a holistic veterinarian in private practice in Denver.

**Wayne Hunthausen, D.V.M.,** is a veterinary behaviorist in Westwood, Kansas, and the author of the *Handbook of Behaviour Problems in Dogs and Cats*.

**Mary Lee Nitschke, Ph.D.,** is a professor of psychology at Linfield College in Portland, Oregon, and an animal behaviorist in Beaverton.

---

out, rewarding all his hard work. Some pets will play with these toys for hours until they collapse in a happy heap.

## The Solutions

**Surround him with familiar sounds.** Cats are better than dogs at amusing themselves and don't get bored as easily. But some cats do get lonely or anxious during the day, says Dr. Nitschke. One way to perk them up is to record some of the family's conversation during dinner, for example, and then put the tape on a timer so that it comes on during the day when you are gone. "This seems to reduce boredom and anxiety," she says. "I don't know exactly how it works, but it clearly does work."

# Breathing Problems

## The Signs

- Your pet is breathing with his mouth open (but he's not panting).
- He is wheezing or coughing.
- He has low energy and doesn't want to eat.
- He can't tolerate exercise.

## The Cause

Cats and dogs may have trouble breathing for some of the same reasons people do: a stuffy nose, asthma, or a lung infection. Then again, breathing problems may be caused by things humans don't get, like kennel cough—a type of bronchitis that can leave dogs, but not cats, with a dry, raspy cough.

In conventional medicine, a breathing problem is ordinarily treated with medications to relieve congestion and open up the airways. The problem with drugs is that they sometimes cause undesirable side effects. That is why veterinarians who practice holistic healing prefer to try other approaches first.

You will want to call your vet at the first sign of breathing problems. In some cases, however, you will find that the problem really isn't serious and that there are an abundance of natural, drug-free remedies that can help. Here is what holistic veterinarians advise.

## The Solutions FOR DOGS & CATS

**Break up the congestion.** Pets with allergies or viral infections sometimes get so congested that they can hardly breathe. For mucus in the nose and sinuses, try a saline solution, says Jeanne Olson, D.V.M., a holistic veterinarian in private practice in North Pole, Alaska. To make a saline solution, dissolve one-quarter teaspoon of salt in one-half cup of warm spring or filtered water and draw some of the mixture into a dropper. Tilt your pet's head up so that his nose points to the ceiling and put three drops in each nostril. Once the drops are in, gently roll your finger across each side of the nose. This will coax the fluid—along with the mucus—out of the nostrils, she explains.

**Let it steam.** Lung congestion caused by bronchitis can be loosened with steam, says Dr. Olson. "Close the bathroom door and turn on the shower, using very hot water. When the room fills with steam, bring in your cat or dog, close the door, and let him breathe the steam for a few minutes."

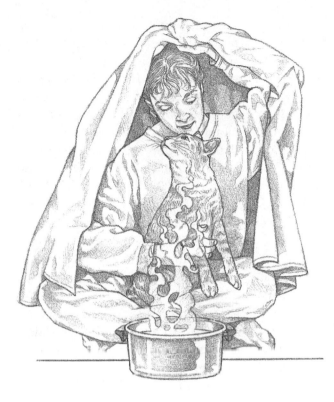

Breathing steam will break up nasal congestion quickly. To make a steam tent, boil a pot of water and put it on the floor or a low table. Hold your pet in front of you and drape a towel over both your heads to trap the steam.

For a more direct steam treatment, boil some pure water, remove it from the heat, and add two tablespoons of fenugreek (*Trigonella foenum-graecum*) seeds, which act as a natural decongestant, says Dr. Olson. Put the pot on the floor or on a low table. Holding your pet in front of you or on your lap, drape a towel over your head to trap the steam, making sure the towel covers your pet. Letting your pet breathe the steam for 5 to 10 minutes will quickly break up mucus so that it is easier to breathe, she explains.

Don't let your pet get too close to the heat. Test it yourself first. Their noses are much more sensitive than yours. If you feel the slightest hint of heat sensation, you are too close.

**Put moisture in the air.** Humidifying the air is an easy way to put healing moisture inside your pet's lungs, says Dr. Olson. Ultrasonic humidifiers are the most effective. "They use a process called nebulization to create tiny droplets of water that get past the upper respiratory system and into the lungs," she adds.

You can humidify a whole room or create a little humidity tent by positioning the humidifier in front of your pet's bed or crate and placing a towel over the bed or crate to trap the moisture. You can leave your pet in the tent for up to 20 minutes, several times a day, Dr. Olson says.

**Add some homeopathy.** Most homeopathic remedies are taken by mouth, but they also seem to be effective when breathed into the lungs, Dr. Olson says. When using a humidifier to relieve upper respiratory problems, she recommends adding Mercurius 30C to the water. Add 10 pellets to one-quarter gallon of distilled water and turn on the humidifier for 20 minutes at a time, three or four times a day, she says.

**Help him breathe with vitamin C.** This powerful vitamin strengthens the immune system and helps it fight infections that can cause breathing problems, says Monique Maniet, D.V.M., a holistic veterinarian in private practice in Bethesda, Maryland. She recommends using a form of vitamin C powder that also contains bioflavonoids, natural compounds that can reduce inflammation in the airways. Pets under 15 pounds can start with 500 milligrams twice a day. Dogs and cats 15 to 50 pounds can take 1,000 milligrams twice a day. Give 3,000 milligrams twice daily to dogs 50 to 100 pounds. Larger dogs can start with 4,000 milligrams twice a day. Under your vet's supervision, gradually increase the dose to a level your pet can tolerate. If he gets diarrhea, go back to the previous dose, says Dr. Maniet.

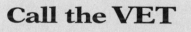

## Call the VET

Most short-term breathing problems are caused by minor bronchial infections or flare-ups of allergies. But shortness of breath can also be a symptom of congestive heart failure, a life-threatening condition in which the heart and lungs aren't able to supply the body with all the oxygen it needs, says Monique Maniet, D.V.M., a holistic veterinarian in private practice in Bethesda, Maryland.

Don't take chances with breathing problems, she advises. You will want to get your pet to the vet right away. This is especially true if your pet has lost his appetite or if you notice a bluish tint in his gums or mouth—a sign that not enough oxygen is getting through.

BREATHING PROBLEMS **173**

**Strengthen the body's defenses.** The herb echinacea (*Echinacea purpurea* or *Echinacea angustfolia*) strengthens immunity and helps the body fight infections, says Dr. Maniet. The amount you give will vary from pet to pet, she adds. A 30-pound dog, for example, would take ¼ of the full human dose, while a 10-pound cat would take ½₁₂ of the full dose.

One problem with echinacea is that many pets don't like the taste, and they certainly don't like swallowing the capsules. Dr. Olson recommends using a brand called Herbs for Kids in liquid form. "It's made with glycerin instead of alcohol, and it's pleasant-tasting," she says.

## The Solutions · FOR DOGS ·

**Soothe them the traditional way.** Dogs with kennel cough often have a dry, scratchy throat along with their bronchitis. You can provide quick relief by giving them a little bit of honey and lemon juice three times a day, says Christina Chambreau, D.V.M., a

## Meet the Experts

**Christina Chambreau, D.V.M.,** is a holistic veterinarian in Sparks, Maryland, and education chairperson for the Academy of Veterinary Homeopathy.

**Monique Maniet, D.V.M.,** is a holistic veterinarian in private practice in Bethesda, Maryland. She is certified in acupuncture.

**Jeanne Olson, D.V.M.,** is a holistic veterinarian in private practice in North Pole, Alaska.

holistic veterinarian in Sparks, Maryland, and education chairperson for the Academy of Veterinary Homeopathy. You don't have to be too precise in measuring the "medicine." For a 30-pound dog, for example, give about one tablespoon of honey and one-half teaspoon of lemon juice at a time. "Some pets will lick it off a spoon," she says. For others, place a needleless syringe, available from pet supply catalogs, in the corner of their mouths and squirt it down their throats.

# CANCER

## The Signs

- Your pet has a lump or sore that won't go away.
- She is eating but is losing weight.
- It is hard for her to chew or swallow.
- There is a discharge or bleeding from any body opening.
- She has a bad smell.
- She tires easily and doesn't want to exercise.

## The Cause

Pets are susceptible to the same types of cancer that people get. Cancer can strike at any age, but it is usually a disease of middle-aged and older dogs and cats. And it is all too common: Cancer causes almost half the deaths of pets older than 10 years.

Veterinarians believe that many cancers are caused by unhealthy things in the environment, such as smog or chemicals. And modern pet foods, according to some holistic vets, may be another problem. "The preservatives and chemical additives in some foods may even promote cancer," says Roger L. DeHaan, D.V.M., a holistic veterinarian in private practice in Frazee, Minnesota.

While you may help prevent some types of cancer by letting your pets drink bottled water, treating your lawn without chemicals, or neutering pets when they are young, often it is just the luck of the draw. If your pet does get sick, she is going to need both traditional and holistic care.

"Even if you do conventional treatment, you have to treat holistically to get rid of whatever caused the cancer in the first place," Dr. DeHaan explains.

Natural remedies do more than battle cancer, adds Carolyn Blakey, D.V.M., a holistic veterinarian in private practice in Richmond, Indiana. They tend to have fewer side effects than mainstream treatments. In addition, they can help pets feel healthier and more energetic while they are battling their illness.

## The Solutions · FOR DOGS & CATS

**BEST BET!** **Focus on nutrition.** Research has shown that some cancer cells thrive on carbohydrates and proteins but don't do as well with fats. Veterinarians sometimes recommend that pets with certain kinds of

## Call the VET

It is not unusual for dogs and cats to lose their appetites now and then. When they quit eating for more than a day or two, however, it is time to call your vet. A reduced appetite is one of the main warning signs of cancer, says Roger L. DeHaan, D.V.M., a holistic veterinarian in private practice in Frazee, Minnesota. "Refusing food isn't normal and could mean there's a problem," he says.

In pets that already have cancer, a reduced appetite can be even more serious because they won't be getting all the nutrients they need to recover. "You have to get food and water into these guys," says Dr. DeHaan. If you have already tried making food more appetizing—by warming it up, for example, or adding tasty liquids or broth—and she still won't eat, you need to call your vet right away, he advises.

cancer be given a diet that is high in fat and lower in protein and carbohydrates, says Gregory K. Ogilvie, D.V.M., professor of oncology and internal medicine at the College of Veterinary Medicine and Biomedical Sciences at Colorado State University in Fort Collins. Every pet (and cancer) is different, however, so be sure to talk to your vet before making major changes in your pet's diet.

**Stimulate her appetite.** Pets with cancer often lose their appetites, but they need to eat in order to heal. One way to renew your pet's interest is to warm the food to about 100°F, suggests Dr. Ogilvie. Doing this releases aromas that pets like, he explains.

**Give them extra enzymes.** Some of the enzymes in raw foods may play a role in killing cancer cells, says Dr. DeHaan. A convenient source of healthful enzymes is raw or very lightly cooked egg yolks. He suggests giving one egg yolk a week to pets under 15 pounds, and two egg yolks a week to larger pets.

**Help with digestion.** Cancer robs the body of key nutrients, so it is essential to make sure that your pet gets every possible benefit from the foods she eats. The beneficial bacteria in acidophilus, available in supermarkets and health food stores, will help pets absorb more nutrients from their food. "Give dogs under 15 pounds and cats a teaspoon of plain, nonflavored acidophilus two to five times a week," says Dr. DeHaan. Dogs 15 to 50 pounds can take two tablespoons of

## SUCCESS

ALTERNATIVE

### A FATEFUL CURE

The lump on Chani's neck didn't look good. Even though her owner, Dusty Rainbolt of Flower Mound, Texas, was about to leave town for a trip, she made time to take the 11-year-old cat to a vet—and the news wasn't good. The lump was a rare, highly aggressive cancer, and Chani was scheduled for surgery the same day.

Chani's veterinarian wasn't optimistic. She said the tumor would almost certainly return, and Chani had only a few weeks to live. In despair, Dusty began looking for alternative treatments. A week later, while attending a cat show in Atlanta, Dusty began talking with an herbalist. "The woman recommended pau d'arco (*Tabebuia impetiginosa*) and red clover (*Trifolium pratense*), and she said that they cured her cat of cancer," Dusty remembers. "I didn't think it would help her, but I was ready to try anything. I started pouring the stuff down Chani."

A month later, she took Chani back to the vet. There was no sign of the tumor. "She said if Chani made it to New Year's, we'd beat the cancer," says Dusty. A year later, the tumor still hadn't returned, and her vet pronounced Chani a miracle cure.

"It's the combination that cured her," says Dusty. "A highly skilled surgeon, the fantastic herbs, and our loving bond. If I hadn't gone on the trip to the cat show, Chani wouldn't be here today."

acidophilus, and larger dogs can have three to six tablespoons a day—both doses given two to fives times a week as well. "They love the flavor, so you can just add it as a garnish to their regular food," he says.

**BEST BET!** **Give them extra vitamins.** The antioxidant vitamins C and E have been shown to slow the growth and spread of some kinds of cancer, and they may help prevent cancer as well. A healthy amount for cats is 250 milligrams of vitamin C twice a day, while dogs can take up to 800 milligrams twice a day, says Dr. Blakey. Check with your vet for the dose that's right for your pet. It is best to use the ester form of vitamin C because it is more digestible, she adds. Since vitamin C can cause diarrhea, you may have to cut back the dose until you find an amount your pet will tolerate.

Vitamin E—given alone or in combination with vitamin C—may also be helpful. Dr. DeHaan recommends giving pets weighing under 15 pounds 30 to 100 international units (IU) of vitamin E a day, while larger pets can take 200 to 400 IU a day.

**Add some algae.** Blue-green algae, available in health food stores, is packed with healthful nutrients, says Dr. DeHaan. He recommends giving cats and dogs under 15 pounds half of a 500-milligram capsule of blue-green algae a day. Pets 15 to 50 pounds can take one to two capsules, and larger dogs can take two to four capsules.

**Protect them with selenium.** The mineral selenium is another antioxidant that helps slow cancer growth, says Dr. DeHaan. "You can give a daily dose of 25 micrograms of methionol selenium to pets under 15 pounds, 100 micrograms to pets 15 and 50 pounds, and up to 200 micrograms a day to dogs over 50 pounds."

**BEST BET!** **Fight cancer with fish-oil supplements.** The omega-3 fatty acids in fish oil act as a natural anti-inflammatory and have been shown to prevent the spread of cancer,

says Susan G. Wynn, D.V.M., a veterinarian in Atlanta and co-editor of *Complementary and Alternative Veterinary Medicine*. Give cats and dogs under 20 pounds 1,000 milligrams a day, she says. Pets 20 to 50 pounds can take 2,000 milligrams. Give 3,000 milligrams to dogs 51 to 80 pounds, and 4,000 milligrams to dogs over 80 pounds. Oils made from the whole fish, like salmon oil, are a good choice because they contain more omega-3 fatty acids than those made from just a part of the fish, like cod-liver oil.

**Surround them with healing sounds.** Soothing music reduces stress, which can help the immune system work more vigorously to battle cancer. "Sound is vibration, and it can have a positive influence on healing," says Deborah C. Mallu, D.V.M., a holistic veterinarian in private practice in Sedona, Arizona. When your pet is ill, she says, fill the house with soothing music—something like classical, New Age, or soft jazz. You can also buy recordings of natural sounds—a water fountain, for example, or the sounds of birds chirping. Sounds from nature will help pets relax and take their minds off their illness, she explains.

**Heal them with color.** All colors contain unique kinds of energy, which some holistic veterinarians believe can help promote healing. "Green is a general healing stabilizer, or you can use red and green together to stimulate the immune system," says Joanne Stefanatos, D.V.M., a holistic veterinarian in private practice in Las Vegas. She recommends placing items containing these colors, such as a sweater or a lamp fitted with a colored lightbulb, near your pet's bed. This way she will absorb the healing colors for many hours a day.

**Try an herbal blend.** A tea made from a packaged blend of burdock root, sheep sorrel, slippery elm, and Indian rhubarb root will help clear toxic substances from the body, which can help prevent and possibly stop cancer, says Dr. Blakey. You can buy this blend, called Essiac, in health food stores.

To make the tea, mix a package of Essiac in about 2½ quarts of spring or distilled water. Bring to a boil and simmer for 10 minutes, stirring occasionally. Then let it stand, covered, for 4 hours. Bring it to a boil again, simmer for 5 minutes, then pour it into a narrow, covered container. Refrigerate for 16 hours to allow the sediment to settle, then pour the resulting amber liquid into a glass or plastic container and store in the refrigerator. "Give pets one to two ounces twice a day," says Dr. Blakey. "Either squirt it in their mouths with a dropper or put it in their drinking water or food—it's not that bitter."

**Strengthen her immunity with herbs.** The immune system normally fights cancer cells just as it fights viruses and bacteria. "The herbs maitake (*Grifola frondosa*) and green tea (*Camellia sinensis*) may stimulate the immune system and have an antioxidant effect," says Dr. Wynn. "And turmeric (*Curcuma longa*) may inhibit the growth of cancerous cells." Health food stores carry these herbs loose or in capsules and tinctures. Whichever form you choose, give pets under 20 pounds one-quarter of the human dose, she says. Pets 20 to 49 pounds can take half the human dose, while those weighing 50 to 80 pounds can take three-quarters. Give larger dogs the full human dose.

**Try a special juice.** Noni juice, available in health food stores, is made from the morinda plant of the South Sea Islands. The juice can relieve pain and may inhibit the growth of cells that can lead to cancer, says Dr. DeHaan. "I usually use the juice for very sick pets with poor digestion," he says. "It tastes like blackberry juice." He recommends giving pets under 15 pounds 10 to 15 drops of the juice each day. Pets 15 to 50 pounds can have one-half teaspoon two or three times a day, and larger dogs can have one teaspoon two or three times a day.

**Cleanse the body with homeopathy.** Cancer cells release large amounts of toxic compounds, says Dr. DeHaan. "I almost always use homeopathic cleansing drops like Theratox and Detoxification to get poisons moving out of the body." Both of these remedies are available from veterinarians.

The homeopathic remedy Nux vomica, in a 30X strength, is good for nausea, and Arsenicum album 30X will help restore energy, Dr. DeHaan adds. You can give your pet one dropperful twice a day. You should use only one homeopathic remedy at a time, and only for short periods, to treat specific symptoms.

**Treat your pet's emotions.** Pets with cancer experience tremendous amounts of physical and emotional stress. A flower essence called Bach Rescue Remedy will help cleanse the body and restore feelings of well-being, Dr. DeHaan. He recommends putting two or three drops of Bach Rescue Remedy in your pet's water dish each day. Or you can put the same amount directly in her mouth. You can give the drops every hour if your pet is severely stressed, he adds.

**BEST BET!** **Stay optimistic.** Dogs and cats have strong powers of intuition and can read our emotions—and even our thoughts—as easily as we understand words, says Dr. Mallu. Maintaining a positive outlook is one of the strongest medicines you can offer. In fact, many pets improve dramatically when their owners stop thinking about worse-case scenarios and instead focus all their energy on good thoughts. "Enjoy your time together and learn to live in the

---

> **Meet the Experts**
>
> **Carolyn Blakey, D.V.M.,** is a holistic veterinarian in private practice in Richmond, Indiana. She is certified in acupuncture.
>
> **Roger L. DeHaan, D.V.M.,** is a holistic veterinarian in private practice in Frazee, Minnesota. He is certified in chiropractic.
>
> **Deborah C. Mallu, D.V.M.,** is a holistic veterinarian in private practice in Sedona, Arizona. She is certified in acupuncture.
>
> **Gregory K. Ogilvie, D.V.M.,** is a professor of oncology and internal medicine at the College of Veterinary Medicine and Biomedical Sciences at Colorado State University in Fort Collins.
>
> **Joanne Stefanatos, D.V.M.,** is a holistic veterinarian in private practice in Las Vegas. She is certified in acupuncture and chiropractic.
>
> **Susan G. Wynn, D.V.M.,** is a veterinarian in Atlanta and co-editor of *Complementary and Alternative Veterinary Medicine*.

---

moment like your pet does," she says. "That's one of the greatest gifts they can teach us."

**Add new treatments slowly.** "When your pet has cancer, her metabolism is out of whack and probably can't handle 10 new things all at once," says Dr. DeHaan. "Start with two or three new things and introduce them over 7 to 10 days. This will help prevent vomiting, diarrhea, or other signs of stress."

If your pet is already being treated for cancer, be sure to talk to your vet before starting natural remedies at home, he adds. Herbs, dietary supplements, and other holistic medicines are quite powerful and may react with other medicines your pet may be taking.

# CAR SICKNESS

## The Signs

- Your pet loses her lunch during or after a ride.
- She pants excessively or drools in the car.
- She has trouble relaxing when riding.

## The Cause

Dogs and cats don't take naturally to riding in cars—they are, after all, designed to travel by paw power alone. While most dogs and some cats learn to enjoy four-wheeled excursions, others hate it so much that that they work themselves into a frenzy, literally making themselves sick.

Emotional stress aside, riding in a car can stimulate the vomiting center in the brain, with predictably messy results.

Veterinarians often recommend behavior-modification techniques, along with medications, to prevent car sickness. There is nothing wrong with this approach in some cases, but it doesn't take into account each pet's emotions and physical needs. That is why veterinarians who specialize in natural healing are more inclined to favor a customized and all-natural plan. "It's all about treating the pet as an individual," says Arthur Young, D.V.M., a holistic veterinarian in private practice in Stuart, Florida.

## The Solutions  FOR DOGS & CATS

**Give your car good energy.** From your pet's point of view, cars are loud and strange, and they take her to scary places, like the kennel or the vet. And if she has gotten sick in the car in the past, it is also a place where she knows that she won't feel very good. It is not surprising that some pets start feeling nauseated as soon as they climb into the backseat.

One way to help your pet adjust is to make the car a fun place to be, says Joanne Hibbs, D.V.M., a veterinarian

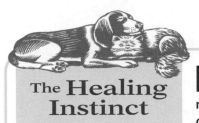

## The Healing Instinct

Deep inside your pet's inner ear is a sensitive, fluid-filled mechanism. When she rides in a car, each bounce of her head causes the fluid to slosh around, which tells the brain exactly how she is moving. Her eyes, however, tell a different story: They say she is standing still. When the signals from the ears don't match signals from the eyes, there is a "sensory disassociation," which is what causes car sickness.

Dogs and cats don't understand the science of car sickness, but they instinctively know how to cope with it, says Joanne Hibbs, D.V.M., a veterinarian in private practice in Powell, Tennessee. Cats, for example, will often dive under a seat or wedge themselves into a dark corner. They do this because they are less likely to get sick when their eyes aren't sending "I'm standing still" messages to the brain.

Dogs have a different strategy: They often ride with their heads out the windows. They aren't just having fun. The wind in their faces and the sight of all the scenery rushing past help the eyes and ears come to an agreement that yes, they are moving. And this results in a happy and healthy ride.

---

in private practice in Powell, Tennessee. She recommends stocking the car with your pet's favorite chew toys, blankets, and treats. "Don't even go anywhere at first," she adds. "Just let her explore, pet her, and make her feel good." If you do this often enough, she will learn that the car is a place where good things happen, and she will be less likely to get sick in the future.

**Press anxiety away.** One acupressure point that can relieve nausea is PC6, located in the small depression on the underside of the front legs just above the pad on the wrists, says Judith Rae Swanson, D.V.M., a holistic veterinarian in private practice in Chicago.

Pressing this point for one minute before you get in the car and, with the assistance of a passenger, as often as necessary while driving, will help keep pets—and their stomachs—calm, she says. Press just hard enough to get their attention and not cause discomfort.

Most pets don't like having their feet handled, Dr. Swanson adds, so try a gentle, whole-body massage for a few minutes before getting in the car. This will help get your pet used to having her feet touched and will also reduce anxiety that can lead to car sickness, she says.

**Give a little ginger.** This traditional remedy works very well for nausea caused by car sickness. "I use the capsules that are sold in health food stores," says John Limehouse, D.V.M., a holistic veterinarian in private practice in Toluca Lake, California. Dogs 15 pounds and over can take 500 milligrams of ginger (*Zingiber officinale*), while smaller pets can take half that amount or less. The easiest way to give ginger is to open a capsule and sprinkle the contents on a tablespoon of baby food. Give it about 20 minutes before going for a drive.

Cats usually won't eat ginger, so you may want to make a tea, says Susan G. Wynn, D.V.M., a veterinarian in Atlanta and co-editor of *Complementary and Alternative Veterinary Medicine*. Add one teaspoon of fresh grated ginger to a cup of hot water. Let it cool, strain it, and add a drop of honey. Squirt a half to a whole dropperful of the tea into the corner of your cat's mouth.

**Try some Chinese herbs.** A traditional Chinese remedy called Pill Curing will help treat and prevent nausea, says Dr. Limehouse. You can put these tiny pills, which are about the size of a pinhead, directly on your pet's tongue, where they will dissolve. About 20 minutes before a car trip, give one vial of pills to dogs over 50 pounds. Pets 15 to 50 pounds can take 10 to 15 pills, and smaller pets can take 10 pills. For very small pets or for pets who won't swallow the pills, dilute them first in a tablespoon of luke-

---

## Meet the Experts

**Joanne Hibbs, D.V.M.,** is a veterinarian in private practice in Powell, Tennessee.

**John Limehouse, D.V.M.,** is a holistic veterinarian in private practice in Toluca Lake, California. He is certified in acupuncture.

**Judith Rae Swanson, D.V.M.,** is a holistic veterinarian in private practice in Chicago. She is certified in acupuncture.

**Susan G. Wynn, D.V.M.,** is a veterinarian in Atlanta and co-editor of *Complementary and Alternative Veterinary Medicine*

**Arthur Young, D.V.M.,** is a holistic veterinarian in private practice in Stuart, Florida. He is certified in homeopathy.

---

warm water and use a dropper to squirt it in their mouths.

**Tame the tummy with Tabacum.** Homeopathic Tabacum will help quell all kinds of nausea, including nausea caused by motion sickness. Dr. Young suggests putting a few pellets of Tabacum 30C on your pet's tongue up to two hours before traveling. "I've had really good luck with this remedy," he adds.

**Ease their emotions.** An effective way to reduce emotional stress—and the nausea that often accompanies it—is with flower essences. Dr. Young recommends putting three drops of premixed scleranthus, which balances the inner ear, into your pet's mouth.

**BEST BET!** **Train the brain.** Even though nausea is caused by physical signals between the inner ear and brain, there are ways to "train" pets to be less sensitive, says Dr. Hibbs. She recommends taking your pet for a short drive once a week or so—just around the block is plenty. After three or four rides, double the distance and go out two or three times a week. Keep taking her for longer and longer drives, with some downtime in between. By gradually getting her used to the motion, her brain will "learn" that the sensations she feels are harmless, and the car sickness should gradually fade, she says.

## The Solutions FOR CATS

**Put out the lights.** A simple way to prevent car sickness in cats is to put them in a small crate or box and cover it with a towel to block out the light, says Dr. Hibbs. Cats feel more secure in the dark, she explains. Don't try this in hot weather, however, because they could overheat, she says.

# CATARACTS

## The Signs
- Your pet's pupils are cloudy or milky white.

## The Cause

It's normal for the eyes to undergo slight changes over time. Dogs and cats don't depend on vision as much as people do, so conditions such as near-sightedness don't slow them down. Pets with cataracts, however, may lose much or all of their vision, making it hard for them to get around.

Cataracts occur when large amounts of proteins in the lenses of the eyes undergo biochemical changes, turning eyes cloudy or milky white. Cataracts are often caused by free radicals, harmful oxygen molecules in the body that gradually damage the delicate tissues in the eyes. Injuries and internal illnesses such as diabetes can cause cataracts as well. Cataracts are most common in older dogs and cats, although younger pets can get them, too. "There really isn't much that conventional medicine can do for cataracts except surgically remove them," says Betsy Walker Harrison, D.V.M., a holistic veterinarian in private practice in Wimberley, Texas.

Even when surgery is the only option, veterinarians who specialize in

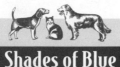

## Shades of Blue

Cataracts aren't the only thing that can cause the eyes to get a bit cloudy. Dogs and cats with a condition called nuclear sclerosis will often develop a slight bluish cast in the eyes that is easily mistaken for cataracts, says Steve Marsden, N.D., D.V.M., a naturopathic physician and holistic veterinarian in private practice in Beaverton, Oregon.

Nuclear sclerosis occurs when tissues in the eyes get harder and more rigid over time. This makes the eyes less transparent and is thought to cause pets to see slight ripples, similar to the ripples in water caused by dropping a stone in a pond.

Any change in the appearance of your pet's eyes is potentially serious and should be checked by a vet. But nuclear sclerosis doesn't have a serious effect on vision and really isn't a problem, says Jeffrey Judkins, D.V.M., a holistic veterinarian in private practice in Portland, Oregon. "Almost every senior dog has it," he adds.

from getting worse, says Jeffrey Judkins, D.V.M., a holistic veterinarian in private practice in Portland, Oregon.

Pets with cataracts always need to be under a veterinarian's care, but there is a lot that you can do at home to keep them under control.

## The Solutions  FOR DOGS & CATS

**Save the eyes with cineraria.** A healing herb called cineraria (*Succus cineraria maritima*) can help reverse cataracts that have already formed and may reduce the need for surgery, says Steve Marsden, N.D., D.V.M., a naturopathic physician and holistic veterinarian in private practice in Beaverton, Oregon. This herb is one of the few things that actually has the potential to clear cataracts, he says. Cineraria eyedrops are available by prescription from veterinarians.

**Fight the free radicals.** Vitamins E and C are known as antioxidant vitamins because they block the harmful oxidizing effects of free radicals, says Dr. Harrison. She recommends giving pets with cataracts 50 international units (IU) of vitamin E for every 10 pounds of weight once a day. "Punch a hole in a vitamin E gel capsule and squeeze some into your pet's food," she advises.

You can give 100 milligrams of vitamin C twice a day for every 10 pounds of body weight, says Dr. Harrison. She recommends buying pow-

natural healing believe it is best to treat cataracts by correcting the underlying problems that are causing them. By countering the effects of free radicals before they damage the eye, it is often possible to prevent cataracts dered vitamin C and adding it to your pet's food. Vitamin C in large amounts can cause diarrhea, she adds, so you may have to experiment a bit until you find an amount that your pet can tolerate.

**Put cod-liver oil to work.** Cod-liver oil contains large amounts of vitamin A, another powerful antioxidant. Dr. Harrison recommends giving about one-quarter teaspoon of cod-liver oil to pets under 15 pounds, one-half teaspoon to pets 15 to 50 pounds, and one teaspoon to larger dogs. Add it directly to your pet's food. Giving too much vitamin A can be harmful, she adds, so it is a good idea to check with your vet to make sure that you are giving the right amount.

**Put vegetables on the menu.** A very nutritious way to boost your pet's supply of antioxidants is to give her more fresh vegetables. Carrots, kale, and other green and yellow vegetables are very rich sources these important substances, Dr. Harrison says. Some pets will eat vegetables raw, but others won't touch them unless they are ground up and mixed in their food.

**Protect the eyes with bilberries.** These European blueberries (*Vaccinium myrtillus*) are rich sources of antioxidants known as flavonoids. When taken in capsule form, these compounds act like armor and help protect the tissues of the eye, Dr. Marsden says. In one human study, Italian researchers found that bilberry

flavonoids mixed with vitamin E were able to stop lens clouding in 97 percent of people with early-stage cataracts. Pet studies haven't been done, but bilberry should be equally effective for them, he says. He recommends mixing the contents of one bilberry capsule (about 50 milligrams) in your pet's food once a day.

**Clear the eyes with homeopathy.** They don't work quickly, but any of the homeopathic Calcarea remedies, Phosphorus, and Silica are very helpful for treating cataracts, Dr. Marsden says. The remedies can't be used interchangeably, he adds. Pets that are also overweight, for example, would benefit most from Calcarea, while timid or shy pets with a tendency to form abscesses might be given Silica.

Whichever homepathic remedy

## Meet the Experts

**Betsy Walker Harrison, D.V.M.,** is a holistic veterinarian in private practice in Wimberley, Texas. She is certified in homeopathy.

**Jeffrey Judkins, D.V.M.,** is a holistic veterinarian in private practice in Portland, Oregon. He is certified in acupuncture.

**Steve Marsden, N.D., D.V.M.,** is a naturopathic physician, licensed acupuncturist, and holistic veterinarian in private practice in Beaverton, Oregon.

your vet recommends, the usual dose is three pellets of 30C strength, given once a day for a week. "Do not expect rapid changes," Dr. Marsden adds. Even though you stop giving the remedy after one week, it might take several weeks before you are able to see any clearing of the lens or an improvement in your pet's ability to get around.

**Help the injuries heal.** Cataracts caused by eye injuries may get better when pets are given homeopathic Conium maculatum, says Dr. Harrison. She recommends giving dogs and cats one or two pellets of Conium maculatum 6X once a day

for three to five days. The easiest way to give the tablets is to crush them and put them in one-half teaspoon of milk. "Most animals will drink it right up," she says.

## The Solutions  FOR DOGS

**Give beta-carotene.** This powerful antioxidant is converted to vitamin A in the body, which helps protect tissues in the eyes, says Dr. Marsden. (Cats can't convert beta-carotene to vitamin A, so this is only an option for dogs.) Check with your vet for the dose that's right for your dog.

# CAT FLU

## The Signs
- Your cat is sneezing a lot.
- He has a stuffy or runny nose.
- There is an eye discharge or sores on the eye, tongue, or mouth.
- He refuses to eat.

## The Cause

That sneezy, sniffly, sick-to-your-stomach feeling is a sure sign that you have the flu—and your cat can sympa-

thize. Cats occasionally get similar viral infections—most commonly, a type of upper respiratory infection known as cat flu.

"Vaccinations can protect cats against the most common causes of cat flu, but even the best vaccines do not provide 100 percent protection," says Alice Wolf, D.V.M., professor of medicine at Texas A&M University College of Veterinary Medicine in College Station. Another problem with the vaccinations, according to holistic veterinarians, is that when repeatedly given over a lifetime, they can affect the immune system, causing it to work abnormally. They feel that a better approach is to supplement vaccinations by strengthening your cat's immune system naturally so that he doesn't get sick in first place.

Even if he does get cat flu, the illness usually isn't serious and will go away on its own within a week, Dr. Wolf adds. To keep your cat more comfortable in the meantime—and to strengthen his defenses so that he is better protected—here are some natural treatments that you may want to try.

## The Solutions

**Help him breathe with aromatherapy.** It is hard for cats to breathe when they are congested. An effective way to break up mucus and open the airways is with a combination of essential oils called Immupower, says Teresa Fulp, D.V.M., a holistic veterinarian in private practice in Springfield, Virginia. "Immupower is fantastic for respiratory infections and is a great decongestant," she says. "Dilute the oil half-and-half with peanut or pure vegetable oil and rub a little bit on the ear tip every four to six hours. Doing this once a day while your cat is sick will keep him breathing easily, says Dr.

Fulp. Immupower is too concentrated to use straight and always should be diluted first.

**Cook a healing meal.** Chicken soup seasoned with garlic has been shown to relieve congestion and strengthen the immune system, says Pat Zook, D.V.M., a holistic veterinarian in private practice in Stone Mountain, Georgia. Homemade soup is best, although canned soup seasoned with garlic may also help. Since cats with cat flu often lose their appetites, the soup can be especially helpful because most cats relish warm broth and will eat it with gusto. You can give four to eight ounces of soup a day for two to three days.

Don't overdo the garlic, Dr. Zook adds. It can cause a type of anemia. For most cats, one-eighth teaspoon a day for up to a couple of weeks is plenty. "If you are smelling garlic on his breath, you are probably getting enough in there." Also, don't use onions in the soup; they can be dangerous for cats.

**Give a tomato chaser.** Another food that's good for congestion is tomato juice. "It helps open the lungs, and some cats really like it," says Dr. Zook. She recommends giving your cat a few tablespoons of warm tomato juice a day.

**Give a vitamin boost.** Even though you can't always prevent upper respiratory viral infections with vitamin C, research has shown that it may shorten their duration and make the symptoms less severe. Dr. Zook recommends adding 125 to 250 milligrams of vitamin C powder to your cat's food every day until he is feeling better. Or you can mix the vitamin C in tomato juice or cool chicken soup, draw it up in a needle-less syringe, and squirt it directly in your cat's mouth.

**Use herbs to boost immunity.** Both echinacea (*Echinacea purpurea*) and goldenseal (*Hydrastis canadensis*) strengthen the immune system, making the body better able to fight infections, says Dr. Zook. She recommends giving your cat an herbal tincture of either one of these herbs. Dilute the tincture by putting two drops in an ounce of water. Give your cat a dropperful of the solution once a day for a week, she advises. It is best to use tinctures that are alcohol-free because alcohol may be harmful for cats.

**Clear the discharge.** A homeopathic remedy called Kali bichromicum can help relieve congestion when there is a sticky, yellow nasal discharge, says Dr. Zook. Dissolve one or two 6X or 15X tablets in water, then use your fingertip to rub the solution on your cat's gums. You can do this every few hours for up to two days, she says.

**BEST BET!** **Keep him clean.** Cat flu often causes a heavy nasal

## Meet the Experts

**Teresa Fulp, D.V.M.,** is a holistic veterinarian in private practice in Springfield, Virginia.

**Carin A. Smith, D.V.M.,** is a veterinary consultant in the state of Washington and the author of *101 Training Tips for Your Cat.*

**Donna M. Starita, D.V.M.,** is a holistic veterinarian in private practice in Boring, Oregon.

**Alice Wolf, D.V.M.,** is a professor of medicine at Texas A&M University College of Veterinary Medicine in College Station.

**Pat Zook, D.V.M.,** is a holistic veterinarian in private practice in Stone Mountain, Georgia. She is certified in acupuncture.

discharge that blocks the nostrils and may irritate the eyes, says Carin A. Smith, D.V.M., a veterinary consultant in the state of Washington and author of *101 Training Tips for Your Cat.* She recommends using a soft, damp cloth to remove the discharge at least once a day. You may have to hold the cloth on the discharge for a while until it softens and easily wipes away.

**Keep an eye on fever.** It's normal for cats to run a fever when they have cat flu (normal cat temperature is 101° to 102.5°F). "I love a fever because it means the body's immune system is working overtime," says Donna M. Starita, D.V.M., a holistic veterinarian in private practice in Boring, Oregon.

You will need to call your vet, however, if the fever is 103.5° or higher or when a lower-grade fever lasts more than a day or two.

**Fill the airways with humidity.** Moist heat is one of the best ways to open up clogged noses and airways, says Dr. Smith. She recommends putting a humidifier near where your cat sleeps. To quickly fill his lungs with moisture, you can also take your cat with you into the bathroom when you bathe or shower, she says.

**BEST BET!** **Keep him eating.** When cats get congested, they lose their sense of smell, and this can cause them to stop eating, says Dr. Wolf. Until your cat's better, she says, it is a good idea to give him foods that are smellier than usual, such as meat baby food, or to add the water from canned tuna or clams. "Most cats will eat more if you talk and sit with them while they eat," adds Dr. Smith.

# CHEWING

## The Signs
- Your shoes are in pieces, or your carpet is ripped.

## The Cause

It is not surprising when a puppy works over your slippers or a kitten is gnawing the drape cords. Young pets have an intense need to chew, if only to relieve teething pain or boredom. It takes them time to learn what they should and shouldn't chew. Adult pets, however, should know the ropes. When they are showing a sudden interest in your possessions—or if they never outgrew the habit—you have to put a stop to it.

The traditional approach to chewing is to stop it with training or, in severe cases, with medications that help control compulsive behavior. There is nothing wrong with these approaches, and in some instances, they are the only ways to stop the habit. But holistic veterinarians believe it is also important to relieve or redirect the nervous energy that often causes misguided chewing.

"Anything that upsets their routine or environment can cause them to act out by chewing on shoes, furniture, or other items that don't belong to them," says Steven Kasanofsky, D.V.M., a holistic veterinarian in private practice in New York City.

Some pets start chewing because they have a deficiency of certain vitamins and minerals, adds Allen M. Schoen, D.V.M., director of the Veterinary Institute for Therapeutic Alternatives in Sherman, Connecticut, and author of *Love, Miracles, and Animal Healing*.

Many behavior problems are difficult to change, but it is usually not that hard to stop pets from chewing, regardless of what's putting their mouths into motion. Here is what holistic veterinarians advise.

## The Solutions *FOR DOGS & CATS*

**Restore their routine.** Dogs and cats don't like frequent changes in their lives. Even small disruptions, like feeding them at different times or taking them for fewer walks, can cause them to chew out of sheer frustration and anxiety. "When your pet suddenly begins to chew, ask yourself what has changed in his environment or routine," advises Dr. Kasanofsky. If you are able to identify and change whatever it is that's making him upset, he will be much less likely to chew.

**Ease their anxieties.** Since pets often chew in order to blow off steam and relieve anxiety, it is worth trying to reduce the stress in their lives. "One of the most successful ways of relieving anxiety is with flower remedies," says Dr. Schoen. There are

dozens of flower remedies that are used for various kinds of emotional problems. The ones that may work best for anxiety-related chewing include the following:

🐾 Aspen. It is used to soothe pets that are edgy because of change, such as when you have moved to a new house or the family's usual schedule has been disrupted.

🐾 Chicory. It may help relieve anxiety that is caused by jealousy.

🐾 Clematis. It is usually given to pets that are anxious because they miss a friend.

🐾 Vervain. It is recommended for pets that have a lot of extra energy.

The easiest way to give flower remedies is to put 10 drops of the liquid in your pet's water twice a day, says Dr. Schoen. Or you can mix the drops in one-quarter cup of water and stir it in your pet's food. "Some pets even take the remedies directly from the dropper," he says.

**Consider a change of diet.** Even though commercial pet foods contain the essential nutrients, some pets aren't able to absorb all the vitamins and minerals that they need. In particular, a deficiency of B-complex vitamins or calcium can lead to chewing problems. Each of these nutrients has a calming effect. Pets that don't get enough calcium or B vitamins may feel edgy and anxious, emotions that they try to dispel with chewing.

Some veterinarians recommend giving dogs and cats dietary supplements, but in most cases, switching your pet to a high-quality, all-natural pet food, such as Innova, Wysong, or PetGuard Premium, will take care of simple nutritional imbalances, says Dr. Schoen. You can buy all-natural foods in some pet supply stores and through mail order.

**BEST BET!** **Provide appropriate chew toys.** Dogs—and to a lesser extent, cats—have a natural need to chew, not only to relieve emotional turmoil but also to keep their teeth and gums healthy. Unless pets have plenty of chewable toys that they can call their own, they are going to turn their attention elsewhere. So it is worth taking a little time to find out what toys your pet enjoys chewing, says Dr. Kasanofsky. For cats, a catnip mouse is hard to beat, and most dogs enjoy fleece toys, tennis balls, Kong toys, or Nylabone chews, available in pet supply stores.

**BEST BET!** **Add excitement to their lives.** Just as humans chew their nails or crack their knuckles when they are bored, dogs and cats sometimes chew as a way of staying entertained, says Wayne Hunthausen, D.V.M., a veterinary behaviorist in Westwood, Kansas, and author of the *Handbook of Behaviour Problems in Dogs and Cats*. The

easiest way to make their jaws less active is to get their paws moving with regular exercise. Dogs and cats that exercise a lot burn off the emotional energy that often leads to chewing, he explains. Exercise also tires them out, and tired pets don't have enough energy left over to destroy your belongings. Most dogs and cats need at least 20 to 30 minutes of exercise twice a day, and high-energy breeds, like Border collies, need a lot more.

**Discourage his attention.** Pet supply stores sell a number of repellents, such as Bitter Apple, which you can apply to the inappropriate objects of your pet's desires—like your shoes or a table leg. Once he takes a lick of the offensive stuff, he may de-

## Meet the Experts

**Wayne Hunthausen, D.V.M.,** is a veterinary behaviorist in Westwood, Kansas, and author of the *Handbook of Behaviour Problems in Dogs and Cats.*

**Steven Kasanofsky, D.V.M.,** is a holistic veterinarian in private practice in New York City. He is certified in acupuncture.

**Allen M. Schoen, D.V.M.,** is director of the Veterinary Institute for Therapeutic Alternatives in Sherman, Connecticut, and the author of *Love, Miracles, and Animal Healing.* He is certified in acupuncture and chiropractic.

cide that his own toys are the best choice after all.

You don't have to spend a lot of money on pet repellents, Dr. Hunthausen adds. Common household products such as Vicks VapoRub or hot-pepper juice will also give pets a "no-chew" message. It is a good idea to test the products in an inconspicuous place to see if they will stain.

# CLAW PROBLEMS

## The Signs
- Your pet clicks when he walks.
- He is limping or licking his feet.
- His nails are split or cracked.
- His toes are swollen, or there is crusty skin around the nails.

## The Cause

Evolution gave dogs strong, blunt toenails for digging, while cats have razor-sharp claws for hunting and climbing trees. For both dogs and cats, life on the wild side naturally kept claws trim. But modern pet pastimes, like clawing the sofa or tunneling into the carpet, do little to shorten the nails. This can be a problem because long claws and nails tend to catch on rough surfaces and tear. Or the nails curl back and grow into the skin.

Trimming your pet's nails will help prevent many problems, but it doesn't necessarily keep the nails healthy. Cats with weakened immune systems, for example, often get nail-bed infections, and mineral deficiencies can cause nails to crack, says George Carley, D.V.M., a holistic veterinarian in private practice in Tulsa, Oklahoma.

Claw problems aren't always easy to treat because they have so many different causes, says Dr. Carley. Once you know what's behind the problem, however, there is a lot that you can do to keep nails and claws healthy. Here is what veterinarians advise.

## The Solutions — FOR DOGS & CATS

**Treat damaged nails with an herbal rinse.** The herb calendula (*Calendula officinalis*), available as a tincture, reduces inflammation and helps damaged nails heal. You can even use it as a styptic to stop bleeding, says Donna M. Starita, D.V.M., a holistic veterinarian in private practice in Boring, Oregon.

You can use calendula by itself or

mix it with St. John's wort (*Hypericum perforatum*). The advantage of using the combination treatment is that St. John's wort reduces swelling and helps kill bacteria and fungi. "Calendula-hypericum rinses are my favorite topical treatment for nail problems," says Dr. Starita. "It brings the tissues together and helps numb the pain."

Add a teaspoon of each tincture to one-quarter cup of water and rinse your pet's nails and nail beds in the solution once a day, she advises.

**Strengthen the body with acupressure.** Dogs and cats sometimes get nail-bed infections when their immune systems are too weak to fight off bacteria or fungi. These infections can make the toes swell or get crusty where the claws grow, explains Dr. Carley. You can strengthen immunity by applying pressure to three acupressure points: SP6, located on the inside of the rear legs just above the hocks (the ankles); LI11, located on the outside of the front legs at the elbow creases; and BL20, a thumb's width down from the spine between the last two ribs. He recommends pressing each of these points for 60 seconds, once or twice a day, until the claws heal.

**BEST BET!** **Keep claws healthy with fatty acids.** Unhealthy nails are often caused by a dietary deficiency, especially an insufficient amount of fatty acids. Giving your pet fatty-acid supplements will help reduce inflammation and boost the immune system, says Dr. Starita. She recommends giving dogs and cats with nail problems a fatty-acid supplement called Eskimo Oil, available from veterinarians. Cats can take one-eighth teaspoon of Eskimo Oil twice a day. Dogs 50 pounds or less can have one-quarter teaspoon, and larger dogs can take one-half teaspoon twice a day.

**Increase body moisture with rehmannia root.** In older pets especially, the body may eliminate too much water, leading to dry, cracked nails. A Chinese herb known as rehmannia root helps the body conserve fluid by strengthening the kidneys, says Dr. Carley. He recommends using a product called Six Flavor Tea Pills, which contains rehmannia root and other ingredients. It is available in some health food stores and catalogs and from veterinarians. Give pets under 15 pounds one-half to one tablet twice a day, he advises. Pets that weigh 15 to 50 pounds can take one to two tablets twice a day, and larger dogs can take as much as three tablets three times a day.

**Keep claws clipped.** One of the best ways to prevent cracked or splintered nails is to give dogs and cats regular pedicures, says Dr. Starita. Nails grow at different rates, but most cats are ready for a trim every week. For dogs, every two to three weeks is plenty. Most pets hate having their

## Meet the Experts

**George Carley, D.V.M.,** is a holistic veterinarian in private practice in Tulsa, Oklahoma. He is certified in acupuncture.

**Donna M. Starita, D.V.M.,** is a holistic veterinarian in private practice in Boring, Oregon.

**Susan G. Wynn, D.V.M.,** is a veterinarian in Atlanta and co-editor of *Complementary and Alternative Veterinary Medicine*.

nails trimmed, so you may want to spread it out over several days, doing a nail or two at a time.

**BEST BET!** **Give them extra zinc.** Dogs and cats that don't get enough zinc will sometimes develop weak nails. You can give pets 20 milligrams of zinc gluconate for every 10 pounds of body weight once a day for two to four weeks, says Susan G. Wynn, D.V.M., a veterinarian in Atlanta and co-editor of *Complementary and Alternative Veterinary Medicine*.

# Coat Dryness

## The Signs
- Your pet's fur has lost its shine.
- The coat is brittle, dry, or stiff.
- She has "fly-away" hair filled with static electricity.
- She is scratching or shedding more than usual.

## The Cause

Whether your pet is curly-coated, short-haired, or blessed with a mane, her coat should always be soft, shiny, and supple. It is for more than just good looks. The appearance of the coat tells a lot about your pet's overall health.

Pet supply stores sell a lot of shampoos, conditioners, and other coat-care products. There is nothing wrong with spending a little money to keep your pet looking good, and in some cases—such as in winter, when the air is unusually dry—a little cosmetic care is all that is needed. But most veterinarians believe that a dry coat, no less than a cough or runny eyes, means something on the inside is affecting how your pet looks on the outside, says Alexander Werner, V.M.D., a veterinary dermatologist in private practice in Studio City, California.

A dry coat usually isn't caused by serious problems, he adds. In most cases, you can keep your pet healthy and restore the shine with a few simple strategies. Here is what veterinarians advise.

## The Solutions FOR DOGS & CATS

**BEST BET!** **Put natural foods on the menu.** The best way to keep your pet's coat healthy is to give her high-quality foods, says Christina Chambreau, D.V.M., a holistic veterinarian in Sparks, Maryland, and education chairperson for the Academy of Veterinary Homeopathy. A homemade diet consisting of meat, grains, and raw vegetables is superior to most commercial foods, she says. In addition, homemade diets don't contain chemical additives or preservatives that can dry the coat, she explains. For more information on homemade diets, see page 61. Or you can switch to an all-natural commercial food like Innova, Solid Gold, PetGuard Premium, or Wysong. You can buy all-natural foods in some pet supply stores and through mail order.

**Improve their digestion.** Every dog and cat digests foods differently, and some pets aren't able to absorb all their nutrients in their food. This can show up as dry, brittle hair. Adding digestive enzymes made specifically for pets, like Vet-Zime, Prozyme, or FloraZyme, to your pet's food will improve digestion and help restore the shine to your pet's coat, says Russell Swift, D.V.M., a holistic

veterinarian in private practice in Dade, Broward, and Palm Beach Counties in Florida.

**BEST BET!** **Shine the coat with fatty acids.** The glow you see in healthy fur comes mainly from fat in the diet. Pets that don't get enough fat—or, more commonly, get the wrong balance of different fats—will often shed more than usual, and the coat will turn dry and dull, says Dr. Werner. "A combination of omega-3 and omega-6 fatty-acid supplements really help a dry coat," he says. Fatty-acid supplements made specifically for pets come in gel capsules or as liquids or granules. Look for supplements containing fish and flaxseed oil because these omega-3-rich oils have been shown to be anti-inflammatory and improve skin health. Read the label to see how much is recommended for your pet.

An alternative to supplements is to drizzle between one-half and one teaspoon of a vegetable oil like olive oil on your pet's food every day. Vegetable oil doesn't contain a lot of omega-3 or omega-6 fatty acids, but adding any fat to your pet's food can help restore shine to the coat, says Dr. Werner. Pets with a history of pancreatitis, however, shouldn't be given extra oils without checking with their vets first.

**Give a coat-healthy vitamin.** Veterinarians have found that vitamin A supplements will help keep the coat healthy, says Nancy Scanlan, D.V.M., a holistic veterinarian in private practice in Sherman Oaks, California. Every pet needs different amounts of vitamin A, so check with your vet before using it at home, she advises.

**Clean her gently.** Human shampoos and detergents are much too strong for your pet's coat, says Steven A. Melman, V.M.D., a veterinarian with practices in Potomac, Maryland, and Palm Springs, California, and author of *Skin Diseases of Dogs and Cats*. It is best to use hypoallergenic shampoos designed for dogs and cats, which actually stimulate the skin to produce more oils, he explains. And unless you are actually treating your pet for fleas, avoid flea shampoos, he adds. They contain insecticides that are too harsh for normal bathing.

**Follow up with a conditioner.** After shampooing your pet, it is a good idea to use a moisturizing coat conditioner, which helps the fur retain moisture. Conditioners are helpful even when you are not shampooing your pet, says Dr. Melman. For cats that will do anything to avoid getting wet, you can use a conditioning spray, he adds. Or take some of the same moisturizer you use for your hands and rub it into her skin and coat.

**Calm the itch.** Pets with dry coats often have itchy skin as well, says Michelle Tilghman, D.V.M., a holistic veterinarian in private practice in

---

## Meet the Experts

**Christina Chambreau, D.V.M.,** is a holistic veterinarian in Sparks, Maryland, and education chairperson for the Academy of Veterinary Homeopathy.

**Steven A. Melman, V.M.D.,** is a veterinarian with practices in Potomac, Maryland, and Palm Springs, California, and the author of *Skin Diseases of Dogs and Cats*.

**Nancy Scanlan, D.V.M.,** is a holistic veterinarian in private practice in Sherman Oaks, California. She is certified in acupuncture and chiropractic.

**Russell Swift, D.V.M.,** is a holistic veterinarian in private practice in Dade, Broward, and Palm Beach Counties in Florida.

**Michelle Tilghman, D.V.M.,** is a holistic veterinarian in private practice in Stone Mountain, Georgia. She is certified in acupuncture.

**Alexander Werner, V.M.D.,** is a veterinary dermatologist in private practice in Studio City, California.

---

Stone Mountain, Georgia. "An effective and fairly common herbal preparation for itchy skin is called TriSnake Pills," she says. Available in Chinese pharmacies and from some holistic veterinarians, this preparation will help soothe a variety of skin problems. There isn't one dose that fits all, however, so ask your vet what dose is right for your pet.

# COLD WEATHER PROBLEMS

## The Signs
- Your pet is biting at his tail or paws.
- His feet, ears, or tail are unusually cold.
- He is shivering or seems lethargic.

## The Cause

When dogs and cats lived in the wild, cold weather was rarely a problem because they evolved to suit the climates in which they found themselves. But people changed nature's plan by bringing thin-coated dogs to New England and desert-dwelling cats to Minnesota. Brrr!

With the exception of pets, such as huskies, that were bred to withstand cold climates, dogs and cats aren't made for frigid conditions. They get just as cold in icy weather as people do. And because they go barefoot all the time, their paws are vulnerable to ice, packed snow, and road salt. In extreme conditions, they can get frostbite, says John F. Sangiorgio, D.V.M., a holistic veterinarian in private practice in Staten Island, New York.

When the thermometer dips below freezing, it is important to protect dogs and cats from the elements, even when they are only spending a short time outside. Here is what veterinarians advise.

## The Solutions — FOR DOGS & CATS

**Nourish the skin.** Cold air is extremely drying, and pets that have spent too much time in the elements will quickly get sore ears and paws, says Katherine Evans, D.V.M., a holistic veterinarian in private practice in Concord, New Hampshire. To moisturize and nourish the skin, apply the gel from a vitamin E capsule, she advises. The juice from an aloe vera plant will also provide quick relief, she says.

Vitamins can protect your pet from the inside out, Dr. Evans adds. Vitamin E and B-complex vitamins will strengthen the tissues and make dogs and cats more resistant to cold. She recommends giving cats and dogs under 15 pounds 100 international units (IU) of vitamin E a day and half a capsule or tablet of B-complex 50 vitamins. Pets 15 to 50 pounds can have between 200 and 300 IU of vitamin E, along with a B-complex 50 vitamin. Dogs over 50 pounds can take 300 to 400 IU of vitamin E and a B-complex 100 vitamin.

**Fortify the coat.** In order to maintain a thick, protective coat, dogs and

# Call the VET

Most dogs and cats can handle winter's chill without experiencing anything worse than a little shiver and shake. But pets that spend a lot of time outdoors in blustery weather could get frostbite, an extremely serious condition in which the body diverts blood away from the extremities—the legs, ears, and tail—in order to preserve core body heat. This can cause tissue in the extremities to break down and die, explains John F. Sangiorgio, D.V.M., a holistic veterinarian in private practice in Staten Island, New York.

Pets with frostbite will often have extremely cold paws, ears, and tails, and the cold will persist even after they have spent time inside, he says. They may bite at their feet and tails as well. Frostbite is always an emergency. But if you can't get to a vet immediately, here is what you should do in the meantime.

- Let them choose their heat. Pets with frostbite need to warm up, but you don't want to warm them up too quickly. The best approach is to put them in a room with a radiator or fireplace and let them move closer or farther away as they see fit. Don't use a heating pad or try to rush the warming process, Dr. Sangiorgio warns.

- Warm the ears and paws with moist heat. When the extremities are extremely cold, it is a good idea to gently dab them with a moist, lukewarm washcloth.

- Let them go hungry. You don't want to feed pets with frostbite because eating will draw circulation into the intestines at a time when it is more important to get circulation to the legs, tail, and ears. "Wait until the body regains its normal temperature before feeding them," says Dr. Sangiorgio. It is fine for them to drink water, however, as long as it is at room temperature.

cats need to get fatty acids in their diets. Dr. Sangiorgio recommends giving fatty-acid supplements, available in pet supply stores, toward the end of summer, which will cause the coat to grow in a bit thicker for the cold months. Follow the instructions on the label.

**Give him extra calories.** Pets that

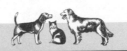

## Cold Weather Comfort

Despite their warm coats, most dogs and cats get a little chilly when the temperature dips. To keep them warm and dry, you may want to invest in winter clothing. Booties and shoes are a must for pets that spend lots of time outdoors in wet, snowy weather. Sweaters keep pets warm while allowing freedom of movement, and a slicker or raincoat shields those pets who just can't bear to be wet.

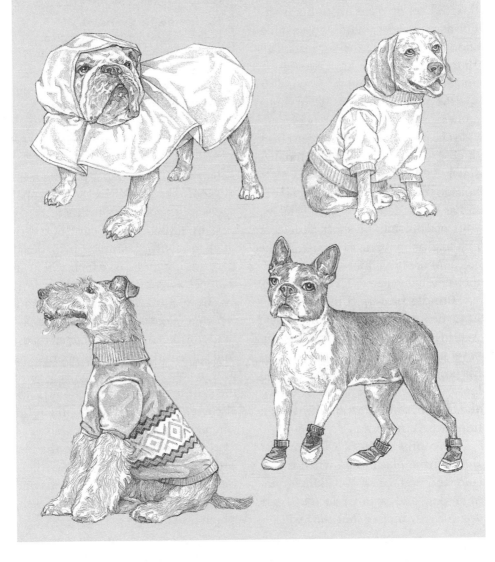

spend time outside need extra calories in the cold months in order to stay warm, says Beatrice Ehrsam, D.V.M., a holistic veterinarian in private practice in New Paltz, New York. "If your pet is on a homemade diet, double the amount of oil and increase the percentage of meat," she advises. "If he's on a commercial diet, add some flaxseed oil or olive oil to his food." For dogs over 50 pounds, give a tablespoon of oil a day, she suggests. Pets 15 to 50 pounds can have a teaspoon, and dogs and cats under 15 pounds.

**Prepare him slowly.** When winter comes on suddenly, your pet's body won't be prepared for the sudden outset of cold. "Animals need to acclimatize slowly," says Nancy Brandt, D.V.M., a holistic veterinarian in private practice in Las Vegas. She recommends taking your pet outside for short periods at first to give him time to get used to the cold. "Make the initial exposure brief, then gradually increase it," she advises.

**Bundle him up.** Unless your pet has a thick coat of fur, he will appreciate wearing a sweater or coat, available in pet supply stores. Just make sure that it fits properly, Dr. Evans adds. "If it's too loose, cold air will get between the coat and his skin, and if it's too tight, it could impede his circulation."

**Give him shelter.** "Outdoor pets should have place to go when it gets cold and wet," says Dr. Sangiorgio. Many dogs and cats are reluctant to use dog (or cat) houses, but they will in-

> ## Meet the Experts
>
> **Nancy Brandt, D.V.M.,** is a holistic veterinarian in private practice in Las Vegas. She is certified in acupuncture.
>
> **Beatrice Ehrsam, D.V.M.,** is a holistic veterinarian in private practice in New Paltz, New York. She is certified in acupuncture.
>
> **Katherine E. Evans, D.V.M.,** is a holistic veterinarian in private practice in Concord, New Hampshire. She is certified in acupuncture.
>
> **John F. Sangiorgio, D.V.M.,** is a holistic veterinarian in private practice in Staten Island, New York.

stinctively curl up under porches or in outdoor sheds. Wherever your pet stays, it is a good idea to create a cozy nest by lining a cardboard box with thick towels, for example. Small "dens" help trap body heat, which will keep your pet warm even on the coldest days.

**Keep him dry.** Damp feet and a wet coat make pets feel a lot colder, no matter what the thermometer reads. And moisture doesn't evaporate as well in cold weather, which can cause the skin to dry and crack. So it is important to thoroughly dry their fur whenever they come inside. On snowy days, you may want to rinse the feet with lukewarm water, then dry them well. This will remove ice shards and packed snow as well as road salt, which is extremely drying.

# CONSTIPATION

## The Signs
- Your pet hasn't had a bowel movement in 48 hours.
- He cries or strains when passing stools.
- The stools are hard and dry.

## The Cause

No one enjoys poop-scooping the yard or litter box, but it is better than the alternative: a pet who is trying to have bowel movements but can't. Occasional constipation is fairly common and doesn't cause problems. When it lasts more than a day, however, stools in the intestine get dry and even harder to pass. Eventually, the lining of the bowel can become inflamed.

Older pets sometimes get constipated because they don't exercise as much as they used to and their abdominal muscles are weaker than they should be. In pets of all ages, constipation may occur when something painful, such as blocked anal sacs or a swollen prostate gland, is making them reluctant to have a bowel movement, says H. Ellen Whiteley, D.V.M., a veterinary consultant in Guadalupita, New Mexico, and consultant for *The Country Vet's Home Remedies for Cats*. Cats sometimes get consti-

pated when they have hair in the digestive tract or, less often, when the litter box is dirty and they refuse to use it, she adds.

Laxatives for pets will relieve constipation, but holistic veterinarians don't like using them too much because they do nothing to correct the underlying problem. A better approach, they say, is to avoid temporary chemical "cures" and to find a long-term, natural solution that will stop the problem that is causing the constipation in the first place. Here is what they advise.

## The Solutions — FOR DOGS & CATS

**Improve the intestines with acupressure.** An acupressure point called ST36, located on the outside of each back leg just below the knee, where the bone meets the muscle, is the master point for the whole gastrointestinal tract, says Kathleen Carson, D.V.M., a holistic veterinarian in private practice in Hermosa Beach, California. She recommends pressing this point for about 30 seconds, two or three times a day, until the constipation goes away. You can press the points on each knee simultaneously or one at a time for 30 seconds each. Once your pet is regular again, repeat

**ALTERNATIVE SUCCESS**

### RELIEF AT LAST

Obie was miserable. A middle-aged Manx cat with chronic constipation, he hadn't had a comfortable bowel movement in months, and nothing his veterinarian tried seemed to help.

"Obie would improve for a while, but then he would reach a plateau and wouldn't get any better," says Kathleen Carson, D.V.M., a holistic veterinarian in private practice in Hermosa Beach, California. "Obie and his owner were getting sick and tired of his being sick," she says.

Finally, Dr. Carson called in a specialist who treated Obie with crystal therapy. "I didn't expect it to be so dramatic," she says, "but the constipation was resolved almost right away. It surprised the heck out of me."

Obie may have been surprised as well, but he didn't show it, says Dr. Carson. He just looked relieved.

---

the treatments every few days to keep him that way.

**Ease discomfort with lavender.** Holistic veterinarians recommend aromatherapy for many types of stress, including stress in the intestines. For pets with constipation, lavender essential oil is a good choice, says Donna M. Starita, D.V.M., a holistic veterinarian in private practice in Boring, Oregon. Dab a little bit of the oil, diluted half-and-half with peanut oil, where your pet can't lick it off—on his ears, for example, or the back of his neck. The oil stays active for four to six hours, so you will need to repeat the treatment several times a day, continuing until the constipation is relieved, she says.

**Increase internal energy.** All of the body's functions require the proper energy balance to work efficiently, and pets with constipation may need a bit of a jump-start. "Crystals focus energy and can be a tremendous healing force inside the body," says Joanne Stefanatos, D.V.M., a holistic veterinarian in private practice in Las Vegas. She recommends hanging a quartz crystal pendant, available in gem or crystal shops, from your pet's collar so that it hangs over the heart. This will allow the crystal to draw healing energy from the surrounding air and transfer it into your pet's body, she explains.

**Lubricate his insides.** To help stools travel more easily through the intestine when your pet is constipated, you may want to add between one-half and one teaspoon of olive or safflower oil to his food, says Dr. Stefanatos.

**BEST BET!** **Calm the gut with Nux vomica.** A homeopathic remedy called Nux vomica will help correct energy imbalances in the intestine that can lead to constipation, says Dr. Carson. She recommends using Nux vomica liquid of 6C strength. Dilute 20 drops of the remedy in an ounce of spring water and give your pet one-half dropperful three times a day until the constipation goes away.

**BEST BET!** **Firm the stools with fiber.** Dietary fiber is one of the best remedies for constipation because it absorbs a tremendous amount of water in the intestine. It makes stools larger and stimulates the colon to work more efficiently. Dr. Stefanatos suggests adding psyllium husks or flaxseeds, both of which are very high in fiber, to your pet's food.

Oat bran and unflavored Metamucil are also good fiber choices, Dr. Whiteley adds. Whichever source of fiber you use, plan on giving about one-half teaspoon per meal to cats and to dogs weighing less than 15 pounds. Dogs 15 to 50 pounds can have a teaspoon, and dogs over 50 pounds can have a tablespoon.

## Call the VET

Dogs and cats can go about 48 hours without a bowel movement and suffer nothing worse than a little cramping and perhaps some gas. Constipation that lasts longer, however, can be serious because the stools get harder, drier, and bigger, until they don't have a chance of moving at all, says H. Ellen Whiteley, D.V.M., a veterinary consultant in Guadalupita, New Mexico, and consultant for *The Country Vet's Home Remedies for Cats.*

"Some pets get so plugged up that they start vomiting," she says. If that happens, or your pet becomes lethargic after being constipated for more than two days, you need to see a veterinarian right away.

**Keep him comfortable with slippery elm.** A healing herb that is often used for throat problems, slippery elm (*Ulmus rubra*) works for intestinal discomfort as well. "The constant straining of constipation can irritate the gut, and slippery elm bark really helps," says Dr. Carson. She recommends diluting 20 drops of slippery elm tincture in an ounce of spring water and giving your pet a dropperful three or four times a day. It is best to use tinctures that are alcohol-free because alcohol may be harmful for cats.

**Restore emotional balance.** Pets that are experiencing a lot of stress will sometimes get constipated, says Dr. Stefanatos. To help them feel calmer and more relaxed, she recommends giving them a flower essence blend called Bach Rescue Remedy. During high-stress times, put a dropperful of the liquid in their water once a day until their bowels are moving normally again, she advises.

**BEST BET!** **Keep them active.** Regular exercise can be used to treat and prevent constipation because it strengthens the abdominal muscles, making them better able to push stools out of the body, says Dr. Whiteley. Most dogs and cats need a minimum of 20 to 30 minutes of exercise twice a day, although older pets or those with physical problems may need less, she says.

**Flush them with fluids.** Dogs and cats may get constipated when there isn't enough water in the in-

---

## Meet the Experts

**Kathleen Carson, D.V.M.,** is a holistic veterinarian in private practice in Hermosa Beach, California.

**Donna M. Starita, D.V.M.,** is a holistic veterinarian in private practice in Boring, Oregon.

**Joanne Stefanatos, D.V.M.,** is a holistic veterinarian in private practice in Las Vegas. She is certified in acupuncture and chiropractic.

**H. Ellen Whiteley, D.V.M.,** is a veterinary consultant in Guadalupita, New Mexico, and consultant for *The Country Vet's Home Remedies for Cats*.

---

testines to help stools move smoothly. "Cats are notorious for not drinking much water," says Dr. Whiteley. One way to encourage pets to get more fluids is to add water to their dry food, or, better yet, to moisten the food with low-salt chicken broth. Canned food is also a good source of fluids.

Dogs will gladly drink water from a bowl, but some cats may have other preferences, Dr. Whiteley adds. "Make sure that your cats have water available the way they like it, by leaving the faucet dripping, for example," she says. "That may encourage them to drink more."

**Ask about enemas.** Most pets won't need heroic measures to relieve constipation, but sometimes stools in the intestine get so dry and hard that they won't come out on their own.

That's when your vet may recommend a natural enema, says Dr. Stefanatos. Enemas can be dangerous to give at home, so you will need to ask your vet for advice.

## The Solutions
FOR CATS

**Groom away constipation.** Cats swallow a lot of hair during their normal grooming. Swallowed hair may form large clogs, causing constipation, says Dr. Stefanatos. You can usually prevent this by combing or brushing your cat every day—or, if he is prone to constipation, by giving him a summer haircut. She recommends the "lion cut," in which you leave a mane and tuft of fur on the tail, and clip the rest of the coat short.

# DANDRUFF

## The Signs
- White flakes are appearing in your pet's coat.
- His skin is peeling.
- He is scratching more than usual.

## The Cause

Dogs and cats are constantly creating new skin cells and shedding the old ones. The reason you don't usually see the flaky castoffs is that there aren't a lot of them floating around at any one time. In pets with dandruff, however, the skin-replacement cycle is vastly accelerated, causing the fur to become littered with a blizzard of little white flakes.

"Skin problems are a wake-up call from the body that something's wrong," says Christina Chambreau, D.V.M., a holistic veterinarian in Sparks, Maryland, and education chairperson for the Academy of Veterinary Homeopathy. Dandruff may be caused by parasites, hormonal imbalances, or even liver disease. It is important to call your vet when dandruff first makes its appearance, she says. But in most cases, it is easy to stop it at home. Here is what veterinarians advise.

## The Solutions
FOR DOGS & CATS

**BEST BET!** **Change his food.** Many skin problems are caused by the chemical additives and preservatives in commercial pet foods, says W. Jean Dodds, D.V.M., adjunct professor of clinical sciences at the University of Pennsylvania School of Veterinary Medicine in Philadelphia and owner

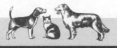

# When Dandruff Walks

The next time your pet's coat is looking a little flaky, and he is so itchy that his hind leg is whirling like a propeller, pick up a magnifying glass and take a close look at one of the flakes. Dandruff doesn't move, but "walking dandruff," the common name for a parasite known as *Cheyletiella*, is plenty mobile. These parasites, which masquerade as flaky skin, are constantly moving from place to place as they search for food—specifically, the lymphatic fluid in your pet's skin.

Walking dandruff usually isn't a serious problem. But the parasites can make pets itchy, and they are contagious—to other pets and to people, says Steven A. Melman, V.M.D., a veterinarian with practices in Potomac, Maryland, and Palm Springs, California, and author of *Skin Diseases of Dogs and Cats*.

Walking dandruff isn't difficult to treat, he adds. One of the best treatments is to use a lime-sulfur dip, available from some mail-order companies. Although it smells like rotten eggs, the dip doesn't use harmful chemicals, and it will eliminate walking dandruff very quickly. Be sure to wash all the bedding in the house, including yours, in hot water and dip (or discard) pet brushes or combs that may be infested. Otherwise, the parasites will walk right back, he explains.

of Hemopet, a national nonprofit animal blood bank in Irvine, California. Feeding your pet a high-quality natural diet, chosen with the help of your vet, will often clear up dandruff within four to six weeks, she says.

There are a number of commercial pet foods that use all-natural ingredients, adds Carolyn Blakey, D.V.M., a holistic veterinarian in private practice in Richmond, Indiana. She recommends a brand called Sojourner Farms, which is a dry mix that contains the proper proportions of grains, herbs, vitamins, and minerals. All you have to do is add fresh meat and vegetables. "It's the Bisquick of pet-food home cooking," she says.

**BEST BET!** **Bring their oils into balance.** Dogs and cats need the proper amounts of fatty acids in order to have healthy, dandruff-free skin, says Dr. Blakey. She recommends supplementing their diets with omega-3 fatty acids formulated specifically for pets. Follow the label directions for the proper dosage.

**Add some vitamin A.** "Vitamin A relieves skin inflammation and helps pets that have dandruff problems," says Nancy Scanlan, D.V.M., a holistic veterinarian in private practice in Sherman Oaks, California. Vitamin A is quite safe, but pets with health problems such as cancer or heart disease shouldn't take large amounts, she adds. Be sure to ask your vet what dose is right for your pet.

**Offer some itch relief.** Since pets with dandruff may get very itchy, veterinarians sometimes recommend a Chinese herbal blend called Skin Balance, which soothes the skin. Skin Balance isn't always easy to find, however. You can buy it in some health food stores and from some holistic veterinarians. The herbal mixture isn't recommended for all pets, Dr. Scanlan adds, so check with your vet before starting it at home.

**Wash away the flakes.** Pet supply stores sell a number of natural shampoos for controlling dandruff. One of the best choices is a shampoo containing salicylic acid, which is chemically similar to the active ingredients in white willow bark, says Steven A. Melman, V.M.D., a veterinarian with practices in Potomac, Maryland, and Palm Springs, California, and author of *Skin Diseases of Dogs and Cats*.

When using an anti-dandruff shampoo, leave the lather on the skin and fur for about 10 minutes to give it time to work, says Dr. Melman. Then rinse your pet thoroughly. "Shampoo your pet whenever the scales come up," he adds. "That should be no more often than every 7 to 10 days."

**Try a vinegar rinse.** It is not uncommon for dogs and cats to develop dandruff when they have mild skin infections, says Dr. Melman. Rinsing their coats with undiluted vinegar will kill a number of common organisms, including yeast, pseudomonas, and

---

## Meet the Experts

**Carolyn Blakey, D.V.M.,** is a holistic veterinarian in private practice in Richmond, Indiana. She is certified in acupuncture.

**Christina Chambreau, D.V.M.,** is a holistic veterinarian in Sparks, Maryland, and education chairperson for the Academy of Veterinary Homeopathy.

**W. Jean Dodds, D.V.M.,** is an adjunct professor of clinical sciences at the University of Pennsylvania School of Veterinary Medicine in Philadelphia and the owner of Hemopet, a national nonprofit animal blood bank in Irvine, California.

**Steven A. Melman, V.M.D.,** is a veterinarian with practices in Potomac, Maryland, and Palm Springs, California, and the author of *Skin Diseases of Dogs and Cats*.

**Nancy Scanlan, D.V.M.,** is a holistic veterinarian in private practice in Sherman Oaks, California. She is certified in acupuncture and chiropractic.

---

staphylococcus, within one to five minutes. The problem with vinegar—for pets as well as people—is its sharp, penetrating smell. A more pleasant alternative is an over-the-counter product called MalAcetic shampoo. It doesn't have the strong smell of vinegar, and it works even better, he says. You can buy it from some vets, groomers, and mail-order companies.

# DEHYDRATION

## The Signs
- Your pet's skin loses elasticity.
- His gums are sticky, and the saliva is stringy.
- His eyes are sunken.

## The Cause

Whether your pet slurps loudly from the toilet or daintily catches drips from a faucet, he is doing more than slaking his thirst. Water lubricates cells, shuttles nutrients through the body, and helps regulate body temperature. Water makes up more than 90 percent of your pet's weight. Dogs and cats that lose as little as 10 percent of their internal water can get extremely ill from dehydration.

Healthy pets drink all the water they need to replace the fluids lost by panting, urinating, or having the occasional bouts of diarrhea and vomiting. But pets with illnesses such as kidney disease or diabetes may lose more fluid than they are able to take in. Severe vomiting or diarrhea can also cause dehydration. So can bacterial infections, which heat the body and speed the loss of essential fluids, says George Carley, D.V.M., a holistic veterinarian in private practice in Tulsa, Oklahoma.

Dehydration is always an emergency. If you suspect that your pet has lost a lot of fluids, you can test for dehydration by lifting and releasing the loose skin over the shoulders. If it doesn't snap back into place right away, your pet is probably dehydrated, and you will need to get him to a veterinarian immediately.

Veterinarians treat dehydration by giving dogs and cats large amounts of fluids, intravenously or under the skin, to replenish what has been lost. Once your pet's fluid levels are back to normal, however, holistic veterinarians look for ways to keep the body's fluids in balance naturally. Here is what they recommend.

## The Solutions — FOR DOGS & CATS

**BEST BET!** **Give him wet foods.** Dry kibble is convenient and inexpensive, but its drawback is that it pulls water from the body to aid in digestion, says Anne Lampru, D.V.M., a holistic veterinarian in private practice in Tampa, Florida. This is more of a problem in cats because they get most of their water from food; they are less likely than dogs to take a long drink of water. Giving your pet moist food or adding water to his kibble will help ensure that he gets all the fluids he needs, she says.

**Slow fluid loss with homeopathy.** Diarrhea and vomiting are common causes of dehydration, so it is worth stopping them quickly. A homeopathic remedy called Nux vomica quickly settles the stomach and intestines, helping ensure that water in the body stays there, says Kathleen Carson, D.V.M., a holistic veterinarian in private practice in Hermosa Beach, California. She recommends diluting 20 drops of Nux vomica 6C in an ounce of water and giving your pet half a dropperful three times a day until he is feeling better.

Many homeopathic remedies can be mixed in drinking water, but pets that are dehydrated probably won't drink enough to get the benefits. It is best to squirt the remedy directly in their mouths using a needleless syringe or a medicine dropper, Dr. Carson says.

**Help the kidneys work better.** In older pets especially, the kidneys don't always work as well as they should, says Dr. Carley. This can be a problem because the kidneys are responsible for regulating the amount of water in the body. One way to improve kidney function is to press the BL23 acupressure point, located on either side of the spine between the second and third lumbar vertebrae. Pressing this point for 60 seconds once a day will strengthen the kidneys and help keep fluids at a healthful level.

**Increase the water energy.** Veterinarians who practice traditional Chinese medicine believe that the herb rehmannia root strengthens a form of energy called *yin*, which, in turn, can increase fluid levels in the body, says Dr. Carley. Pets that are dehydrated because of kidney disease can be given a product called Six Flavor Tea Pills. Available in health food stores, it contains rehmannia root and other herbs that strengthen the yin of the kidneys and liver and help them work more efficiently. Cats and dogs under 15 pounds can take one-half to one whole tablet

## Meet the Experts

**George Carley, D.V.M.,** is a holistic veterinarian in private practice in Tulsa, Oklahoma. He is certified in acupuncture.

**Kathleen Carson, D.V.M.,** is a holistic veterinarian in private practice in Hermosa Beach, California.

**Anne Lampru, D.V.M.,** is a holistic veterinarian in private practice in Tampa, Florida. She is certified in acupuncture and homeopathy.

**Jory Olsen, D.V.M.,** is a veterinary internal-medicine specialist in private practice in Marietta, Georgia.

**James R. Richards, D.V.M.,** is director of the Cornell Feline Health Center at Cornell University in Ithaca, New York.

twice a day. Pets weighing 15 to 50 pounds can take one to two tablets twice a day, and dogs over 50 pounds can take up to three tablets three times a day.

**BEST BET!** **Restore their appetites.** Pets that are dehydrated often refuse to eat, and this can make the problem worse, says James R. Richards, D.V.M., director of the Cornell Feline Health Center at Cornell University in Ithaca, New York. He recommends warming your pet's food before putting it in his bowl. Warming food makes it smell stronger, and the smellier it is, the more likely your pet will eat it.

**BEST BET!** **Encourage him to drink.** Mild dehydration can often be reversed by encouraging your pet to drink plain water. One way to do this is to add a little low-salt chicken broth to his water or give him ice cubes. Many pets enjoy crunching ice, which will get more water into their systems, says Jory Olsen, D.V.M., a veterinary internal-medicine specialist in private practice in Marietta, Georgia. If your pet refuses to drink, your vet may recommend using a needleless syringe, loaded with plain water or a rehydration fluid such as Pedialyte, to put the water directly in his mouth.

# DENTAL PROBLEMS

## The Signs
- Your pet has terrible breath.
- The teeth are yellow or brown.
- The gums are red or bleed easily.
- He is chewing only on one side.
- He is drooling a lot or refusing to eat.

## The Cause

There's a lot to be said for catching dinner on the run. At one time, dogs and cats ate mainly live—or at least recently killed—prey. Chewing through tough skin and bones scrubbed their teeth like a natural toothbrush, and their dental health was probably a lot better than it is today. The food we pour in their bowls may be nutritious, but it doesn't require a lot of tooth action. So perhaps it is not surprising that almost all dogs and cats three years and older develop dental problems.

Most dental problems occur when a thin, bacteria-packed film called plaque accumulates on the teeth. Plaque is a common cause of periodontal, or gum, disease. It can also lead to cavities, especially in cats, says

Ihor Basko, D.V.M., a holistic veterinarian in private practice in Honolulu and Kilauea, Hawaii. More worrisome is the fact that bacteria in the mouth sometimes slip into the bloodstream, damaging the heart or kidneys, he adds.

Veterinary dentists can repair some of the damage caused by dental disease, but the procedures are uncomfortable as well as expensive. They may not be necessary, however, if you practice regular dental care. Unlike many health threats, dental disease can often be stopped entirely with natural home care. It is not enough only to keep the teeth clean, Dr. Basko adds. You also have to strengthen the whole body so that your pet can fight dental disease from the inside out. Here's what veterinarians advise.

## The Solutions FOR DOGS & CATS

**Give them foods with the perfect crunch.** Dry kibble is supposed to cut down on dental problems because it gently scrubs the teeth. It probably helps a little, but most pets eat kibble in gulps without a lot of chewing. It also tends to shatter when pets bite, so it doesn't really clean the teeth, says Anne Lampru, D.V.M., a holistic veterinarian in private practice in Tampa, Florida.

A better choice is to give your pet tartar-control foods and treats along with his regular food. They contain tough vegetable fibers, so when your pet takes a bite, the food particles literally wrap around the teeth, cleaning

them with each bite, says Susan G. Wynn, D.V.M., a veterinarian in Atlanta and co-editor of *Complementary and Alternative Veterinary Medicine*. One good choice for a tartar-control treat is TartarChek. Tartar-control foods are available from vets.

**Give a healing enzyme.** Pets with dental disease often have red, swollen, or bleeding gums. A naturally occurring enzyme called coenzyme $Q_{10}$ will help gums heal more quickly, says Dr. Basko. He recommends giving cats and dogs weighing up to 20 pounds 10 milligrams of coenzyme $Q_{10}$ a day. Dogs weighing 21 to 50 pounds can take up to 30 milligrams once a day, and dogs over 50 pounds can take 30 milligrams twice a day. You can stop the supplement when your pet's gums return to normal. Coenzyme $Q_{10}$ is available in health food stores.

**Increase immunity with vitamin C.** The immune system is designed to fight bacteria throughout the body, including in the mouth. Giving your pet vitamin C will help keep the immune system strong, says Dr. Basko. He recommends giving cats 100 to 250 milligrams of vitamin C a day. Dogs up to 50 pounds can take between 250 and 500 milligrams a day, and those over 50 pounds can take 500 milligrams two or three times a day. Since vitamin C can cause diarrhea, you may have to cut back the dose until you find an amount your pet will tolerate.

**Help them chew away plaque.** A bone is nature's toothbrush, says Dr.

Lampru, who recommends giving dogs and cats a bone to chew every day. It is important to use raw or lightly cooked (steamed for 15 to 30 seconds) bones because bones that are well-done splinter too easily, she adds.

For dogs, large knuckle bones are the best choice, and lightly steamed chicken necks are fine for cats, says Dr. Basko. A large dog or a determined cat may splinter even a tough bone, so make sure that the bone is too large to swallow and too tough to break down into fragments. Watch your pet chew. If he seems bent on destruction, give him a Kong or Nylabone instead.

Raw vegetables also rub away plaque, Dr. Basko adds. He recommends giving dogs and cats small bits of carrots, broccoli, or other vegetables and fruits several times a week. Many pets won't eat raw vegetables, so it is fine to lightly steam them, he adds.

**BEST BET!** **Keep the teeth clean.** It is not always convenient, but brushing your pet's teeth at least twice a week is one of the best ways to remove plaque along with the harmful bacteria it contains, says Dr. Lampru. Pet supply stores sell a variety of toothbrushes, but a soft baby toothbrush works fine. Or you can simply rub the outer surfaces of your pet's teeth with a piece of gauze. The insides of the teeth are less important because the motion of the tongue naturally keeps them clean.

**Use a natural toothpaste.** Toothpastes designed for pets may contain antibacterial additives like chlorhexidine. While these additives do kill harmful bacteria, they can be hard on the liver, says Dr. Basko. A safer alternative is to use a mixture of hydrogen peroxide and baking soda, adding just enough hydrogen peroxide to make a paste.

**Give them steak instead of hamburger.** Many holistic veterinarians recommend giving pets raw meat as part of their daily diet. The problem with hamburger or chopped meat, however, is that it doesn't do a lot to keep the teeth clean. The next time meat is on the menu, says Dr. Basko, give your cat a large piece. You can also give your cat chicken gizzards to clean his teeth. For dogs over 15 pounds, give them a large, tough cut of beef that can't be swallowed whole. As pets chew off swallowable bits, they will scour their teeth at the same time.

Some vets recommend lightly steaming the meat in order to kill harmful organisms such as salmonella, says Allen M. Schoen, D.V.M., director of the Veterinary Institute for Therapeutic Alternatives in Sherman, Connecticut, and author of *Love, Miracles, and Animal Healing*.

## The Solutions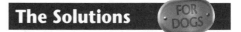

**Choose the right toys.** Dogs love to chew, and you can use this

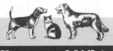

# Clean and White

The best way to keep your pet's breath fresh is to remove plaque from the teeth as soon as it appears. There are many dental-care products to choose from. Here are a few that veterinarians recommend.

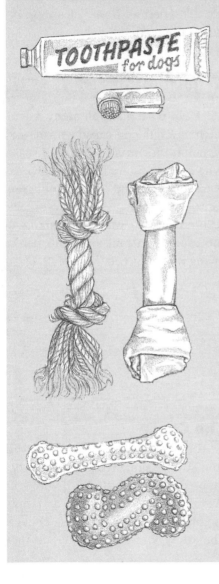

**Toothpaste.** Pet toothpastes come in a variety of tasty flavors, like chicken, fish, liver, and malt, and they won't upset your pet's stomach the way human toothpastes can.

**Finger brushes.** They look like thimbles with bristles. Because they slip over the end of a finger, they are much easier to use than a regular toothbrush.

**Dental floss chew.** Made of durable nylon strands that have been wrapped and tied in a knot, these are chew toys that remove plaque from between the teeth and at the gum line—and many dogs love them.

**Rawhide chews.** These rugged chew toys often last for weeks, and the scraping action helps keep the teeth clean. Some rawhide chews are basted in spearmint for additional bad-breath control. Supervise your pet while he chews these so that he doesn't swallow large pieces.

**Rubber-studded chews.** Made of extra-strong rubber, these toys are covered with rubber teeth, which clean your pet's teeth and massage the gums while your pet chews.

## Meet the Experts

**Ihor Basko, D.V.M.,** is a holistic veterinarian in private practice in Honolulu and Kilauea, Hawaii, and the creator of the video *The Healing Touch for Your Dogs*. He is certified in acupuncture.

**Anne Lampru, D.V.M.,** is a holistic veterinarian in private practice in Tampa, Florida. She is certified in acupuncture and homeopathy.

**Allen M. Schoen, D.V.M.,** is the director of the Veterinary Institute for Therapeutic Alternatives in Sherman, Connecticut, and the author of *Love, Miracles, and Animal Healing*. He is certified in acupuncture and chiropractic.

**Susan G. Wynn, D.V.M.,** is a veterinarian in Atlanta and co-editor of *Complementary and Alternative Veterinary Medicine*.

natural behavior to keep their teeth clean by providing them with dental toys, says Dr. Basko. Toys such as Hercules and Rhino are covered with small rubber nubs that rub against and clean the teeth and gums every time your dog chews. Some toys even act like dental floss, cleaning between the teeth.

## The Solutions · FOR CATS ·

**Help with a supplement.** Lactoferrin, available in capsule form, may be helpful for cats with gum disease. When the gums are inflamed, give between one-half and one 350-milligram capsule once a day, says Dr. Wynn. She recommends mixing the contents of the capsule in milk or syrup before giving it to your pet.

# DEPRESSION

## The Signs
- Your pet is sleeping more than usual.
- She is always eating or maybe refusing to eat.
- She hides or seems lethargic.

## The Cause
Dogs and cats get depressed for some of the same reasons people do. They don't understand divorce or death or the fact that a family member has gone away to college. They only know that someone they

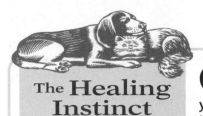

## The **Healing Instinct**

**O**n sunny days, dogs and cats gravitate to bright patches of sunlight, either in the yard or under a window in the house. "We know pets are comfort-seeking beasts," says Mary Lee Nitschke, Ph.D., professor of psychology at Linfield College in Portland, Oregon, and an animal behaviorist in Beaverton. "But I think there is more to it than just thermal comfort."

Many veterinarians believe that dogs and cats instinctively use sunlight to help recharge their emotional batteries and, of course, to warm up when they are feeling cold. "Given a choice between a heating pad and a sunny tabletop, cats choose the sun," Dr. Nitschke adds.

love and depend on isn't around anymore, and this can leave them profoundly depressed, says Pam Johnson Bennett, a feline behavior consultant in Nashville and author of *Twisted Whiskers*.

On the other hand, some pets get depressed when someone new—a person or a pet—joins the family, and they realize that they are not the center of attention anymore. Even moving to a new home can put them in a funk, Bennett says.

Depression is a natural emotion, but when it lasts too long, it can lead to physical problems, making pets more susceptible to illness. In fact, pets who are sick may have many of the same symptoms as those who are depressed, so you will want your vet to take a look, says Susan G. Wynn, D.V.M., a veterinarian in Atlanta and co-editor of *Complementary and Alter-*

*native Veterinary Medicine*. But as long as your pet is healthy, there are natural treatments that can battle depression without the need for powerful drugs. Here is what alternative practitioners advise.

## The Solutions  FOR DOGS & CATS

**Lift their spirits with music.** Not every pet responds to music, but some get deeply engaged when they hear their favorite melodies, especially when the music is associated with something they love and trust. "Music can be very effective for healing the emotions," says Donna M. Starita, D.V.M., a holistic veterinarian in private practice in Boring, Oregon.

**Shine away the blues.** During the cold, dark months especially, giving dogs and cats some extra light can help ease depression. "Light and the functioning of the pituitary and endocrine glands are intimately tied together," says Mary Lee Nitschke, Ph.D., professor of psychology at Linfield College in Portland, Oregon, and an animal behaviorist in Beaverton. Light stimulates the body to release hormones that can have an uplifting effect on mood, she explains.

All you really need is a place where your pet can bask a little—on a sunny back porch, for example, or on a window perch. Giving her an extra 20 to 30 minutes of sunlight a day may be all it takes to help her feel better.

**Stimulate her mind.** A fun way to counter depression is to give pets something interesting to think about, says Dr. Nitschke. For dogs, an easy and always-entertaining game is to hide treats throughout the house, then sit back and watch as their noses go to work. Cats don't get as excited by hide-and-seek, but they will show spark when you tempt them with pounce-able feathers or fishing-pole-style toys, she says.

Games can be especially helpful when pets are jealous and depressed because there is someone new in the family, Bennett adds. "They are a sure-fire way for them to bond, and that can help eliminate the depression."

**Give her a fresh start.** "Sometimes when pets are in deep mourning for another pet, they refuse to play," says Dr. Nitschke. You can help reduce your pet's grief by temporarily taking away some of the familiar items she associates with her lost friend. Or take

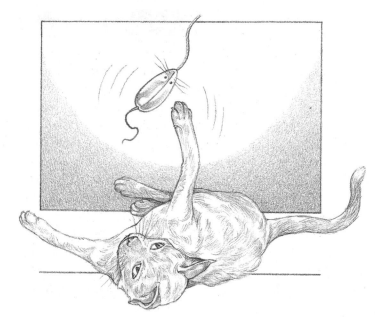

Cats can't resist moving objects, even when they are feeling blue. And once they start playing, their spirits will naturally rise. Fishing-pole-style toys, available in pet supply stores, are inexpensive and can provide years of fun.

your pet on a weekend trip to get her out of the house for a while. The combination of new sights and smells and getting away from a "sad" place will help your pet get over the emotional hump and start the healing process, she says.

**Relieve grief with homeopathy.** Pets who are depressed because of grief may feel better when given homeopathic Ignatia amara, says Kathleen Carson, D.V.M., a holistic veterinarian in private practice in Hermosa Beach, California. Give one or two drops of liquid or one or two pills of 30C-strength Ignatia amara. If your pet doesn't seem to be feeling better after one dose, give another dose the following day, she suggests. Consult your holistic veterinarian before going to the next higher dose.

**Help her recover with flower essences.** "Gentian is very good for general depression," says Dr. Carson. "If your pet suffers extreme depression, give her gorse. And for pets mourning the loss of a loved one, star-of-Bethlehem helps with sorrow. Honeysuckle helps with the nostalgia and sorrow that your pet may feel after a loss, and walnut eases her pain during the transition."

You can use any one of these essences or combine up to six of them in equal amounts, diluting six to eight drops of each essence in an ounce of spring water. Give between one-half and one dropperful four times a day,

says Dr. Carson. You can mix the remedy with food or water or put a drop on your finger and rub it into the hairless area inside your pet's ear.

**Communicate honestly.** Dogs and cats have impressive powers of intuition, and when you are feeling discouraged and depressed, they may feel bad, too. "It's important to have positive thoughts around your pets," says Dr. Carson. "But you have to be honest and tell them what is going on. Just saying out loud, 'I'm upset, but it's not your fault,' can help."

**Touch away depression.** A massage technique called TTouch has been widely used to reduce stress,

## Meet the Experts

**Pam Johnson Bennett** is a feline behavior consultant in Nashville and the author of *Twisted Whiskers* and *Psycho Kitty*.

**Kathleen Carson, D.V.M.,** is a holistic veterinarian in private practice in Hermosa Beach, California.

**Mary Lee Nitschke, Ph.D.,** is a professor of psychology at Linfield College in Portland, Oregon, and an animal behaviorist in Beaverton.

**Donna M. Starita, D.V.M.,** is a holistic veterinarian in private practice in Boring, Oregon.

**Susan G. Wynn, D.V.M.,** is a veterinarian in Atlanta and co-editor of *Complementary and Alternative Veterinary Medicine*.

anxiety, and other negative emotions. "I find TTouch to have a really powerful effect on depression," says Dr. Nitschke. TTouch is performed by gently using your fingertips to move the skin in a clockwise direction, taking one to two seconds to complete 1¼ circles in each place. Pay particular attention to the ears, face, and neck.

# DIABETES

## The Signs
- Your pet is eating or drinking a lot more than usual.
- He needs to urinate all the time.
- His urine or breath smells sweet.
- He is losing weight.

## The Cause

When your pet eats the kibble in his bowl, his body begins transforming it into a sugary fuel called glucose. Glucose gives cells the energy they need to survive. The only way for glucose to get into cells, however, is with the help of a hormone called insulin. When pets don't produce enough insulin—or the insulin they do produce doesn't work efficiently—they may develop a serious condition called diabetes.

Dogs' genes may make them prone to developing diabetes, or the disease may occur, less commonly, following an illness that causes severe inflammation and damage to the pancreas, says Jory Olsen, D.V.M., a veterinary internal-medicine specialist in private practice in Marietta, Georgia. Cats are also at risk for developing diabetes based on their genes, but they also develop symptoms when they are overweight because fat can make the body resistant to the effects of insulin. In all cases, the symptoms are the same: fatigue, weight loss, and an insatiable appetite and thirst accompanied by excessive urination. Most internists around the country treat diabetes on a fairly regular basis.

Many pets with diabetes will need daily injections of insulin to replenish their natural supplies. Even when they are taking medications, however, there are a number of natural remedies that can reduce the amount of insulin they need. And in some pets, especially cats, it is sometimes possible to reverse diabetes with simple dietary changes.

## Call the VET

Even though diabetes is potentially serious, it can often be controlled with a combination of home remedies and insulin. But sometimes the treatment itself causes problems. Pets that get more insulin than the body needs may have a sudden and dangerous drop in blood sugar called insulin shock.

"If your pet is lethargic, wobbly, and weaving like he is drunk, or if he goes into a coma, give him a simple sugar like Karo syrup—just rub it on his gums if he can't swallow," says Jory Olsen, D.V.M., a veterinary internal-medicine specialist in private practice in Marietta, Georgia. "Then take him to the vet immediately."

## The Solutions *FOR DOGS & CATS*

**BEST BET!** **Improve insulin with vanadium.** A trace mineral called vanadium can help make your pet more responsive to the insulin he produces naturally, says Dr. Olsen. This means that a pet taking vanadium may need less synthetic insulin to control diabetes. "It also has some insulin-like effects of its own," he adds. Vanadium is available in liquid, tablet, or capsule form and is sold in health food stores. Cats can take four to eight milligrams a day, he says. Dogs can take five to eight milligrams a day for every 10 pounds of weight.

**BEST BET!** **Put them on a diet.** "A lot of cats are obese, and if you can slim them down, the diabetes may go away," says Pat Zook, D.V.M., a holistic veterinarian in private practice in Stone Mountain, Georgia. Dogs will also benefit from losing weight, although not as much as cats, she adds.

The best way to help pets lose weight is to keep them active and switch to a food that contains a fairly low-fat protein source, such as chicken or turkey, says Dr. Olsen. Your vet may also recommend that you cut back the amount you feed your pet by 25 percent for a few weeks to see if it helps. Diabetes can be tricky to control, however, so be sure to talk to your vet before making changes in your pet's diet.

**Slow food absorption with fiber.** Increasing the amount of fiber in your pet's diet will help food be absorbed more gradually so that even small amounts of insulin may be able to handle the load, says Dr. Zook. Start by giving your pet a tablespoon of a high-fiber food, such as canned pumpkin or wheat bran, with every meal, she suggests.

Increasing fiber will sometimes cause loose stools, she adds, so you may have to experiment a bit to find an amount that doesn't cause problems.

**BEST BET!** **Control blood sugar with vegetables.** To give your pet extra fiber as well as high levels of vitamins and minerals, slip some raw vegetables into his bowl. "It's hard to convince some cats to eat their vegetables, but you may find some they like," Dr. Olsen says. Many dogs and cats like cantaloupe and string beans, he adds.

You can try giving your pet fresh chopped vegetables, but you will probably have more success if you run them through a blender or food processor, then mix them in the food.

**Give them supplements.** "Antioxidants like vitamin E and fish oils im-

---

**Meet the Experts**

**Jory Olsen, D.V.M.,** is a veterinary internal-medicine specialist in private practice in Marietta, Georgia.

**Pat Zook, D.V.M.,** is a holistic veterinarian in private practice in Stone Mountain, Georgia. She is certified in acupuncture.

---

prove insulin response and may even increase insulin production," says Dr. Olsen. He recommends giving cats with diabetes about one-third of a 1,000-milligram fish-oil capsule—preferably salmon oil or fish-body oil, rather than cod-liver oil—once a day. Pets under 15 pounds can take one-half capsule, and larger pets can taken between one and two capsules. For vitamin E, give pets weighing under 15 pounds 100 international units (IU) twice a day. Pets 15 to 50 pounds can take 200 IU, and dogs over 50 pounds can take 400 IU twice a day, says Dr. Olsen.

---

# Diarrhea

## The Signs
- Your pet's stools are soft or watery.
- She is having accidents in the house.

## The Cause

The amount of water that dogs and cats drink is roughly equivalent to the amount they excrete—not only in urine but also in stools. When they have diarrhea, however, they can lose tremendous amounts of fluid very quickly, along with food in the intestines that wasn't absorbed by the body.

Anything that upsets the digestive tract, from eating garbage to having intestinal parasites, can cause diarrhea. In addition, some pets are allergic to ingredients in popular pet foods, which can also cause loose stools, explains Kathleen Carson, D.V.M., a holistic veterinarian in private practice in Hermosa Beach, California. And in some cases, pets can't digest properly because the foods don't contain the same enzymes that are found in natural whole foods.

Veterinarians occasionally use medications to stop diarrhea, although they usually recommend letting it run its course. The problem, however, is that diarrhea may come back again and again. That is why holistic veterinarians try to get to the source of the problem. For many pets, this may be as simple as changing what goes in the food bowl. Along with a variety of natural remedies, changes in diet will often stop diarrhea and prevent it from coming back.

## The Solutions 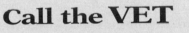 FOR DOGS & CATS

**BEST BET!** **Start with a fast.** The quickest way to stop diarrhea is to put your pet on a food fast for 24 hours. When food isn't going into the intestines, nothing will come out, says H. Ellen Whiteley, D.V.M., a veterinary consultant in Guadalupita, New Mexico, and consultant for *The Country Vet's Home Remedies for Cats*.

## Call the VET

Diarrhea that comes on suddenly usually goes away just as quickly. But sometimes diarrhea is a sign of serious problems like distemper, parvovirus, or even poisoning, says H. Ellen Whiteley, D.V.M., a veterinary consultant in Guadalupita, New Mexico, and consultant for *The Country Vet's Home Remedies for Cats*.

When diarrhea is accompanied by blood in the stool or lasts more than 24 hours, you will need to call your vet. "Puppies and kittens can get dehydrated very quickly, and they may need fluid therapy and other supportive care," she adds.

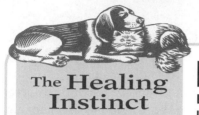

## The Healing Instinct

Dogs and cats will eat just about anything, which is why they get diarrhea so often. But sometimes their wide-ranging appetites lead them to more healthful—if less appetizing—choices. "Eating dirt—a condition called pica—is common in dogs and cats," says H. Ellen Whiteley, a veterinary consultant in Guadalupita, New Mexico, and consultant for *The Country Vet's Home Remedies for Cats*.

They don't do it because they love the taste. Researchers have found that certain soils can absorb harmful toxins in the intestine, buffer acidic foods, and replace essential minerals—all of which can be very helpful for pets with diarrhea.

Dogs and cats aren't the only animals that instinctively eat what their bodies need. Chimpanzees suffering from diarrhea, for example, will often eat soils that contain absorbent minerals similar to those used in Kaopectate. So if your pet just occasionally snacks on soil, she is probably just trying to keep her insides calm. A pet who does it all the time, however, probably has a problem and needs to see a vet.

After a daylong fast, give your pet bland foods, such as skinless, boneless chicken breasts for cats and hamburger and rice for dogs. Keep the meals very small and give them often, up to five or six times a day, she says. Fasting doesn't include taking away water, so be sure to keep the water bowl full. And check with your vet before putting young or diabetic pets on a fast.

**Stop the discomfort with Nux vomica.** A homeopathic remedy called Nux vomica is good for the entire digestive tract and will help stop diarrhea, says Dr. Carson. She recommends using a 6X potency, mixing 20 drops in an ounce of spring water.

Give your pet half a dropperful three times a day.

**Stop the cramps.** Dogs and cats with diarrhea often have painful cramps when the intestines expand and contract. A quick way to stop cramping is with aromatherapy, using an antispasmodic oil such as basil or peppermint, says Joanne Stefanatos, D.V.M., a holistic veterinarian in private practice in Las Vegas. She recommends diluting either of these essential oils half-and-half with vegetable oil and rubbing the mixture on the tips of your pet's ears until she is feeling better.

**Give intestinal energy.** A quick way to ease digestive problems is with acupressure. There are three acupressure points that vets often stimulate to relieve diarrhea.

🐾 LI4, located in the web of skin between the dewclaw and the first long toe on the front feet.

🐾 LI11, located on the outside of the front legs at the elbow creases.

🐾 ST25, located just below the last rib.

Until your pet is feeling better, it is a good idea to stimulate each of these points for about 30 seconds once a day, says Dr. Stefanatos.

**Put bacteria to work.** The digestive tract always has a mixture of good and bad bacteria—and sometimes the bad wins, causing diarrhea. You can restore the body's natural balance by giving your pet additional beneficial bacteria. One way to do this is with pet supplements containing *Lactobacillus acidophilus*, available in pet stores. Follow the instructions on the label. Or you can give your pet live-culture yogurt, which contains the same organisms, Dr. Whiteley explains. Cats can have one to two teaspoons of yogurt a day, spread over several feedings. Dogs can take one to two tablespoons, depending on their size, she says.

**Feed your pet a natural diet.** "Changing to a good-quality food relieves some of the stress on the gut," says Dr. Carson. It also allows you to alter the ingredients according to your pet's needs. Your best strategy is to prepare your pet's meals at home, using whole ingredients, like chicken, beef, rice, and fresh vegetables. Or buy an all-natural commercial food, like PetGuard Premium, she suggests. You can find all-natural foods in some pet supply stores and through mail order.

**Give your pet Kaopectate.** Available in drugstores and supermarkets, Kaopectate contains a mineral found in clay called attapulgite, which absorbs diarrhea-causing bacteria and toxins in the digestive tract. For pets under 15 pounds, Dr. Stefanatos recommends giving one-half teaspoon of Kaopectate every hour for four hours. Pets 15 to 50 pounds can take a teaspoon every hour, and dogs over 50 pounds can take a tablespoon every hour.

**Firm the stools with fiber.** Dietary fiber absorbs a lot of water in the

## Meet the Experts

**Kathleen Carson, D.V.M.,** is a holistic veterinarian in private practice in Hermosa Beach, California.

**Joanne Stefanatos, D.V.M.,** is a holistic veterinarian in private practice in Las Vegas. She is certified in acupuncture and chiropractic.

**H. Ellen Whiteley, D.V.M.,** is a veterinary consultant in Guadalupita, New Mexico, and consultant for *The Country Vet's Home Remedies for Cats*.

digestive tract, which can help stop diarrhea, Dr. Stefanatos says. She recommends giving about one-half teaspoon of fiber-rich foods, such as canned pumpkin or flaxseeds, with every meal to cats and dogs weighing less than 15 pounds. Dogs 15 to 50 pounds can take a teaspoon of high-fiber foods, and larger dogs can take a tablespoon.

# DIGGING

## The Signs
- Your dog is trying to get to China through the backyard.

## The Cause

Your dog's instinct to dig is a lot older than the invention of lawns and gardens. When dogs lived in the wild, they would dig holes in which to sleep or to bury things. And in hot weather, they would dig down a few inches to get to cooler ground. But what worked thousands of years ago can be a problem in today's world since your dog's urge to dig is likely to clash with your instinct to have a nicely manicured yard.

"We have civilized dogs and have made them do things that are different from their instincts," explains Jeanne Olson, D.V.M., a holistic veterinarian in private practice in North Pole, Alaska. "There's going to be a throwback once in a while."

Dogs dig not only because of blind instinct, she adds. From a canine point of view, there are many good reasons for digging. (Cats, on the other hand, rarely dig except for bathroom purposes.) You can get a good sense of why your dog is digging by the type of hole he leaves.

🐾 A dog who wants a comfortable place to rest usually will dig a shallow hole that's large enough for him to stretch out in.

🐾 A large, deep hole is a sign that your dog is trying to make his great escape. A dog usually does this when something interesting—the dog next door, for example—is beckoning from the other side.

🐾 A dog will dig a lot of small holes when he is feeling frustrated or bored or when he is bursting with pent-up energy. A dog will also dig when he is feeling lonely. "Dogs are very social animals," says Robin Cannizzaro, D.V.M., a holistic veterinarian in private practice in St. Petersburg, Florida. "If they are

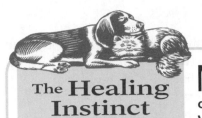

## The **Healing Instinct**

Most dogs dig to blow off steam or just because it is fun, but some do it because they are preparing their next meal. Veterinarians have found that dogs—along with cats, horses, and cattle—will sometimes eat soil when they aren't getting all the minerals they need from their diets. Digging and eating dirt is their way of taking a multi-supplement.

Even though soil-eating, known as pica, can temporarily replace missing nutrients, it is not something to ignore, says Pat Bradley, D.V.M., a holistic veterinarian in private practice in Conway, Arkansas. Pets usually eat dirt because there is an underlying problem, such as anemia, that is causing them to run short on essential nutrients. Your pet has the right idea, but he will still need a checkup to make sure that nothing serious is wrong.

left alone without much attention or interaction, they need to find something to do, and digging is a way of acting out."

Veterinarians sometimes recommend that inveterate diggers be given some extra training and, in some cases, mood-altering drugs like fluoxetine (Prozac) to stabilize their emotions. But digging usually doesn't require a dramatic response. Here are some easier, more-natural ways to end the excavations.

## The Solutions FOR DOGS

**Communicate positively.** "Dogs do better at listening to what you want them to do as opposed to what you don't want them to do," says Deborah C. Mallu, D.V.M., a holistic veterinarian in private practice in Sedona, Arizona. Rather than telling your dog,

"Don't dig here," she suggests showing him a place where he can dig and tell him, "You can have this nice place to dig in and lie in the cool dirt."

**BEST BET!** **Spend more time together.** Dogs often dig because they don't have enough to occupy their time, says Dr. Cannizzaro. "Take walks, go to the park, and just keep your dog active on a regular basis," she says. "Dogs need interaction and stimulation during the course of the day, just like we do."

**BEST BET!** **Give him lots of exercise.** Some dogs put their paws to work simply because they have too much energy and not enough outlets for it, says Pat Bradley, D.V.M., a holistic veterinarian in private practice in Conway, Arkansas. "It's not that your dog is being bad," she explains. "It's just that the energy has to come out somewhere." Most dogs need a minimum of two 20-minute walks each day, and some dogs need a lot more. A tired dog is much less likely to be a digging dog, she explains.

**Calm his emotions.** Since dogs may dig when they are anxious or frustrated, it is worth trying to calm your dog with flower essences, says Adriana Sagrera, D.V.M., a holistic veterinarian in private practice in New Orleans. She recommends putting four or five drops of the essence Bach Rescue Remedy in his water once a day. "Or put two drops directly into his mouth twice a day," she adds.

**BEST BET! Keep him cool.** In hot weather, dogs will often dig holes so that they can lie down in cool dirt, just like their ancestors did. "Make sure that your dog has shady areas to go to and plenty of water to drink," advises Dr. Mallu.

**Limit the damage.** If it is not the digging itself that bothers you, but the bottomless holes you have to patch up, you may want to put down a barrier to limit the damage. "Lay down some wire fencing or chain mesh and put an inch or two of topsoil over it," suggests Dr. Olson. Your dog will still be able to dig, but the wire will prevent him from doing serious damage.

**Give a gentle reminder.** Dogs usually have favorite places to dig and will keep returning to those places no matter how many times you fill them in. "Get a nontoxic spray that dogs stay away from, like bitter apple, and spray it on the area," suggests Allen M. Schoen, D.V.M., director of the Veterinary Institute for Therapeutic Alternatives in Sherman, Connecticut, and author of *Love, Miracles, and Animal Healing*. Another possibility is to place a large tarp over the area and cover it with stones. This will help your dog get out of the habit of digging in that area.

## Meet the Experts

**Pat Bradley, D.V.M.,** is a holistic veterinarian in private practice in Conway, Arkansas. She is certified in homeopathy.

**Robin Cannizzaro, D.V.M.,** is a holistic veterinarian in private practice in St. Petersburg, Florida. She is certified in acupuncture and homeopathy.

**Deborah C. Mallu, D.V.M.,** is a holistic veterinarian in private practice in Sedona, Arizona. She is certified in acupuncture.

**Jeanne Olson, D.V.M.,** is a holistic veterinarian in private practice in North Pole, Alaska.

**Adriana Sagrera, D.V.M.,** is a holistic veterinarian in private practice in New Orleans.

**Allen M. Schoen, D.V.M.,** is the director of the Veterinary Institute for Therapeutic Alternatives in Sherman, Connecticut, and the author of *Love, Miracles, and Animal Healing*. He is certified in acupuncture and chiropractic.

**Put yourself in his position.** Dogs sometimes dig for the same reason the chicken crossed the road—to get to the other side. If you can figure out what your dog is trying to accomplish and then help him get it, he may not feel the need to dig, says Dr. Mallu. For instance, he might be digging because he wants to play with the dog in the next yard. Arranging play sessions so that the two dogs can get together may be all it takes to get him to ditch the digging, she says.

# DROOLING

## The Signs
- Your pet is dripping on the floor.
- She is breathing hard or seems listless.
- She is pawing at her mouth or shaking her head.

## The Cause

All dogs drool a little, and some breeds, especially those with heavy lips like bloodhounds and Newfoundlands, drool a lot because the loose skin around their mouths traps saliva and overflows. Even cats will drool occasionally, mainly when they are feeling happy and affectionate.

Drooling itself isn't a problem, but any change in your pet's drooling usually means that she isn't feeling well. Drooling increases when dogs or cats are nauseated or when something gets stuck beneath the gums or between the teeth. Serious conditions such as liver disease can also cause drooling.

The idea isn't to stop the drooling, but to solve the underlying problem that is creating the extra moisture, says Susan G. Wynn, D.V.M., a veterinarian

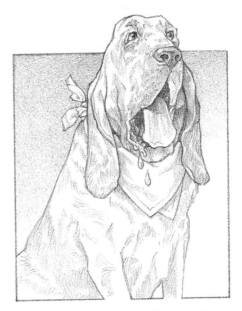

It won't stop him from drooling, but a bandanna tied around your dog's neck will catch most of the moisture before it soaks the floor. Bandannas look smart, and most dogs won't even know they are wearing them.

## Call the VET

Some dogs and cats never drip a drop, while others drool so much that you may be tempted to call a plumber. Whether your pet is usually dry or drippy, a sudden increase in moisture is an important warning sign, says Anna Maria Scholey, Vet.M.B. (bachelor of veterinary medicine, a British equivalent of D.V.M.), a holistic veterinarian in private practice in Carrollton, Texas.

The most serious cause of sudden drooling—and, fortunately, one of the rarest in dogs and cats—is rabies, she says. Tonsillitis and other infections can also cause pets to drool much more than usual, as can serious conditions like liver disease or poisoning. Don't take chances when your pet is getting unusually wet around the mouth. Call your vet right away, she advises.

in Atlanta and co-editor of *Complementary and Alternative Veterinary Medicine*. Here are a few natural ways to keep your pets a little drier.

## The Solutions FOR DOGS & CATS

**Do a mouth check.** Dogs and cats with something stuck between their teeth—a piece of string or a bit of bone, for example—will often drool heavily. They will also drool when they have gum or tooth disease, says Jane Laura Doyle, D.V.M., a holistic veterinarian in private practice in Berkeley Springs, West Virginia. It is often easy to spot and remove foreign objects, she says. To check for gum disease, smell your pet's breath. If it smells truly awful, your pet may have a bad

tooth or a bacterial infection in the gums that should be treated by your vet, she says.

**Try a Chinese cure.** Many dogs and cats will drool heavily during car trips because the motion upsets their stomachs, says Junia Borden Childs, D.V.M., a holistic veterinarian in private practice in Ojai, California. A Chinese herbal remedy called Pill Curing, available from health food stores, is very helpful for preventing nausea and the drooling that may accompany it. Dr. Childs recommends giving 10 pills to pets weighing under 15 pounds, 10 to 15 pills to pets 15 to 50 pounds, and one vial of pills to dogs over 50 pounds. Pill Curing works best when it is given about 20 minutes before traveling, she adds.

## Meet the Experts

**Junia Borden Childs, D.V.M.,** is a holistic veterinarian in private practice in Ojai, California.

**Jane Laura Doyle, D.V.M.,** is a holistic veterinarian in private practice in Berkeley Springs, West Virginia. She is certified in acupuncture and homeopathy.

**Linda East, D.V.M.,** is a holistic veterinarian in private practice in Denver. She is certified in homeopathy.

**Anna Maria Scholey, Vet.M.B.,** is a holistic veterinarian in private practice in Carrollton, Texas. She is certified in acupuncture and homeopathy.

**Susan G. Wynn, D.V.M.,** is a veterinarian in Atlanta and co-editor of *Complementary and Alternative Veterinary Medicine.*

**BEST BET!** **Give homeopathic relief.** The homeopathic remedies Ipecacuanha and Cocculus are often recommended for stopping nausea, says Linda East, D.V.M., a holistic veterinarian in private practice in Denver. The remedy Tabacum is also helpful, adds Dr. Wynn. Whichever remedy you use, look for a strength of 30C and give your pet three to five pellets, or two or three drops, up to two hours before traveling, she says.

**Press for dryness.** To stop the drooling and nausea fast, Dr. Wynn recommends stimulating the PC6 acupressure point, located in the depression on the underside of your pet's front legs just above the pad on the wrists. Stimulating this point for about 30 seconds will help correct energy imbalances in the body that create extra moisture.

# DUNG EATING

## The Signs
- Your dog is eating his own stools or the stools from other animals.

## The Cause

It's hard for humans to understand, but many dogs eat dung as a matter of course. Mother dogs eat the stools of their puppies in order to keep the nest clean and, in the wild, to prevent predators from homing in on the smell. And some dogs may simply like the taste, says Jane Laura Doyle, D.V.M., a holistic veterinarian in private practice in Berkeley Springs, West Virginia.

Veterinarians aren't sure why some dogs eat dung all the time while others never seem to develop a taste for it. (Cats rarely eat dung.) They do know that some dogs eat stools because they are not getting all the nutrients they need from their regular food. In addition, specialists in Chinese veterinary medicine suspect that dung eating may be a symptom of "stomach fire," a condition in which there is an imbalance of energy between the liver, spleen, and stomach, says Junia Borden Childs, D.V.M., a holistic veterinarian in private practice in Ojai, California.

Dung eating isn't dangerous, although dogs that indulge are more likely to get worms than those that don't. But it is an unpleasant habit, to say the least. Here are a few ways to help your dog turn his appetite to more wholesome things.

## The Solutions

**Correct the energy flow.** Dogs have two acupressure points, LI4 and LIV2, that can help correct energy imbalances that can lead to strange appetites, says Dr. Childs. To stimulate LI4, located in the web of skin between the dewclaw and first long toe on the front feet, massage the area in a downward motion for 30 seconds once a day. To stimulate the LIV2

point, located on the rear feet, just above where the inside toe meets the foot bone, massage the point and stroke downward for about 30 seconds once a day, she says.

**BEST BET!** **Cook naturally.** Some commercial pet foods are nutritious and well-balanced, but others are made with inferior ingredients that aren't easily absorbed by the body, says Dr. Doyle. When your dog isn't getting all the nutrients he needs from his food bowl, he is going to forage elsewhere, she explains. One of the best ways to stop dung eating is to give dogs a high-quality, homemade diet consisting of fresh meats, grains, and vegetables. For more information on homemade diets, see page 61. Or ask your veterinarian to recommend a commercial natural food that will provide all the wholesome ingredients that your dog needs.

**Give him a supplement.** Every dog digests his food differently, which means that even high-quality foods don't always provide all the nutrients dogs need. This is why it is a good idea to give your dog vitamin and mineral supplements made for pets, says Anna Maria Scholey, Vet.M.B. (bachelor of veterinary medicine, a British equivalent of D.V.M.), a holistic veterinarian in private practice in Carrollton, Texas. One supplement, called Missing Link, provides a

## Meet the Experts

**Junia Borden Childs, D.V.M.,** is a holistic veterinarian in private practice in Ojai, California.

**Jane Laura Doyle, D.V.M.,** is a holistic veterinarian in private practice in Berkeley Springs, West Virginia. She is certified in acupuncture and homeopathy.

**Anna Maria Scholey, Vet.M.B.,** is a holistic veterinarian in private practice in Carrollton, Texas. She is certified in acupuncture and homeopathy.

**David Spiegel, V.M.D.,** is a veterinary behaviorist in private practice in Wilmington, Delaware.

**Susan G. Wynn, D.V.M.,** is a veterinarian in Atlanta and co-editor of *Complementary and Alternative Veterinary Medicine*.

number of essential nutrients that can help reduce a dog's desire for dung, she says. Giving your dog a digestive enzyme, available in pet supply stores, can also reduce dung eating by helping your dog digest his food more completely, she adds. Follow the directions on the label.

**BEST BET! Keep him active.** Dogs will occasionally eat dung merely as a way of passing the time. Keeping your dog busy by giving him fun toys to play with, for example, and by taking him for extra walks will make him less likely to seek other less-tasteful sources of amusement, says David Spiegel, V.M.D., a veterinary behaviorist in private practice in Wilmington, Delaware.

**BEST BET! Add Adolph's meat tenderizer.** Adolph's meat tenderizer contains an enzyme that may improve digestion and give stools a taste dogs find objectionable, says Susan G. Wynn, D.V.M., a veterinarian in Atlanta and co-editor of *Complementary and Alternative Veterinary Medicine*. Dogs under 15 pounds can take one-quarter teaspoon of Adolph's with every meal, says Dr. Wynn. Give dogs 15 to 30 pounds one-half teaspoon. Dogs weighing 31 to 50 pounds can take three-quarters teaspoon, and dogs over 50 pounds can take one teaspoon.

# EAR INFECTIONS

## The Signs
- Your pet shakes her head or holds it to one side.
- She is scratching or rubbing her ears, or she is rubbing her head against the furniture or carpet.
- There is a yellow, brown, or black discharge in one or both ears.
- The ears smell bad or are tender or red.

## The Cause

Humans can hear sound waves traveling at 20,000 cycles per second, while dogs hear sound waves traveling at 100,000 cycles per second. Cats can hear even higher frequencies; it is what enables them to detect the ultrasonic squeaks of mice.

To protect this exquisite sense of hearing, their ear canals are L-shaped, which helps prevent damage to the eardrum. The problem with this design is that it also allows the ears to trap moisture, debris, earwax, and parasites—any one of which can lead to ear infections. Cats often get infections because of ear mites, and up to 80 percent of ear problems in dogs are linked to allergies, adds Allen M. Schoen, D.V.M., director of the Veterinary Institute for Therapeutic Alternatives in Sherman, Connecticut, and author of *Love, Miracles, and Animal Healing*.

The traditional treatment for ear infections is to give antibiotics, antifungal drugs, or other medications. The problem with this approach is that medications upset the normal chemistry inside the ear, possibly turning a simple infection into a complicated, long-term problem, says Ihor Basko, D.V.M., a holistic veterinarian in private practice in Honolulu and Kilauea, Hawaii. It makes more sense, he says, to deal with underlying allergies and strengthen the immune system so that it is able to battle bacteria and other germs before they cause infection. In addition, there are many natural treatments for cleaning the ears and stopping infections without using drugs.

## The Solutions FOR DOGS & CATS

**BEST BET!** **Clean the ears with vinegar.** If your pet's ears are filled with brownish-pink wax, there is a good chance that allergies

## Call the VET

Ear infections can look and smell awful, but they usually affect only the outer part of the ear and aren't too serious. You will still want to see your veterinarian, however, to find out what is causing the problem, particularly if your pet is doing a lot of scratching. Vigorous scratching can break blood vessels in the earflap, causing the entire ear to swell like a balloon. This condition, called a hematoma, must be drained by a veterinarian to prevent permanent damage.

Other symptoms to watch out for include head tilting, clumsiness, walking in circles, or drooping eyes. These are signs of an inner-ear infection, which must be treated by a vet. Your pet will probably need antibiotics to knock out the infection. In addition, your vet may need to drain pus and other fluids from inside the ear.

have triggered a yeast infection. You can clear up yeast infections by cleaning the ears thoroughly. Veterinarians often recommend using white vinegar, also called acetic acid, because it removes dirt and debris and helps restore a healthful chemical balance in the ears, says Anne Lampru, D.V.M., a holistic veterinarian in private practice in Tampa, Florida.

Diluted vinegar works well, but veterinarians often recommend a prescription product called Alocetic. It contains acetic acid along with aloe vera to soothe inflammation. When using either vinegar or Alocetic, pour a small amount into the ear canal, massage the area, then gently wipe the inside of the ear with a cotton ball. Do this once a day until the ear is better.

**Stop infections with pau d'arco.** Also called Inca Gold, the herb pau d'arco, which comes from the inner bark of a South American tree, is a natural antibiotic that quickly kills fungi and bacteria, says Joanne Stefanatos, D.V.M., a holistic veterinarian in private practice in Las Vegas. Mix equal parts pau d'arco (*Tabebuia impetiginosa*) tincture and mineral oil and put several drops in your pet's ears at the first sign of infection, she says. You can give the drops two or three times a day for several days.

**Reduce inflammation with vitamin C.** The adrenal glands produce a natural steroid that can help reduce inflammation when ears get infected. Giving pets vitamin C can help the adrenal glands work more efficiently. Cats and dogs weighing under 15 pounds can take between 100 and 250 milligrams of vitamin C a day. Pets 15 to 50 pounds can take 250 to 500 milligrams a day, and larger dogs can take 500 milligrams two or three times a day, says Dr. Basko. Vitamin C can cause diarrhea, so you may have to cut back the dose until you find an amount that your pet will tolerate.

**Eliminate toxins with a healthful diet.** Giving your pet a healthful, homemade diet or high-quality commercial food that doesn't contain additives or preservatives can vastly reduce the amount of wax that the ears produce, while also helping the immune system work well, explains Dr. Basko. For more information on all-natural diets, see page 61.

**Air out the ears.** Increasing air circulation inside the ears can control the growth of bacteria, yeast, and fungi, says Dr. Lampru. Periodically trimming or plucking hair inside the ears will allow more air to get inside, she says.

**Strengthen the digestive tract.** Supplements such as bromelain and quercetin can help prevent an allergic response in the gastrointestinal tract, making food allergies less of a problem, says Dr. Schoen. While your

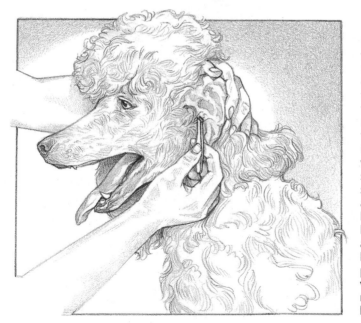

Bacteria thrive in warm, moist environments, which is why dogs with hairy ears tend to get ear infections. One way to reduce the risk is to trim around the opening of the ear canal with blunt-nosed scissors or electric clippers so that the hair is about one-half inch long. Plucking excess hair inside the ears will also allow air to circulate. Plucking can be painful, however, so veterinarians recommend having it done by a groomer.

## Meet the Experts

**Ihor Basko, D.V.M.,** is a holistic veterinarian in private practice in Honolulu and Kilauea, Hawaii. He is certified in acupuncture.

**Anne Lampru, D.V.M.,** is a holistic veterinarian in private practice in Tampa, Florida. She is certified in acupuncture and homeopathy.

**Allen M. Schoen, D.V.M.,** is director of the Veterinary Institute for Therapeutic Alternatives in Sherman, Connecticut, and the author of *Love, Miracles, and Animal Healing.* He is certified in acupuncture and chiropractic.

**Joanne Stefanatos, D.V.M.,** is a holistic veterinarian in private practice in Las Vegas. She is certified in acupuncture and chiropractic.

pet has the infection, give a 250-milligram quercetin/bromelain combination capsule (like Doctor's Best) 15 to 30 minutes before each meal. You can give pets weighing less than 15 pounds one-quarter capsule. Pets weighing 15 to 50 pounds can take one-half to one whole capsule. And larger dogs can take one to two capsules, he says.

**Stop ear mites with oil.** When an infection is caused by ear mites, putting a few drops of almond or olive oil in each ear will smother the mites and may allow the infection to heal, explains Dr. Lampru. You usually need to continue the oil treatments for three to four weeks, putting three to seven drops of oil into the ear canals each day. Cleaning wax and other debris from the ears before using oil will help the treatment work more efficiently.

**Try an over-the-counter remedy.** One of the best ways to stop ear mites is with over-the-counter products containing pyrethrins, like Natural Animal and Pet Gold herbal powders. Made from chrysanthemums, pyrethrins are natural insecticides that are very safe to use, says Dr. Lampru. Just follow the directions on the label.

# EAR MITES

## The Signs
- Your pet is scratching her ears all the time.
- There is dark, dry debris in the ears.
- Her ears are inflamed or swollen.

## The Cause

It probably isn't what nature intended, but the insides of your pet's ears, which are warm, moist, and well-protected, provide a perfect environment for mites. These annoying creatures are so small that you can barely see them, but your pets can certainly feel them. Ear mites—and the nonstop scratching they cause—can result in sores, infections, or even hearing loss, says Carolyn Blakey, D.V.M., a holistic veterinarian in private practice in Richmond, Indiana. Dogs occasionally get ear mites, but it is generally more of a problem in cats, she adds.

You can eliminate ear mites with medications, but the mites may come

## Call the VET

Ear mites are itchy, uncomfortable, and unpleasant, but they rarely cause serious problems—unless your pet scratches her ears so vigorously that she damages the skin or gets an infection.

It is fine to try home remedies for about a month, says Michele Yasson, D.V.M., a holistic veterinarian in private practice in New York City and Rosendale, New York. If your pet is still scratching, make an appointment to see your vet. There is a good chance that your pet will need more powerful treatments to kill the mites and stop the itching.

Don't wait a month, however, if your pet also has swelling inside the ear or a pus-filled or discolored discharge, she adds. These are signs of infection, and she will need to see the vet right away.

back, usually when the body's natural defenses are weaker than they should be. "A healthy animal won't have the ear environment that is conducive to mites setting up house," says Michele Yasson, D.V.M., a holistic veterinarian in private practice in New York City and Rosendale, New York. Mites are merely the "messenger" telling you that there is a problem, she explains. "If you kill the messenger, the message still hasn't changed."

There is nothing wrong with using medications to get rid of mites, she adds. In most cases, however, there are gentle, more natural ways to get rid of them and to keep them from coming back.

## The Solutions   FOR DOGS & CATS

**Start with a tea rinse.** Green tea is a natural antiseptic that helps remove "mite mess" from the ear canal, says Dr. Yasson. Steep a tablespoon of green tea leaves in a cup of hot water for three to four minutes, strain it, then let it cool to room temperature. Using a small dropper, flush your pet's ear canal with the tea. Massage the outside of the ear to circulate the tea, then stand back: When your pet shakes her head, the tea—along with the grit in the ear—will come flying out. Then dry the outer part of the ear canal with a tissue or cotton ball, says Dr. Yasson. Do this once a day for a month.

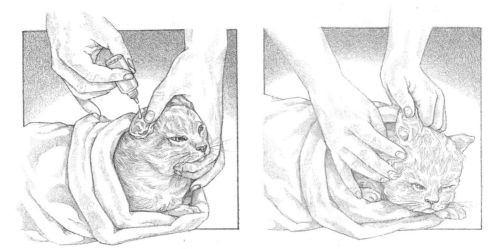

To give your cat ear drops without getting scratched, wrap her entire body, including the feet, securely in a small bath towel. Leave her head unwrapped and make sure that the towel is loose enough for her to breathe. Circle her head with your hand, putting your fingers under her chin and your thumb over the top of her head to hold her steady. With the other hand, hold the ear dropper so that the opening is just above the ear canal. Put in the drops and massage the base of her ear to circulate the liquid.

**BEST BET!** **Foil them with oil.** A traditional, all-natural remedy for mites is to put three to five drops of oil in the ear canal. The oil smothers the mites and also helps soothe the ears, says Dr. Yasson. Generally, it doesn't matter what kind of oil you use, although some holistic vets recommend almond or olive oil. (Don't use tea tree oil, which can be dangerous for cats.) For a double benefit, soak a few crushed garlic cloves in the oil overnight. Garlic helps kill bacteria that can lead to ear infections in pets with ear mites, says Dr. Yasson. You will need to give the oil treatments once a day for at least a month, she adds.

For the oil to be effective, it is a good idea to clean your pet's ears first. Otherwise, the accumulated discharge may protect the mites from the oil.

**Help the body help itself.** Once you have gotten rid of ear mites, you need to make sure that they don't come back. Some holistic veterinarians recommend giving pets echinacea (*Echinacea purpurea* or *Echinacea angustifolia*), an herb that strengthens the immune system and makes it harder for parasites to thrive. You can give echinacea for about two weeks after treating your pet for mites.

Dogs and cats will usually take echinacea liquid without putting up a fuss, but some pets dislike the taste. An alternative is to give them echi-

---

## Meet the Experts

**Carolyn Blakey, D.V.M.,** is a holistic veterinarian in private practice in Richmond, Indiana. She is certified in acupuncture.

**Michele Yasson, D.V.M.,** is a holistic veterinarian in private practice in New York City and Rosendale, New York. She is certified in acupuncture.

---

nacea capsules. Whether you are using capsules or liquid, give dogs over 50 pounds the full human dose, says Dr. Yasson. Pets 20 to 50 pounds can take one-half of the human dose, and pets under 20 pounds should take one-quarter of the human dose.

**Feed them well.** Giving pets high-quality foods—or preparing nutritious, homemade foods—will keep the immune system strong and help prevent mites from getting established, says Dr. Yasson. For more information on natural diets, see page 61.

**BEST BET!** **Treat all your pets.** One reason mites are so hard to get rid of is that they are readily passed from pet to pet, says Dr. Yasson. Even if you successfully treat one pet, she may get reinfected the next time that she rubs heads with one of her friends. The only way to get rid of mites for good is to treat all your pets—not only the one who is doing the scratching.

# EYE IRRITATION

## The Signs
- Your pet's eyes are red, itchy, or inflamed.
- There is a yellow or green discharge in the corner of the eye.
- Her eyes continually water.
- She squints or won't open one eye.
- The skin around the eyes is swollen.

## The Cause

The eyes are a lot tougher than they look. Dogs and cats are always coming into contact with something—from the sharp tip of a foxtail to irritating pollen in the air—that causes one or both eyes to swell, water, or redden, a condition called conjunctivitis.

Most eye irritations aren't serious and will go away on their own within a few days. But it is impossible to tell at home which irritations are minor and which are scary. "Conjunctivitis can exist by itself, or it can signal a much more serious eye problem," says Steve Marsden, N.D., D.V.M., a naturopathic physician and holistic veterinarian in private practice in Beaverton, Oregon. A red eye with a discharge can point to acute early glaucoma (a serious eye disease), an ulcer on the cornea, food

allergies, or a foreign body in the eye, he explains. You really need to call your vet when you notice any problems with the eyes, he adds.

In some cases, however, eye irritation is easy to treat at home. Veterinarians who specialize in holistic medicine have developed a number of simple, drug-free strategies that will stop pain and inflammation quickly. Here are a few tips that you may want to try.

## The Solutions   FOR DOGS & CATS

**Brighten the eyes with eyebright.** The herb eyebright (*Euphrasia officinalis*) is an antioxidant and anti-inflammatory that nourishes and eases irritated eyes, says Betsy Walker Harrison, D.V.M., a holistic veterinarian in private practice in Wimberley, Texas. She recommends mixing five drops of eyebright extract in a cup of saline solution and putting a few drops in each of your pet's eyes. Or you can soak a gauze pad in the solution and use it to gently swab her eyes once or twice a day.

Eyebright also works as a compress. Steep an eyebright tea bag in a cup of warm water for five minutes. Let it cool, then use the tea to moisten a soft, clean cloth. Gently hold the damp cloth across your pet's eyes. You

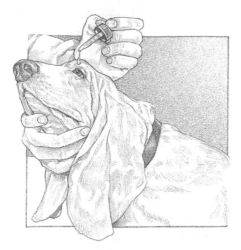

To give eyedrops, hold your pet's head securely and place the dropper directly over her eye. Hold the eye open with one hand while squeezing in the drops with the other.

can apply the compress twice a day for three to five minutes at a time.

**Stop the sting.** A quick way to reduce eye pain and swelling is to combine equal parts eyebright and goldenseal eyedrops, both of which can be purchased, and put one or two drops of the solution in your pet's eyes three times a day, says Dr. Marsden.

**Coat the eyes.** Another way to ease irritation quickly is to put one drop of almond or cod-liver oil in your pet's eyes one to four times a day, says Dr. Harrison.

**Help injuries heal.** Dogs and cats sometimes get minor eye injuries that can cause painful irritation, says Dr. Harrison. There are a number of homeopathic remedies that can be very effective.

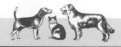

## Help for Dry Eyes

Dogs and cats produce tears just as much as people do. Tears lubricate the surface of the eyes and wash away irritants such as dust, pollen, or bacteria. But some pets, especially dogs, may develop a condition called dry eye, or keratoconjunctivitis sicca, in which there aren't enough tears to keep the eyes lubricated.

Veterinarians have always believed that there isn't a cure for dry eye. The main treatment was to use artificial tears, a sterile fluid that resembles the body's natural tears, or to give a drug called cyclosporine, which increases tear production and can slow the destruction of the tear gland. But some holistic veterinarians believe that dry eye is associated with liver problems, says Steve Marsden, N.D., D.V.M., a naturopathic physician and holistic veterinarian in private practice in Beaverton, Oregon. When the liver problems are taken care of, either with Western or alternative medicine, the eyes will often take care of themselves, he explains.

🐾 Arnica is recommended when tissues surrounding the eye are inflamed or swollen.

🐾 Symphytum is good when the eyeball has taken a direct hit.

🐾 Belladonna stops inflammation and is often recommended for pinkeye.

🐾 Pulsatilla is used when pets have pinkeye as well as thick yellow or greenish discharge.

🐾 Euphrasia will help pets that are tearing heavily.

Whichever remedy you use, veterinarians usually suggest giving two 30C pellets. Give one dose and wait a half-hour, advises Dr. Harrison. If the eye still isn't better, you can give a second dose.

**Give them chrysanthemum.** Any species of chrysanthemum sold as the Chinese remedy juhua is your best bet for relieving eye irritation, Dr. Marsden says. He recommends giving cats and dogs under 15 pounds one-quarter teaspoon of the powdered herb twice a day. Pets 15 to 50 pounds can take one-half teaspoon, and larger dogs can have up to one tablespoon.

**Press the eye points.** There are several acupressure points that can help stop pain and redness caused by conjunctivitis. The main points are as follows.

## Call the VET

Even minor eye problems can look pretty ugly, and it is hard to tell which ones you need to worry about. Here are four signs that *always* mean that you should call the vet, says Steve Marsden, N.D., D.V.M., a naturopathic physician and holistic veterinarian in private practice in Beaverton, Oregon.

- The eye is clearly painful, and your pet is shaking her head or pawing her eye to get relief.
- The blood vessels in the whites of the eyes (the sclera) are unusually swollen.
- The main part of the eye, the cornea, has unusual lines or circles, or it appears to be layered.
- The entire eye suddenly becomes cloudy.

If you see any of these symptoms, don't bother with home care," says Dr. Marsden. "Go straight to your vet."

🐾 ST2, located in the middle of the bony ridge below the lower eyelid.

🐾 GB1, located at the outer corner of the eye.

🐾 GB41, located on the rear feet just below the ankle.

If your pet will let you work on her and seems comfortable, Dr. Marsden recommends pressing any one of these points for one to three minutes as many as five times a day.

---

## Meet the Experts

**Betsy Walker Harrison, D.V.M.,** is a holistic veterinarian in private practice in Wimberley, Texas. She is certified in homeopathy.

**Steve Marsden, N.D., D.V.M.,** is a naturopathic physician, licensed acupuncturist, and holistic veterinarian in private practice in Beaverton, Oregon.

---

# FEAR OF BEING ALONE

## The Signs
- Your cat hides when you leave the house.
- Your dog cries, howls, or gets destructive when he is alone.
- Your dog or cat has "accidents" when you are gone.

## The Cause

Dogs and cats have been domesticated for thousands of years. They depend on their owners for everything—not only food but also love and attention. Most pets can handle being alone as long as they get plenty of attention the rest of the time. But some pets start getting panicky the moment their owners leave the house or even when they hear the keys jingling.

Dogs who get frightened when they are alone will sometimes destroy shoes or furniture or even jump through closed windows in their desperate attempts to allay their fears. Cats don't get as visibly nervous; they are more likely to stay in hiding until their owners return.

It is not only being alone that triggers fears, says Pam Johnson Bennett, a feline behavior consultant in Nashville and author of *Twisted Whiskers*. Some pets get insecure and anxious when "competitors," such as a new baby or boyfriend, enter their lives. They may respond by not eating for days at a time. Or they will mark your possessions with urine to let you know they are afraid, she says.

Severe fears can be difficult and time-consuming to treat. Conventional therapy has relied on training or behavior modification and, in the worst cases, on tranquilizers or mood-altering drugs. These aren't your only choices, however. Holistic veterinarians have developed a number of alternative therapies that can make pets more comfortable and secure—without using symptom-masking drugs.

## The Solutions FOR DOGS & CATS

**Minimize the fear with flower essences.** The flower essences aspen, mimulus, and Rescue Remedy can be often used to help soothe and relax pets who get anxious when they are alone. Combine eight drops of each in one ounce of distilled water, says Jeanne Olson, D.V.M., a holistic veterinarian in private practice in North Pole, Alaska. The easiest way to give flower essences is to put a dropperful in your pet's water once a day. Or you can put two to four drops in his mouth, between the lips and gums, two or three times a day. It works well when you give it an hour before you leave the house.

**Calm them with music.** "My cats stay very calm when I put on classical music because it is the same music they hear when I'm home," Bennett says. Any music can work, she adds, although it is best to choose music with a slow, even rhythm rather than hard-driving rock 'n' roll.

**Help them sleep.** Dogs and cats can't get very upset when they are sleepy, which is why some veterinarians recommend giving them a little warm milk before you leave the house. Milk contains tryptophan, a natural chemical that plays a role in promoting sleep, says Mary Lee Nitschke, Ph.D., professor of psychology at Linfield College in Portland, Oregon, and an animal behaviorist in Beaverton. Dogs and cats love milk, so you won't have any trouble getting them to take their "medicine." You can give pets about one-quarter cup of milk at a time, she says.

**Relax them with magnets.** "The best relaxation technique for your pets, especially those suffering severe stress or anxiety attacks, is magnet therapy," says Joanne Stefanatos, D.V.M., a holistic veterinarian in private practice in Las Vegas. Available from some holistic veterinarians and in catalogs, small "healing" magnets change the body's energy fields and are often used for emotional healing. All you have to do his hold the "north pole" end of the magnet on your pet's forehead until he is feeling calmer. It may take about 20 minutes, so make sure that you get comfortable before starting, she adds.

**Stop fear with touch.** Many pets crave human touch, especially when they are scared. A specialized kind of touch called TTouch, which involves using your fingertips to trace small clockwise circles on your pet's body, can be particularly helpful. Pay particular attention to the ears, face, and neck, taking a second or two to complete each circle. Holistic veterinarians have found that TTouch not only calms frightened animals but also can help them be more calm and relaxed in the future.

**Encourage independence.** Dogs and cats are accustomed to asking for attention, and we are accustomed to giving it. Problems may arise when pets get so dependent for love, amusement, attention, or anything else that they forget how to function normally when you are not around. For them, being alone for 15 minutes can seem like a lifetime of abandonment.

The way to prevent this emotional dependency is to give them limited—or at least planned—attention, says Wayne Hunthausen, D.V.M., a veterinary behaviorist in Westwood, Kansas, and author of the *Handbook of Behaviour Problems in Dogs and Cats*. This means giving them attention when you feel like it, not when they demand it. If you do this consistently, they will learn how to entertain themselves without any help from you. Pets that are emotionally self-sufficient are much less likely to get anxious when they are left alone, he explains.

**BEST BET!** **Help them overcome their fears.** Pets know in advance when you are leaving because they recognize all the little cues that precede the actual event, like opening the closet, picking up your briefcase, jingling car keys, and so on. So, they start getting nervous before you are out the door. By the time the big event finally happens, they are almost beside themselves.

You can interrupt the entire process by changing your pet's expectations, says Dr. Hunthausen. It takes a little work, but it is worth it. Start doing your "leaving ritual" when you are *not* leaving. Jingle the keys while watching TV. Walk to the door, open it—and don't leave. Put on your coat, walk around for a while, then take it off. If you keep doing this, repeating the cues 15 to 20 times a day for a few weeks, your pet will gradually realize that the cues that once made him frantic don't mean much. "Picking up your keys or going toward the closet loses the scary meaning that it used to have," he explains.

When your pet is getting less frantic before you leave, it is time to take things a little further and practice leaving. In other words, go out the door, shut it behind you, and then come right back in. You will probably get a pretty big greeting. A little later, go out the door and don't come back for a few minutes. This time you will get a much bigger greeting. So you do

## Meet the Experts

**Pam Johnson Bennett** is a feline behavior consultant in Nashville and the author of *Twisted Whiskers* and *Psycho Kitty*.

**Wayne Hunthausen, D.V.M.,** is a veterinary behaviorist in Westwood, Kansas, and the author of the *Handbook of Behaviour Problems in Dogs and Cats*.

**Mary Lee Nitschke, Ph.D.,** is a professor of psychology at Linfield College in Portland, Oregon, and an animal behaviorist in Beaverton.

**Jeanne Olson, D.V.M.,** is a holistic veterinarian in private practice in North Pole, Alaska.

**Joanne Stefanatos, D.V.M.,** is a holistic veterinarian in private practice in Las Vegas. She is certified in acupuncture and chiropractic.

it again and again, always varying the time you are gone, from 1 or 2 minutes to 15 or 20. After a while, your pet will get the idea that leaving doesn't mean going away for a long time. Once he understands that you are always coming back, and possibly very soon, he will be less likely to get frantic when you are gone, says Dr. Hunthausen.

**BEST BET!** **Make hellos and goodbyes routine.** Making a big deal out of comings and goings gets your pet excited and makes the anxiety worse, says Dr. Hunthausen. "Keep homecomings and departures really low-key—just say goodbye and leave."

## The Solutions *FOR DOGS*

**BEST BET!** **Keep him occupied.** Most dogs will gladly sleep the day away, including dogs who get frightened when they are alone. Problems tend to occur within an hour after you leave, when the anxiety is highest. If you can help your dog get through that first hour, there is a good chance that he will be fine the rest of the day, says Dr. Hunthausen. One way to do this is with toys that are designed to hold food, like Kong, Goody Ship, Buster Cube, or Bite a Bone. "They not only give your pet something to do during the first hour when his anxiety is the worst but also teach him to look forward to seeing you go," he says.

# FELINE IMMUNODEFICIENCY VIRUS

## The Signs

- Your cat has a fever that comes and goes.
- The lymph nodes—under the jaw and elsewhere—are swollen.
- He has sores in his mouth.
- He refuses to eat and is losing weight.
- He keeps getting infections.

## The Cause

It has been called feline AIDS because the virus that causes it is closely related to the human virus. Cats that get feline immunodeficiency virus, or FIV, often have no symptoms at all. "Just like HIV in humans, there is a long, silent period before cats with FIV develop signs of illness," says Alice Wolf, D.V.M., professor of medicine at Texas A&M University College of Veterinary Medicine in College Station. In fact, it often takes up to six years before cats with FIV get sick, if they get sick at all.

It is not the virus itself that makes this condition potentially serious. The real problem is that the virus weakens the entire immune system. This makes cats vulnerable to secondary illnesses, in which otherwise minor conditions like diarrhea or runny eyes begin causing problems.

There isn't a cure for FIV, but there is a lot you can do to ensure that your cat has a long, healthy life. "The best treatment is to keep their immune systems as healthy and strong as possible," says Pat Zook, D.V.M., a holistic veterinarian in private practice in Stone Mountain, Georgia.

## The Solutions   FOR CATS

**BEST BET!** **Give your cat wheat sprouts.** Usually given as supplements, wheat sprouts contain compounds that act as antioxidants—that is, they neutralize harmful oxygen molecules in the body that can weaken the immune system, says Dr. Zook. She recommends giving cats with FIV a product called Feline Support, which contains wheat sprout derivatives along with a variety of antioxidants. "It really seems to give cats some bounce," she says. You can give your cat one wheat sprout supplement a day. Some cats will crunch them right down, but others won't touch them unless you crush them first and mix them in their food.

**Give an herbal boost.** An herb called astragalus (*Astragalus mem-*

*branaceus*), available as a tincture, gives the immune system a long-term boost, says Dr. Zook. She recommends giving cats four drops of the tincture twice a day. Most herbal tinctures contain alcohol, she adds, so it isn't good for long-term use. Look for glycerin-based tinctures in health food stores.

**Build immunity with acupressure.** There are three acupressure points that can be stimulated to keep the immune system strong.

🐾 ST36, located on the outside of the rear leg just below the knee joint.

🐾 SP6, located on the inside of the rear leg just above the ankle.

🐾 LU7, located just above the wrist joint on the inside of the front leg.

Pressing each of these points for about 30 seconds once a day will help keep your pet strong and better able to fight infections, Dr. Zook says.

**Cool fevers with alcohol.** Fever is one of the body's tools for fighting infections, but it can be dangerous for cats with FIV because they are already weaker than they should be. One way to lower fever is to dab a little rubbing alcohol on the pads of the feet. Alcohol stings, says Dr. Wolf, so don't use it if your cat has cuts or sores on his feet.

 **Feed him well.** Good nutrition is vital for cats with FIV. Holistic veterinarians recommend giving cats a homemade diet consisting of one-half meat, one-quarter raw vegetables, and one-quarter cooked carbohydrates, like brown rice. Or give your cat a high-quality, all-natural pet food like Innova or Solid Gold, says Carolyn Blakey, D.V.M., a holistic veterinarian in private practice in Richmond, Indiana. You can buy natural pet foods in some pet supply stores and through mail order. For more information on homemade diets, see page 61.

**Give natural enzymes.** To help your cat get the most nutrients from his food, give him a raw egg yolk once a week and a teaspoon of nonflavored live-culture yogurt five days a week. These foods may contain natural enzymes, which will help the digestive system work more efficiently, says

---

## Meet the Experts

**Carolyn Blakey, D.V.M.,** is a holistic veterinarian in private practice in Richmond, Indiana. She is certified in acupuncture.

**Roger L. DeHaan, D.V.M.,** is a holistic veterinarian in private practice in Frazee, Minnesota. He is certified in chiropractic.

**Alice Wolf, D.V.M.,** is a professor of medicine at Texas A&M University College of Veterinary Medicine in College Station.

**Pat Zook, D.V.M.,** is a holistic veterinarian in private practice in Stone Mountain, Georgia. She is certified in acupuncture.

Roger L. DeHaan, D.V.M., a holistic veterinarian in private practice in Frazee, Minnesota. You can also give your cat a commercial digestive enzyme for pets, such as Prozyme or FloraZyme, following the directions on the label.

**Provide extra vitamins.** Give cats with FIV vitamins C, E, and A, says Dr. Blakey. "Antioxidants help boost the immune system and are incredibly safe." She recommends using a combination supplement, available from veterinarians, called Cell-Advance 440. It contains the proper mix of nutrients. Give your cat one capsule a day, she advises.

**Keep your cat safe.** Cats with FIV are not only contagious to other cats but also very vulnerable to viruses and other germs. "Cats that are kept indoors will live longer," says Dr. Wolf. And while many mainstream veterinarians feel that yearly vaccines are important for cats with FIV, some holistic vets believe that they put unnecessary stress on the body. Your vet will help you decide whether vaccines are a good option for your cat.

# FEVER

## The Signs
- Your pet is panting even when he is resting.
- The ears are hot and may be red inside.
- His appetite is off.
- His energy levels are low.

## The Cause

In pets (as in people), fever is usually caused by a bacterial or viral infection, such as from a cold or a bout of the flu. While prolonged high temperatures can be a problem, most fevers aren't dangerous. In fact, they may help pets recover because they make it more difficult for germs to thrive inside the body. "Fever is not a disease," says Linda East, D.V.M., a holistic veterinarian in private practice in Denver.

The conventional approach—at least in modern medicine—is to give medications that fight infection and lower fever. But vets who practice natural healing feel that it is equally important, if not more so, to bolster the immune system at the same time. "The idea is to treat the whole pet, to strengthen him in such a way that he can deal with whatever is causing the fever," Dr. East explains. Of course, even a slight fever can make pets feel

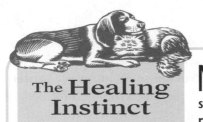

The **Healing Instinct**

**M**aybe you wake up one morning, and your pet isn't in his favorite spot by the side of the bed. Or maybe he doesn't come running at the sound of kibble hitting his bowl. You look around and finally find him, looking weak and miserable, inside the bathtub or stretched across a cold linoleum floor.

Pets with fevers will instinctively seek out cold surfaces to help lower their temperatures, says Maria H. Glinski, D.V.M., a holistic veterinarian in private practice in Glendale, Wisconsin. Spending as little as a half-hour in a cool place can lower their temperatures by one-half to one degree, which can make a big difference in how they feel.

Of course, pets with fever don't always feel warm—sometimes they get chills as well. So don't be surprised if you find your pet curled up in the bathtub in the morning and next to the radiator at night. "The body's natural wisdom will draw them from one to the other, depending on what they are feeling," Dr. Glinski explains.

hot and miserable. Here are a few ways to lower the heat and help your pet fight off the underlying problem.

## The Solutions FOR DOGS & CATS

**Press away the heat.** To lower fever in a hurry, gently press the GV14 acupressure point for about 60 seconds. You will find this fever-reducing point on your pet's back where the neck meets the shoulder blades. Repeat the pressure every 5 to 10 minutes for up to an hour, says Maria H. Glinski, D.V.M., a holistic veterinarian in private practice in Glendale, Wisconsin.

**Boost his immunity.** While you are doing hands-on care, take a little time to stimulate the ST36 acupres-sure point, located on the outside of the hind leg just below the knee. Pressing this point once or twice a day for up to 60 seconds will stimulate the immune system so that it battles the underlying infection more effectively, says Dr. Glinski.

**Cook some comfort food.** Pets with fevers often lose their appetites, which means they are not getting all the nutrients they need to keep their immunity strong. They also tend to quit drinking fluids, which raises the risk of dehydration. Putting a little sodium-free chicken or beef broth in their bowls will encourage them to lap up critical fluids. They will also get essential vitamins and minerals, says Dr. Glinski.

For cats, who are more finicky about their food than dogs, a bowl of tuna juice is hard to resist. Squeeze the juice from a can of tuna into a bowl and dilute it half-and-half with water, says Susan G. Wynn, D.V.M., a veterinarian in Atlanta and co-editor of *Complementary and Alternative Veterinary Medicine*.

**Put herbs to work.** Echinacea (*Echinacea angustifolia* or *Echincacea purpurea*) has been called the superherb because of its ability to help the body fight infection, says herbalist Gregory L. Tilford, co-owner of Animals' Apawthecary in Conner, Montana, and author of *Edible and Medicinal Plants of the West*. He recommends giving pets with a fever 12 to 20 drops of a low- or non-alcohol echinacea tincture for every 20 pounds of weight. Giving the drops two or three times a day will help the immune system battle both fever and infection, he says.

Another herb that can boost immunity is astragalus (*Astragalus membranaceus*). When your pet has a fever, you can use it in the same amounts as echinacea, Tilford says.

**Try some Hepar sulphuris calcareum.** Also known as Hepar sulph, this homeopathic remedy will help reduce fevers caused by a variety of infections, says Dr. Glinski. She recommends using a 6C or 30C pellet. Give one pellet to pets under 50 pounds and two pellets to larger dogs.

Repeat the treatment once an hour for four hours, she advises.

**Provide some puncture protection.** It is not uncommon for pets to develop fevers from infected puncture wounds caused by fighting, for example, or from stepping on a nail. The homeopathic remedy for this type of infection is Ledum—one dose of either 6C or 30C pellets. When pets are given the remedy immediately after their injuries, germs are much less likely to cause infections, abscesses, or fever, Dr. East explains. You can give two pellets of Ledum to dogs over 50 pounds and one pellet to smaller pets.

**Relieve the aches and pains.** Fever can make pets feel sore all over. To ease the aches, Dr. Glinski recommends the homeopathic remedy Arnica. Give one 30C pellet to pets under 15 pounds and two pellets to larger pets. Repeat the treatment once an hour for up to four hours. It is not a good idea to mix homeopathic remedies, so be sure to use Arnica only after stopping Hepar sulph or Ledum.

**Try Dr. Bach's 39th Remedy.** Also called Rescue Remedy, this combination of five flower essences can help relieve stress and discomfort in pets with fevers. Place one or two drops on your pet's tongue or inside his cheek as often as every 15 minutes for up to four hours, suggests Dr. Glinski.

**Make him stronger with vitamin C.** This powerhouse nutrient can help stimulate your pet's immune system so that it is better able to fight off viral and bacterial infections, says Dr. Glinski. She recommends mixing a little buffered, powdered vitamin C in a dollop of yogurt or cottage cheese. Most pets will gulp it right down.

Dogs over 50 pounds can be given 1,000 milligrams twice a day, while smaller pets should only take 500 milligrams once a day. Just be sure not to give straight vitamin C, she warns. It contains ascorbic acid, which may upset your pet's stomach. In addition, large amounts of vitamin C may cause diarrhea, so it is a good idea to give smaller doses at first to give the body time to adjust.

**BEST BET!** **Give them plenty of water.** Pets that are overheating can lose essential fluids and become dehydrated very quickly. Make sure to keep their water bowls full, preferably with spring or filtered water. If your pet re-

## Call the VET

Even though fever is a natural part of the body's healing process, it may be a sign of serious problems—anything from feline leukemia to Lyme disease to cancer, says Maria H. Glinski, D.V.M., a holistic veterinarian in private practice in Glendale, Wisconsin. "We worry most when the fever is in a very young or very old animal because they are more fragile and dehydrate more easily," she adds.

The normal temperature for dogs is between 100° and 102.5°F. For cats, it is between 101° and 102.5°. Unfortunately, you can't tell your pet's temperature by feeling his nose—you have to check it the old-fashioned way, with a rectal thermometer. Lubricate the end of a pet thermometer with petroleum jelly and gently twirl it into the rectum. Insert it no more than one inch in cats and small dogs, two inches in medium and large dogs. Hold your pet still for about two minutes, then remove the thermometer and check the reading. A fever of 103.5° or higher is potentially dangerous, and you should call your vet right away.

If your pet has other symptoms—he is vomiting, for example, or hasn't eaten for 24 hours or more—don't wait to see whether the temperature is rising or not. Call your vet right away.

## Meet the Experts

**Linda East, D.V.M.**, is a holistic veterinarian in private practice in Denver. She is certified in homeopathy.

**Maria H. Glinski, D.V.M.**, is a holistic veterinarian in private practice in Glendale, Wisconsin. She is certified in acupuncture.

**Gregory L. Tilford** is an herbalist and co-owner of Animals' Apawthecary in Conner, Montana, and the author of *Edible and Medicinal Plants of the West*.

**Susan G. Wynn, D.V.M.**, is a veterinarian in Atlanta and co-editor of *Complementary and Alternative Veterinary Medicine*.

fuses to drink, you may want to give him a helping hand. Fill an eyedropper or turkey baster with water and squirt a little into the side of his mouth. (Don't squirt the water toward the back of his mouth because it might get into the lungs.) For an added boost, you can offer your pet a bowl of electrolyte solution, such as Pedialyte, which restores essential minerals called electrolytes that often run low in pets with fevers, Dr. Glinski says.

**Soothe them with soup.** "I treat feverish pets at home with my homemade soup," says Dr. Glinski. She makes her healing soup by boiling four cloves of garlic, along with broccoli and some carrots, in organic beef or chicken stock mixed with filtered or spring water. Strain off the liquid, let it cool, and add it to your pet's food or give it as a broth. You can also blend the boiled ingredients together and give them as a snack. Just don't add onions to the soup, she warns, because they can be harmful for cats.

## The Solutions — FOR DOGS

**Brew some herbal pain relief.** Willow bark tea (*Salix alba*), which acts like aspirin, can reduce fever and help ease aches and pains, Tilford says. (Aspirin and related substances may be harmful for cats and should never be used without a veterinarian's supervision.) Stir a teaspoon of shredded willow bark in eight ounces of hot water and simmer for about three minutes. Let it cool to room temperature and give a tablespoon or two for every 20 pounds of pooch twice a day, he suggests.

# FIGHTING

## The Signs
- Your pet's play is getting too rough.
- You are hearing more growling or hissing than usual.
- Your pet has been snapping at or biting other pets.

## The Cause

Almost all pets occasionally get into spats. It is their way of settling differences or just letting other pets know that they are having a bad day. But when fights are happening all the time and the fur is really flying, you need to act quickly before someone gets hurt.

"When you have a household with more than one pet, you are blending personalities," says Pat Zook, D.V.M., a holistic veterinarian in private practice in Stone Mountain, Georgia. "Just like people, animals don't always get along with each other." Add jealousy, frustration, possessiveness, poor social skills, health problems, or raging hormones into the mix, and you have all the ingredients for a good fight.

Mainstream veterinarians sometimes treat combative behavior with antidepressants or other drugs, says Jean Hofve, D.V.M., a holistic veterinarian in private practice in Denver. While medications can be useful, especially when they are combined with training or behavior-modification therapy, they only treat the symptoms of emotional unrest. A better (and drug-free) approach is to support your pet's emotions while improving his behavior so that he is happier and more confident—and less likely to look for trouble.

## The Solutions FOR DOGS & CATS

**Adjust his energy.** Pets have two acupressure points—LI4 and LIV2—that can help correct energy imbalances that can lead to aggression, says Junia Borden Childs, D.V.M., a holistic veterinarian in private practice in Ojai, California. To stimulate LI4, located in the web of skin between the dewclaw and first long toe on the front feet, massage the area in a downward motion for 30 seconds once a day. To stimulate the LIV2 point, located on the rear feet, just above where the inside toe meets the foot bone, massage the point and stroke downward for about 30 seconds once a day, she says.

**Calm them with Chinese herbs.** The herbs shou wu pian and xiao yao, which are available in pill form from some holistic veterinarians and in traditional Chinese medicine supply stores, can make pets less hostile and moody, says Dr. Childs. Every pet will need a different dose, so check with your vet before using this treatment at home, she says.

**Make peace with flower essences.** Holistic veterinarians use flower essences to treat many emotional imbalances, including those that lead to fighting and aggression. The essence holly, for example, can help make pets less jealous, and vine helps make them less bossy, says Dr. Hofve. When pets are upset after a fight, the essence mixture called Bach Rescue Remedy can be very helpful, she adds.

To prepare a flower remedy, put two drops each of one or more essences in a one-ounce brown bottle filled with spring water, says Dr. Hofve. (When using Bach Rescue Remedy, add four drops instead of two.) Give your pet four drops of the remedy three or four times a day. You can put them directly in his mouth or mix them in his food or water. Doing this every day for two to six weeks will usually cause a noticeable change for the better in his behavior, she says.

**BEST BET!** **Keep them separate.** Even pets that get along will sometimes indulge in rough play that can escalate into real aggression. To prevent problems, Dr. Zook recommends keeping fight-prone pets separate when

## Call the VET

Most dogs and cats settle their disagreements without resorting to violence—or at least without getting hurt. But dogs and cats that are true fighters aren't so lucky. When they tangle, they are sure to be on the receiving end of a quick snap of teeth or raking of claws, either of which can cause painful wounds that often get infected. An out-and-out brawl can leave both combatants seriously injured.

Talk to your vet as soon as you notice aggressive behavior, advises Pat Zook, D.V.M., a holistic veterinarian in private practice in Stone Mountain, Georgia. Fighting is usually caused by emotional problems, but in some cases it is simply a result of not feeling well. "Some pets start to get really grouchy as they get older," she says.

you aren't around to supervise them. This is especially important while they are eating meals or when there is a big size difference, she adds. "If a Great Dane is trying to play with a Chihuahua, and the Great Dane is crushing him, put the Dane in a separate area to play and exercise," she says.

**Have your pet neutered.** In male dogs and cats particularly, the onset of puberty can bring higher levels of aggression. Neutering your pet while he is still young will help reduce aggressive behavior before it becomes part of his personality, says Dr. Zook. Pets should be neutered at six months or when they first begin to show signs of aggression.

## The Solutions

**FOR DOGS**

**BEST BET!** **Keep him under control.** Even dogs that are naturally aggressive will act more appropriately when they understand that you, their

## Meet the Experts

**Junia Borden Childs, D.V.M.,** is a holistic veterinarian in private practice in Ojai, California.

**Jean Hofve, D.V.M.,** is a holistic veterinarian in private practice in Denver.

**Pat Zook, D.V.M.,** is a holistic veterinarian in private practice in Stone Mountain, Georgia. She is certified in acupuncture.

natural leader, don't approve of their behavior. "You have to teach them, 'Hey, that's not cool,'" says Dr. Zook.

Taking your dog to obedience school—or, if he has already been, to a refresher course—is often the easiest way to help him learn to take his cues from you. Whether or not you take him to school, however, it is up to you to show your disapproval every time he acts up by telling him "No!" and pulling him back by the collar.

# FLATULENCE

## The Signs
- Your pet is passing gas every day.
- The odor is ruining your relationship.

## The Cause

Social implications aside, flatulence isn't a serious problem. "It is your pet's way of telling you that there is something indigestible in his diet," says Susan G. Wynn, D.V.M., a veterinarian in Atlanta and co-editor of *Complementary and Alternative Veterinary Medicine.*

Many pet foods supply the majority of their protein from nonmeat sources, like corn and wheat, which are difficult for some pets to digest, she explains. When food isn't completely digested, it provides a rich source of nourishment for bacteria in the large intestine. The undigested portion begins to ferment, causing gas and sometimes uncomfortable pressure in the abdomen.

Happily for their owners, cats are much less flatulent than dogs. "Cats have a shorter digestive tract, and things tend to move through quickly," explains Russell Swift, D.V.M., a holistic veterinarian in private practice in Dade,

Broward, and Palm Beach Counties in Florida. Cat foods also contain more meat and less of the gas-producing ingredients that are in dog foods.

Even though occasional flatulence is normal, holistic veterinarians believe that too much gas is a sign that your pet's diet and overall health aren't as good as they could be. Here are a few ways to clear the air and keep your pet more comfortable.

## The Solutions — FOR DOGS & CATS

**BEST BET!** **Feed him the wild way.** Your pet's digestive tract hasn't changed much since his wild ancestors were foraging for food thousands of years ago. Some holistic vets believe that giving dogs and cats a

## Call the VET

Some intestinal gas is a normal part of digestion. When it occurs all the time, however, or is accompanied by other symptoms like diarrhea, weight loss, or blood or mucus in the stool, there may be a problem in the digestive tract.

Severe flatulence is often a sign of parasites, says Jeffrey Feinman, V.M.D., a holistic veterinarian in private practice in Fairfield County in Connecticut. It can also be caused by a serious condition called inflammatory bowel disease. When flatulence flares and doesn't go away within a day or two, you need to call your vet, he says. This is especially true for cats since they are much less likely than dogs to be gassy in the first place.

"wild" diet will improve their digestion while curtailing the fumes. Dr. Swift recommends a diet that includes raw meat and vegetables, bonemeal, digestive enzymes (which are similar to the enzymes found in the stomachs of their traditional prey), and beneficial bacteria such as acidophilus. Every pet has different nutritional needs, so you will need to ask your vet to help plan a healthful, low-gas diet.

**BEST BET!** **Switch to a different food.** Your pet will probably be less gassy if you give him a food that contains a higher percentage of meat-based protein, says Dr. Wynn. Look for foods in which proteins from meat sources constitute at least two of the first three ingredients listed on the label, she advises.

**Put yogurt to work.** Changing your pet's diet will often change the balance of bacteria in the intestine, causing a sudden increase in flatulence. To keep him smelling sweet, Dr. Wynn advises adding a little plain, live-culture yogurt to his food. This will reduce gas by replacing some of the good bacteria in the digestive tract. Give him yogurt for several days after changing his diet, she adds. You should give one to two teaspoons of yogurt a day to pets under 15 pounds, working your way up to the maximum of three tablespoons a day to dogs over 80 pounds.

**Use a yogurt substitute.** While yogurt is good for most pets, some dogs and cats are sensitive to lactose, a sugar found in milk, yogurt, and other dairy foods. If your pet gets diarrhea after eating yogurt, you can use acidophilus supplements instead to boost his levels of beneficial bacteria, says Jeffrey Feinman, V.M.D., a holistic veterinarian in private practice in Fairfield County in Connecticut. You can give pets over 15 pounds the human dose that is listed on the label. Smaller pets can take half of the human dose, he says. Acidophilus supplements are available in supermarkets and health food stores.

**Add a little water.** Dry pet foods contain enormous amounts of air. When the air gets into the digestive tract, it has to go somewhere—and out it goes, many times a day. Soaking dry food in water until it triples in size—you will see air bubbles escaping—will remove the air before it gets into the digestive tract, which will often help reduce flatulence, Dr. Feinman says.

The one drawback to soaking dry food is that it loses some of its ability to scrape the teeth clean. A compromise is to soak most of the food, but sprinkle a little dry food on top, Dr. Feinman suggests.

**Curb it with charcoal.** Activated charcoal, available in health food stores and drugstores, can absorb tremendous amounts of gas in the digestive tract, says Dr. Swift. He recommends giving cats and small dogs

## ALTERNATIVE

## ✱SUCCESS

# A BREATH OF FRESH AIR

Labrador retrievers are lovable, affectionate dogs, and Duncan was no exception. But despite his good manners and wonderful temperament, he had a rather serious problem—serious enough that his owners boarded him in a kennel whenever guests came to town.

Duncan was unbelievably—unbearably—gassy. His owners had tried everything to fight the fumes, including putting him on a special diet, but nothing seemed to help. Duncan's veterinarian was beginning to suspect that he had an intestinal problem. He scheduled a procedure called endoscopy to take a look at Duncan's insides.

But before performing the test, Jeffrey Feinman, V.M.D., a holistic veterinarian in private practice in Fairfield County in Connecticut, decided to try one more thing. He started giving Duncan papaya enzymes and acidophilus supplements to improve his digestion.

The results, Dr. Feinman says, were dramatic. Within three days, Duncan literally ran out of gas. "He continues to be socially acceptable," he says.

under 15 pounds one-quarter of the dose listed on the label. Pets 15 to 50 pounds can take one-half of the recommended dose, and dogs over 50 pounds can take the full amount.

**Try the power of flowers.** Dogs and cats sometimes get gassy because they ate something that is upsetting their systems. To bring the body back into balance, holistic veterinarians recommend using the flower essence crab apple. Put two or three drops directly on your pet's tongue or in his drinking water each day, says Dr. Swift.

## The Solutions
FOR DOGS

**Purge it with papaya.** Dogs aren't at all fussy about what they eat. Yesterday's garbage is just as tempting as today's kibble—and a lot smellier when it comes out in the form of gas. To relieve flatulence caused by dietary indiscretions, Dr. Feinman recommends giving them papaya enzyme once a day for several days. Available in health food stores, papaya enzyme helps break down gas-producing particles in the digestive tract. A dog that weighs

50 pounds can take the dose for adults, he says. You can give more or less of the enzyme to larger or smaller dogs, depending on their weight.

Digestive enzymes can be helpful even if your pet hasn't been foraging, Dr. Swift adds. He often recommends giving pets "broad-spectrum" digestive enzymes such as Prozyme, available from holistic veterinarians and pet supply stores. These enzymes help break down proteins, carbohydrates, fats, and fiber. Dr. Swift recommends sprinkling the enzyme on your pet's food, following the instructions on the package.

---

## Meet the Experts

**Jeffrey Feinman, V.M.D.,** is a holistic veterinarian in private practice in Fairfield County in Connecticut.

**Russell Swift, D.V.M.,** is a holistic veterinarian in private practice in Dade, Broward, and Palm Beach Counties in Florida.

**Susan G. Wynn, D.V.M.,** is a veterinarian in Atlanta and co-editor of *Complementary and Alternative Veterinary Medicine*.

---

# FLEAS

## The Signs
- Your pet is scratching a lot or is losing patches of fur.
- There is pepperlike debris in his fur.
- His skin is red or sore, or there is a scabby rash.
- He has been getting tapeworms.

## The Cause

Young fleas emerge from their cocoons when they sense in their vicinity heat and vibration from a passing pet, for example. These signals act like dinner bells, and fleas will leap up to 150 times their body length in order to get on board. Once they have made themselves at home, they will dig in for a good blood meal.

Flea bites are painless and by themselves aren't always itchy. But many dogs and cats are allergic to flea saliva. A bite can trigger a scratching frenzy that can last as long as a week. Some pets get so itchy and scratch so hard that they damage the skin, causing a painful infection.

Most veterinarians have begun recommending medications to fight fleas. These products are very effective,

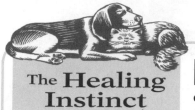

## The **Healing Instinct**

**D**ogs and cats spend a lot of time grooming, and they go through all sorts of contortions to lick and nibble itchy spots. All this mouth motion does more than scratch itches and spit-shine the fur. Veterinarians have found that normal grooming can remove enormous numbers of fleas. In fact, cats can remove at least 50 percent of their fleas by grooming, and dogs are pretty good at it, too. This is one reason that pets can have fleas for months, but you will never see a single one.

While rigorous grooming helps remove fleas, it causes other problems at the same time. Fleas often harbor tapeworms, which get into your pet's system when he swallows the fleas, says Carin A. Smith, D.V.M., a veterinary consultant in the state of Washington and author of *Get Rid of Fleas and Ticks for Good!* You can tell that your pet has tapeworms by looking at his stool: If you see what look like grains of white rice, he probably has tapeworms—and, in most cases, fleas as well.

but they aren't necessary because you may be able to control the problem without resorting to drugs or spray-on pesticides. "The holistic approach takes longer, but it uses less-toxic approaches," says Nancy Scanlan, D.V.M., a holistic veterinarian in private practice in Sherman Oaks, California. "Sick pets tend to have lots more fleas than healthy pets do, so we try to improve their health as well."

## The Solutions FOR DOGS & CATS

**Use a natural repellent.** Rather than fighting fleas that are already in place, you can keep them off to begin with. A supplement called Body Guard Powder, available from some vets, repels fleas from the inside out, says

Joanne Stefanatos, D.V.M., a holistic veterinarian in private practice in Las Vegas. During flea season, pets weighing under 20 pounds can have 1 teaspoon twice a day, mixed in their food. Pets weighing 20 to 50 pounds can take 1½ teaspoons twice daily, and larger pets can take up to a tablespoon twice a day.

**Repel them with bad taste.** A combination of brewer's yeast and garlic changes the flavor of your pet's blood, says Dr. Scanlan. Most dogs and cats love the pungent taste, but fleas take one bite and say "ugh." She recommends sprinkling about a tablespoon of brewer's yeast on your pet's food each day. Dogs over 50 pounds can have as much as two teaspoons of garlic a day, and smaller dogs can have one-quarter to one-half teaspoon a day. Garlic can be a problem for cats, so don't give them too much. A safe limit is one-eighth teaspoon or less a day for up to two weeks at a time. As an added benefit, brewer's yeast contains B vitamins that can improve your pet's overall health, making him better able to resist fleas. Some dogs are allergic to yeast, however, so it is a good idea to check with your vet before using it at home.

**Drive them off with bad smells.** Fleas don't like the smell of citrus, and you can often keep them away by washing floors and baseboards with Lemon Fresh or cleaners that contain citronella, says Dr. Stefanatos.

Other aromatic herbs that repel fleas include pennyroyal (*Mentha pulegium* or *Hedeoma pulegioides*), peppermint (*Mentha piperita*), or spearmint (*Mentha spicata*), says Pat Zook, D.V.M., a holistic veterinarian in private practice in Stone Mountain, Georgia. Make an herbal tea by putting one-quarter cup of the dried herb in a quart of hot water and letting it steep in a covered pot for 15 minutes. Strain the tea, let it cool, and mop it on your floors and baseboards.

Aromatic cedar is another natural flea repellent, which is why many pet beds are made with cedar chips, says Carin A. Smith, D.V.M., a veterinary consultant in the state of Washington and author of *Get Rid of Fleas and Ticks for Good!*

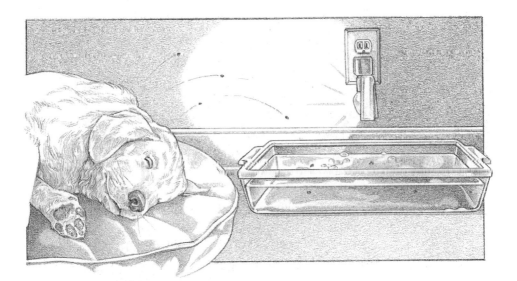

The one thing that fleas like almost as much as a warm pet is a warm light. You can use this against them by filling a cake pan with soapy water and putting it under a night-light near where your pet sleeps. Fleas are attracted to light and will make a leap for it—and land in the water and drown.

**BEST BET!** **Comb them out.** "The safest and most natural flea treatment is to use a flea comb to remove fleas from your pet every day," says Dr. Smith. "Comb your pet over a hard floor so that you can see and catch the fleas. Keep a bowl of soapy water nearby and drop in the fleas to drown them."

**Fill the tub.** Another way to eliminate fleas is to drown them, says Dr. Smith. Fill a tub or sink with water and give your pet a good dunking all the way up to his neck. The fleas will quickly head for dry ground above the neck, and you can pick them off as soon as they appear.

To make the bath even more effective, lather up your pet's neck with a flea shampoo containing pyrethrins, a natural insecticide made from chrysanthemums. Leave the lather on for about 10 minutes. When the fleas run uphill, they will get trapped in the suds and die, Dr. Smith explains. Then rinse your pet thoroughly, which will send the remaining fleas down the drain.

**Hit them when they are down.** A bath kills fleas, but it won't keep them off for good. So it is a good idea to dust or spray your pet with a flea product containing pyrethrins, following the instructions on the label, Dr. Smith advises.

**Dust with diatomaceous earth.** Despite its earthy name, diatomaceous earth consists of the skeletons of mi-

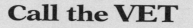

# Call the VET

Fleas are more than just itchy aggravations. "Each flea drinks 15 times its body weight in blood every day," says Carin A. Smith, D.V.M., a veterinary consultant in the state of Washington and author of *Get Rid of Fleas and Ticks for Good!* When your pet has a lot of fleas—100 or more at a time isn't unusual—he can lose up to a milliliter of blood a day. This isn't a problem for grown, healthy pets, but it can cause anemia in puppies and kittens as well as in older pets that have other health problems.

You can recognize anemia by looking in your pet's mouth. The gums and tongue should be a healthy, bubble-gum pink. If they are pale or white, he could be losing large amounts of blood, and you will need to call your vet right away.

croscopic algae that contain trace minerals. It can help keep your pet's skin healthy so that it naturally repels fleas, says Dr. Scanlan. Liberally sprinkle it on your pet once a day during flea season and rub it into the skin, she says.

You can buy diatomaceous earth in pet supply stores. Be sure to buy the kind called amorphous, Dr. Scanlan adds. Another type, called glassified, is used as a filter in swimming pools and can be dangerous for pets.

**Stop the itch with homeopathy.** To stop itching caused by fleas, give one to three pellets of the homeopathic remedy Ctenocephalidae nosode 12X three times day for one week, says Dr. Stefanatos.

**Run an oatmeal bath.** Washing pets with an oatmeal shampoo is one of the best ways to relieve itching, says Steven A. Melman, D.V.M., a veterinarian with practices in Potomac, Maryland, and Palm Springs, California, and author of *Skin Diseases of Dogs and Cats*. Be sure to use cool water because warm water makes itching worse, he adds. You can use the oatmeal shampoo once a day for three to four days.

**BEST BET! Suck up the problem.** For every adult flea that is dining on your pet, there may be a hundred more eggs, larvae, and cocoons in the house, waiting to take their turn. "Get rid of them by vacuuming your house at least once a week," says Dr. Smith. Be sure to vacuum the furniture, cracks in the baseboards, and other dark places where flea larvae wait to mature. Throw out the vacuum cleaner bag each week, she adds. Otherwise, the eggs inside the bag will hatch and start the problem all over again.

**BEST BET! Wash his bedding.** "Wash fabrics that your pet lies on at least once a week because normal washing in hot water and soap will remove flea eggs and larvae," says Dr.

## Meet the Experts

**Steven A. Melman, D.V.M.,** is a veterinarian with practices in Potomac, Maryland, and Palm Springs, California, and the author of *Skin Diseases of Dogs and Cats*.

**Nancy Scanlan, D.V.M.,** is a holistic veterinarian in private practice in Sherman Oaks, California. She is certified in acupuncture and chiropractic.

**Carin A. Smith, D.V.M.,** is a veterinary consultant in the state of Washington and the author of *Get Rid of Fleas and Ticks for Good!* and *101 Training Tips for Your Cat*.

**Joanne Stefanatos, D.V.M.,** is a holistic veterinarian in private practice in Las Vegas. She is certified in acupuncture and chiropractic.

**Pat Zook, D.V.M.,** is a holistic veterinarian in private practice in Stone Mountain, Georgia. She is certified in acupuncture.

Smith. If your pet likes lounging on the furniture, you can make life a little easier by covering it with towels, which you can change every day.

**BEST BET!** **Salt the carpet.** An all-natural substance called borax salts causes adult fleas to dry out and die. It also kills flea larvae when they eat or inhale the dust, says Dr. Scanlan. The ingredient you are looking for on the label is sodium polyborate, which is found in products such as Rx for Fleas. Dr. Scanlan recommends working the powder deeply into the carpet and leaving it in place. Then vacuum up the residue. "Wear a mask when applying borax salts, and don't let pets onto the carpet until you have vacuumed up the excess," she adds. Borax salts are very effective, but the benefits are temporary: As soon as you shampoo the rug, you will have to powder it again.

**Put worms to work.** Fleas that live in the yard don't always stay in the yard since every time your pet goes outside he acts like a flea magnet. To get rid of fleas outdoors, Dr. Scanlan recommends using nematodes, microscopic worms that you can get from garden supply stores. When mixed in water and sprayed on the yard, nematodes eat immature fleas as well as other insects, she explains.

**Take away their hiding places.** Fleas thrive in moist shaded areas—in tall grass, for example, or in weeds underneath trees. "One way to control fleas is to keep the grass mowed short," says Dr. Scanlan.

# Food Allergies

## The Signs
- Your pet is licking or biting her skin or scratching her face.
- Her ears or "armpits" look red and irritated, or the ears contain a gooey discharge.
- She is vomiting or has diarrhea or gas.
- Your cat has small scabs around her ears and neck.

## The Cause

Pets are adventuresome eaters. Given a chance they will gobble trash, spoiled meat, or old, dead mice with the same lip-smacking gusto they show for the finest canned cuisine. Beyond a little gas or an upset stomach, they will be none the worse for the experience.

For dogs and cats with food allergies, however, even normal eating can

# Call the VET

Food allergies are often difficult to treat at home because it's hard to know what your pet is allergic to. Even when your vet puts your pet on a scientifically designed diet, it may take two months or more before the problems go away. In the meantime, she will continue scratching, sometimes damaging the skin in the process.

"Any time a dog or cat is itchy enough that she is injuring her skin, it is time to see your vet," says Karen Komisar, D.V.M., a holistic veterinarian in private practice in Lynn, Massachusetts. Your pet may need antibiotics to treat skin infections, and possibly other medications to control the itching until the more natural, holistic remedies have time to work.

be a problem. When they eat the wrong food, they may get extremely itchy. Any ingredient can potentially cause allergies, with beef and soy protein being common offenders. Unless you suspect that there is a problem and change foods, your pet will just get itchier and itchier, possibly scratching herself raw, says Adriana Sagrera, D.V.M., a holistic veterinarian in private practice in New Orleans.

The best way to stop food allergies is to identify the problem ingredient and avoid it in the future. Veterinarians also recommend trying to make the immune system more "accepting" so that it doesn't react to harmless substances.

## The Solutions FOR DOGS & CATS

**BEST BET!** **Find the problem ingredient.** The only way to find

out if your pet has food allergies is to put her on an elimination diet. This means taking her off her old food and snacks and switching her to a hypoallergenic food—one that contains ingredients that she has never had before, says Anne Lampru, D.V.M., a holistic veterinarian in private practice Tampa, Florida. You will also need to replace the tap water in her bowl with distilled water. If her symptoms go away in six to eight weeks, you can be pretty sure that she was allergic to something in her food. Then you will be ready for the next step: figuring out what, exactly, she is allergic to.

Your veterinarian will recommend reintroducing one of the old ingredients—this could be a meat, a grain, or a vegetable—in her diet. If she doesn't start scratching or having other reactions within three days, you will know

**ALTERNATIVE**

# ❀SUCCESS

## TROUBLE WITH CHEESE

Ruff's owner was at her wit's end. For years the poor dog, a seven-year-old Lhasa apso, had been suffering from low energy, a chronic cough, and a yellow discharge from his nose, and no one could say what was wrong. Finally, Ruff's owner took him to Wanda Vockeroth, D.V.M., a holistic veterinarian in private practice in Calgary, Alberta, Canada.

"No one had considered food allergies," Dr. Vockeroth says. "I took Ruff off commercial food and put him on a duck and potato diet, with carrots for snacks." Her goal was to give Ruff foods he'd never had before, which would make the allergies go away. The new diet worked, but Ruff was still having problems. So Dr. Vockeroth started asking more questions.

She discovered that Ruff's owner had been giving him medications by slipping them inside pieces of cheese—and Ruff, it turned out, was allergic to cheese. So Dr. Vockeroth suggested that Ruff take his pills in a "safe" canned food, instead. "After two weeks, Ruff was perkier than he had ever been, and the nasal discharge and coughing essentially disappeared," she says.

that ingredient is fine, and you can add it to your "okay" list. If, on the other hand, she suddenly starts scratching up a storm, you may have identified one of her allergens. By continuing this process—trying out new foods and watching for reactions—you will develop a list of acceptable foods. With this knowledge, you can begin preparing nutritious, home-cooked or commercial meals that you know won't cause any problems.

Elimination diets are very effective at identifying allergens, but you have to be sure that your pet is get-

ting all the nutrients she needs, Dr. Lampru says. It is important to work with your veterinarian when planning and following an elimination diet, she says.

**Shop for natural foods.** Some dogs and cats are sensitive to the chemical preservatives, dyes, or artificial flavorings used in many commercial pet foods. "You may have to keep searching for a food they respond well to," says Dr. Lampru. Holistic veterinarians often recommend foods such as Innova, PetGuard Premium, Wysong, Solid Gold, and Flint River

Ranch, which are made with all-natural ingredients. You can buy natural foods in some pet supply stores and through mail order.

**BEST BET!** **Give them raw foods.** Your pet's digestive tract, which evolved over thousands of years, isn't really designed for commercially prepared foods that are cooked during processing. When there's a problem with allergies, switching to raw foods, preferably organic, may help, says Christina Chambreau, D.V.M., a holistic veterinarian in private practice in Sparks, Maryland, and education chairperson for the Academy of Veterinary Homeopathy. (The exceptions are grains such as brown rice, which need to be cooked.) In some cases, just switching to a raw food diet will eliminate the allergies, she says. For more on natural- and raw-food diets, see page 61.

Snacks should also be raw or lightly cooked, adds Arthur Young, D.V.M., a holistic veterinarian in private practice in Stuart, Florida. "Cooked broccoli and string beans, raw zucchini, raw carrots, alfalfa sprouts, and baby carrots are much better treats than things that come off the shelf," he says.

**Give the intestines some downtime.** Putting pets on a "modified fast" will help eliminate substances from the body that may be triggering the allergies, Dr. Sagrera says. She recommends taking pets with allergies off their regular food and giving them only one tablespoon of raw meat a day, along with pure water. Large pets can fast for three days, while smaller pets, including cats, can go one day. "If they seem very unhappy about not eating, you can give them some homemade chicken or beef broth," she adds. Be sure to talk with your vet before beginning a fast.

**Soothe them with a spritz.** Eliminating food allergies can be a time-consuming process. To keep your pets comfortable and itch-free in the meantime, holistic veterinarians sometimes recommend spraying the skin with flower essences. Combine two or three drops each of agrimony, beech, cherry plum, crab apple, olive, and walnut in a spray bottle filled with spring or purified water, says Wanda Vockeroth, D.V.M., a holistic veterinarian in private practice in Calgary, Alberta, Canada. Then spritz the itchy spots or dab some of the mixture on a cloth and wipe it on, she says.

**BEST BET!** **Try the chamomile solution.** Another way to soothe scratchy skin is with a solution made from chamomile (*Matricaria recutita*) and colloidal oatmeal shampoo, says Sandra Priest, D.V.M., a holistic veterinarian in private practice in Knoxville, Tennessee. Add two to four drops of chamomile herbal extract to eight ounces of the shampoo. Lather your pet thoroughly, let it sit for a few minutes, then rinse it off, she advises. Many pets won't hold still for baths, of course. An alternative is to spray itchy areas with a solution made from two to four drops of chamomile extract and two ounces of pure water, Dr. Priest suggests.

**Detoxify with herbs.** There are a number of herbs that promote healing by clearing your pet's body of harmful substances and making the body more resistant to food allergens. Burdock (*Arctium lappa*) is always a good choice, says Greig Howie, D.V.M., a holistic veterinarian in private practice in Dover, Delaware. If that doesn't help, you may want to try dandelion (*Taraxacum officinale*), yellow dock (*Rumex crispus*), or goldenseal (*Hydrastis canadensis*).

Dr. Howie recommends following the instructions on the label, giving dogs over 50 pounds the full human dose. Pets that weigh 15 to 50 pounds can take one-half the human dose, and smaller pets can take one-quarter of the human dose.

## The Solutions FOR CATS

**Make the switch gradually.** Cats don't always take well to elimination diets because they dislike having their routines interrupted. Suddenly changing your cat's diet could cause her to stop eating entirely. That can lead to a serious liver disorder called hepatic lipidosis, says Dr. Lampru. She recommends gradually replacing some of your cat's regular food with the new food over a period of several

## Meet the Experts

**Christina Chambreau, D.V.M.,** is a holistic veterinarian in Sparks, Maryland, and education chairperson for the Academy of Veterinary Homeopathy.

**Greig Howie, D.V.M.,** is a holistic veterinarian in private practice in Dover, Delaware. He is certified in acupuncture and homeopathy.

**Karen Komisar, D.V.M.,** is a holistic veterinarian in private practice in Lynn, Massachusetts. She is certified in homeopathy.

**Anne Lampru, D.V.M.,** is a holistic veterinarian in private practice in Tampa, Florida. She is certified in acupuncture and homeopathy.

**Sandra Priest, D.V.M.,** is a holistic veterinarian in private practice in Knoxville, Tennessee. She is certified in chiropractic.

**Adriana Sagrera, D.V.M.,** is a holistic veterinarian in private practice in New Orleans.

**Wanda Vockeroth, D.V.M.,** is a holistic veterinarian in private practice in Calgary, Alberta, Canada. She is certified in acupuncture.

**Arthur Young, D.V.M.,** is a holistic veterinarian in private practice in Stuart, Florida. He is certified in homeopathy.

weeks. Keep making the change slowly even if the allergy symptoms continue to appear. It may take several months before all the offending molecules leave your cat's system.

# FUR LOSS

## The Signs
- Your pet's fur is thinning, and the skin is visible.
- There are bald patches in his coat.
- His skin is hot, itchy, or inflamed.

## The Cause

It is normal for dogs and cats to lose some of their fur as the seasons change, but except for the hairy evidence on floors and carpets, you shouldn't really be aware of it. When the coat is getting so thin that you can see skin underneath, your pet has gone beyond normal fur loss, and there is probably something wrong.

Hair loss is usually caused by skin problems, such as ringworm, flea allergies, or hot spots, says Lowell Ackerman, D.V.M., a veterinary dermatologist in Mesa, Arizona, and author of the *Guide to Skin and Haircoat Problems in Dogs*. Pets that are losing fur are often itchy and scratch a lot. The skin may look red and sore as well.

In dogs, fur loss may be caused by hormonal problems, such as when the thyroid or adrenal glands are producing too much or too little hormone.

Cats are less likely than dogs to have hormone problems, but they do get allergies that make them itch. And when they scratch a lot, they can wear away the fur, says Dr. Ackerman. In addition, cats that are experiencing stress will groom themselves as a way of using up anxious energy. Their persistent licking will sometimes barber their hair into something resembling a buzz cut.

There are dozens of medications for treating allergies, hormone imbalances, and emotional problems such as stress. Drugs are sometimes necessary, but they aren't perfect solutions because they treat only the symptoms and not the underlying problems. That is why many holistic veterinarians prefer a different approach. Their goal is to find ways to get your pet's body back into balance. This will help keep the skin and even the glands healthier, which, in turn, can restore a healthy-looking coat.

## The Solutions FOR DOGS & CATS

**Clear away stress with crab apple.** Pets that are anxious and stressed will sometimes lose fur not only because they lick their coats more than they should but also because emotional turmoil can disrupt

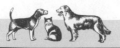

## Pet Pattern Baldness

Most dogs and cats have a full coat of fur, but some have been bred to have spare hair. The Chinese crested dog, for example, has tufts of fur only on the head, feet, and tail. Sphynx cats barely have any hair at all. They are covered with velvet fuzz that makes them look completely bald.

Even though some breeds are born bald, baldness usually comes as a surprise—for the owners if not the pets themselves. As with humans, baldness in pets may be a hereditary condition, especially in dachshunds. And it follows a certain pattern: The hair starts to thin on the ears, chest, or belly, and eventually it disappears entirely.

Pets aren't very sensitive about their pale pates, of course, so you don't need to invest in Rogaine or toupees. During the cold months, however, a sweater is always appreciated.

their bodies' hormones. The flower essence crab apple can "rebalance" their bodies' emotions and help keep pets calm.

"Crab apple can also be used as a cleansing remedy, and it calms itchy skin," says Carolyn Blakey, D.V.M., a holistic veterinarian in private practice in Richmond, Indiana. She recommends giving your pet two to four

drops of crab apple essence twice a day until his hair starts coming back. You can put the drops directly in his mouth or squeeze a dropperful of the essence in his water bowl once a day.

**Try a homeopathic skin remedy.** Holistic veterinarians often use homeopathy to relieve stress as well as skin problems. You may want to try an itch-relief remedy such as HomeoPet Miliary Eczema Male or Miliary Eczema Female, available in some pet stores, says Dr. Blakey. Dogs can take 10 drops and cats 3 drops, both three times a day, she advises. If the problem doesn't clear up in a few days or clears up and quickly returns, you will want to call your vet.

**Stop itching with fatty acids.** Veterinarians have found that fatty-acid supplements will help many skin problems, including itching and fur loss. "They are just fabulous," says Donna M. Starita, D.V.M., a holistic veterinarian in private practice in Boring, Oregon. She recommends a liquid supplement called Eskimo Oil because pets love the flavor. Give one-eighth teaspoon twice a day to cats, she says. Dogs weighing 50 pounds or less can have one-quarter teaspoon twice a day, and larger dogs can have one-half teaspoon twice a day. Eskimo Oil is available from veterinarians.

Another source of fatty acids is fish oil. It contains omega-3 fatty acids, which can help relieve skin problems that lead to fur loss, says Susan G. Wynn, D.V.M., a veterinarian in Atlanta and co-editor of *Complementary and Alternative Veterinary Medicine*. Give cats and dogs under 20 pounds 500 milligrams a day, she says. Pets that weigh 20 to 49 pounds can take 1,000 to 2,000 milligrams. Give 3,000 milligrams to dogs 50 to 79 pounds and 4,000 milligrams to dogs 80 pounds and over. Oils made from the whole fish, such as salmon oil, are a good choice because they contain more omega-3 fatty acids than those made from just a part of the fish, such as cod-liver oil.

**Help the hormones with lavender.** Pets that are losing hair because of nerves or a hormonal imbalance will benefit from the scent of lavender essential oil, says Dr. Starita. "Lavender has a calming effect, and it soothes and supports the adrenal glands so that they can heal," she explains. She recommends dabbing a little lavender on the fur on the back of your pet's neck once a day, which will allow him to breathe the healing aroma.

**Calm anxiety with St. John's wort.** The herbal remedy for stress is St. John's wort (*Hypericum perforatum*). "When a pet is in a state of fear or anxiety for a long period of time, the adrenal glands bottom out, and the pet can go into depression," says Dr. Starita. St. John's wort can turn things around fairly quickly. St.

---

### Meet the Experts

**Lowell Ackerman, D.V.M.,** is a veterinary dermatologist in Mesa, Arizona, and the author of the *Guide to Skin and Haircoat Problems in Dogs*.

**Carolyn Blakey, D.V.M.,** is a holistic veterinarian in private practice in Richmond, Indiana. She is certified in acupuncture.

**Donna M. Starita, D.V.M.,** is a holistic veterinarian in private practice in Boring, Oregon.

**Joanne Stefanatos, D.V.M.,** is a holistic veterinarian in private practice in Las Vegas. She is certified in acupuncture and chiropractic.

**Susan G. Wynn, D.V.M.,** is a veterinarian in Atlanta and co-editor of *Complementary and Alternative Veterinary Medicine*.

---

John's wort can cause side effects in some pets, however, so be sure to talk to your vet before using it at home.

**Build the body with supplements.** It is essential for pets to get the right balance of vitamins and minerals in order to keep the skin healthy and the hormones in balance. A nutritional supplement called Gerizyme, available from veterinarians, can be very helpful, says Joanne Stefanatos, D.V.M., a holistic veterinarian in private practice in Las Vegas. Pets weighing under 15 pounds can take one tablet a day. Pets 15 to 50 pounds can take two to three tablets, and larger pets can take four tablets.

# FUSSY EATING

## The Signs
- Your pet picks at her food or refuses to eat.
- She eats human food but ignores her own.

## The Cause

Dogs and cats aren't naturally choosy. Their instincts, formed at a time when a good meal was hard to find (or catch), told them to eat whatever they could, whenever they got the chance. But pets today have more culinary choices and opportunities than their ancestors ever did. We indulge them with fat- and flavor-rich commercial foods, along with tasty scraps from the dinner table. They soon learn that if they ignore their food and serenade us with a cacophony of cries and whines, something better will come their way.

A reluctance to eat pet food isn't always caused by finicky tastebuds, adds Thomas Van Cise, D.V.M., a holistic veterinarian in private practice in Norco, California. So it is a good idea to get your pet checked by the vet to rule out any physical causes. Stress can also be a factor, especially in multi-pet households where competition and bullying for food can get intense. Some pets get so anxious that they don't eat well, he explains.

Mealtime stress usually isn't a difficult problem to solve because you can always feed your pets separately. Teaching pets to enjoy what is in front of them, however, can take a little more work. Here is what veterinarians advise.

## The Solutions — FOR DOGS & CATS

**Boost the flavor.** Dogs and cats don't appreciate subtlety. If their food doesn't have a powerful aroma, they will lose interest and beg for something else. That's why veterinarians recommend buying the smelliest food you can find when you want to test your pet's appetite. If the smell is unusually pungent for you, it is probably just right for your pet.

You may not have to switch foods to find tastes and aromas that your pet likes, adds Susan G. Wynn, D.V.M., a veterinarian in Atlanta and co-editor of *Complementary and Alternative Veterinary Medicine*. Most dogs like garlic, for example. Adding fresh garlic to their food will substantially boost the aroma and stimulate their appetites. Dogs over 50 pounds can have as much as two teaspoons of

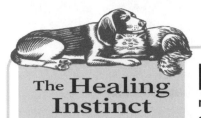

## The **Healing Instinct**

In the days when food was often in short supply, every bite was precious. That's why nature created an internal mechanism to ensure that dogs and cats always devoured what they caught.

During the hunt, their bodies released torrents of digestive juices. This prepared the digestive tract for the gamy meal to come and stimulated their appetites so that they ate as much as they could hold.

Today, of course, their food just sits there—and, in many cases, so do dogs and cats. To stimulate their appetites, you may want to duplicate nature's plan by making sure that they get plenty of regular exercise. This will reawaken their ancient instincts along with their hearty appetites.

garlic a day, and smaller dogs can have one-quarter to one-half teaspoon a day. Cats like garlic, too, but they can't have too much because it can cause a certain type of anemia. You can give them up to one-eighth teaspoon a day for two weeks at a time. Another way to make your pet's food more appetizing is to add some chicken or beef broth to her food, which will satisfy her natural craving for meat flavors.

**Switch to a natural food.** Even though commercially prepared pet foods are designed with taste in mind, many pets prefer foods that more closely resemble what their ancestors ate: raw meat, with a smattering of vegetables and grains, says Dr. Van Cise. A "whole" diet, prepared with fresh, organic ingredients, is not only flavorful but also a lot better for them, he says.

The problem with homemade diets is that they are not as convenient as scooping kibble from a bag. That is why you may decide to prepare a week's worth of food at one time, then store it in the freezer. At mealtimes, heat the food to slightly more than room temperature. (Be careful if you use a microwave, which can create hot spots in the food that could burn your pet's mouth.) This will give your pet the taste and aromas she craves with some of the convenience of packaged foods. For more information on preparing natural diets at home, see page 61.

**BEST BET!** **Put away the buffet.** Many owners fill the bowl with food in the morning and leave it out the whole day. This eat-when-you're-hungry approach, called free-choice feeding, is convenient, but it is not a good idea when there is a finicky eater

## ALTERNATIVE

## 🐾 SUCCESS

### UNLEASHED FROM FEAR

Some pets are fussy eaters because they have been spoiled. Some have trouble finding foods they like. And some are reluctant to eat because a near-disaster scared them right out of their appetites.

That's what happened to Smoky, an elegant gray cat who was out on his deck one day enjoying a little alfresco dining. Smoky was wearing a long leash, which was attached to a lawn chair. He had just settled down to his dinner when a car door slammed nearby.

Smoky panicked and bolted—over the side of the deck. He nearly hanged himself before his owner could rescue him. "After that, Smoky wouldn't eat or go near his food bowl because he associated this horrible experience with eating," says Pam Johnson Bennett, a feline behavior consultant in Nashville and author of *Twisted Whiskers*, who counseled Smoky and his nearly frantic owner.

Bennett recommended changing everything associated with the trauma, from switching food bowls to feeding Smoky in a new, safe place. She also recommended giving him a little playtime before meals to release tension and relax him. Finally, she treated Smoky with the flower essence aspen, which helped reduce his anxious feelings. "The treatments worked," says Bennett. "It took a couple of days, but he was soon back to normal."

in the family. Food that is left out all day gradually gives up its tempting aromas. It also teaches pets to take their food for granted, so they are not as excited about eating. "If you snacked all day long, you probably wouldn't sit down and eat a good meal either," says Pam Johnson Bennett, a feline behavior consultant in Nashville and author of *Twisted Whiskers*.

Holistic veterinarians recommend feeding pets in a way that is more in harmony with nature's plan. Feeding pets twice a day and taking the food away after 20 to 30 minutes more closely duplicates their natural eating schedule. It also teaches them that if they are going to eat, they had better do it right away, or they will lose the chance until their next feeding.

**Reduce mealtime stress.** If your pet seems reluctant to approach her food, the problem is more likely to be anxiety than a sudden loss of interest. Food is a common source of conflicts in multi-pet households, and pets that have had one bad experience may continue to be nervous and reluctant to eat. A flower essence called rock water can be very helpful for relieving this type of stress, says Dr. Van Cise. He recommends putting two drops of rock water essence in an ounce of spring water. Mix the solution well, then put four drops on your pet's tongue or next to her gums four times a day. Or you can put a dropperful of the solution in her water once a day.

Other flower essences that you may want to try are crab apple and hornbeam, which are often recommended for pets with eating disorders, says Dr. Van Cise. Another essence, aspen, is helpful for dogs and cats that associate eating with a previous traumatic experience, he says. You can give the essences separately or mix them together in an ounce of spring water, using about four drops of each essence. Then administer as described above.

Another way to reduce mealtime stress is with aromatherapy, using the essential oils lavender and orange, says Dr. Van Cise. You can dilute the oils half-and-half with vegetable oil and apply a few drops of the mixture to the fur on your pet's neck. Or you can put a few drops of undiluted oil— two to three drops for cats and up to five drops for dogs—on a bandanna and tie it around your pet's neck. The oils don't stay active indefinitely, so you will need to repeat the treatment once or twice a day, he says.

**Separate feuding pets.** If conflicts occur at mealtimes between pets in a multi-pet household, you can ease the tension by feeding them in different rooms, says Dr. Wynn. This gives pets the chance to eat in peace and may reduce anxiety associated with food.

## The Solutions

**Hold the tuna.** Even though cats love the taste of tuna, you don't want to give it too often because they may

---

## Meet the Experts

**Pam Johnson Bennett** is a feline behavior consultant in Nashville and the author of *Twisted Whiskers* and *Psycho Kitty*.

**Thomas Van Cise, D.V.M.,** is a holistic veterinarian in private practice in Norco, California. He is certified in acupuncture.

**Susan G. Wynn, D.V.M.,** is a veterinarian in Atlanta and co-editor of *Complementary and Alternative Veterinary Medicine*.

refuse to eat anything else, Dr. Wynn says. Another problem with tuna is that it can leach vitamin E from the body. It is fine to give tuna on rare occasions, but only if you mix it with your pet's regular food, she says. This will prevent her expectations from rising to unrealistic levels.

**Keep the bowl clean.** Cats are sensitive to odors and will sometimes refuse to eat if something isn't to their liking. It is a good idea to avoid plastic food dishes because they retain smells that cats may find objectionable, Bennett says. It is better to use stainless steel, glass, or ceramic dishes and wash them thoroughly after each meal.

Don't bother with the side-by-side food and water bowls sold in pet supply stores, Bennett adds. This type of feeding arrangement allows water and food to slosh back and forth, creating tastes and consistencies that some cats find unpleasant.

**Keep an eye on her appetite.** Dogs can easily go a day or two without food, so their occasional bouts of fussy eating aren't a problem. But cats can get extremely ill if they go without food for even a short time, says Dr. Van Cise. So don't take fussy eating or other appetite changes lightly. If your cat has quit eating for more than a day, call your vet right away.

# Hair Balls

## The Signs
- Your pet is throwing up wads of fur.

## The Cause

Cats can spend hours a day busily engaged in grooming. What's good for their coats, however, isn't so good for their insides. With every lick, loose fur sticks to their rough tongues, so they swallow it. Some of the hair is eliminated in the stools, but some stays in the stomach, forming a gooey wad.

When enough hair accumulates, cats chuck it up, leaving an unpleasant hairy mess—usually on your best carpet.

Hair balls occur mainly in cats, especially the long-haired breeds, but dogs can get them, too. "Even my Pomeranian has problems with hair balls," says Kathleen Carson, D.V.M., a holistic veterinarian in private practice in Hermosa Beach, California.

Veterinarians sometimes advise giving pets an oily remedy, available in pet supply stores and from veterinarians, that lubricates the hair and helps it slide through the intestines. The problem with these types of products is that they often contain artificial flavors and preservatives. That is why holistic veterinarians prefer to use natural methods both for preventing hair balls and for eliminating those that have already formed.

## The Solutions  FOR DOGS & CATS

**BEST BET!** **Help them pass with petroleum jelly.** An inexpensive strategy is to place about one-quarter teaspoon of petroleum jelly on your pet's front paws. When he licks his paws, he will swallow the petroleum jelly, which will lubricate hairs in the stomach so that they move gently into the digestive tract. Apply the petroleum jelly once a day for about four days when your pet is hacking, says Craig N. Carter, D.V.M., Ph.D., head of epidemiology at the Texas Veterinary Medical Diagnostic Laboratory at Texas A&M University in College Station.

**BEST BET!** **Give them extra fiber.** The dietary fiber found in foods like oat bran and green beans passes largely intact through the stomach and intestines. Along the way, it will grab hair and carry it out of the body, says H. Ellen Whiteley, D.V.M., a veterinary consultant in Guadalupita, New Mexico, and consultant for *The Country Vet's Home Remedies for Cats*. Dogs and cats don't like the taste of bran any more than most people do,

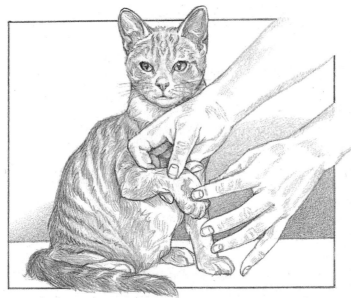

Petroleum jelly is one of the best hair-ball remedies. The easiest way to give it is to rub a little bit on the top of your pet's paw. They dislike the sticky sensation and will quickly lick it off.

and many pets don't care for whole green beans either. They do like canned pumpkin, however, which is very high in fiber, says Dr. Whiteley. She recommends giving small pets between one-half and one teaspoon of canned pumpkin with every meal. Medium-size and large dogs can have between a teaspoon and two tablespoons of pumpkin with meals.

Another way to get more fiber in pets' diets is to mix flaxseeds or psyllium husks, which are available in natural food stores, in their food, says Joanne Stefanatos, D.V.M., a holistic veterinarian in private practice in Las Vegas. Psyllium and flaxseeds act as natural laxatives, which will help stools—and hair—move through the system more quickly. You can give small pets about one-quarter teaspoon of flaxseeds or psyllium with every meal. Larger dogs can take up to a tablespoon, she says.

**Speed it through the system.** Another way to eliminate hair from the intestines is to give pets a natural laxative. Combine raw oatmeal, honey, and olive oil into a paste and offer one to two tablespoons as a treat when hair balls are a problem, suggests Dr. Carson. For pets that experience hair balls regularly, you can give the mixture two or three times a week.

Giving pets one-half teaspoon of olive or safflower oil twice a day will have a similar effect, adds Dr. Stefanatos.

**Reduce the discomfort.** Hair balls can irritate the stomach and intestines, causing constipation or an upset stomach, says Dr. Carson.

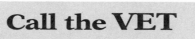

## Call the VET

Hair balls are usually nothing more than a nasty nuisance. But sometimes they get so large that they can't move in either direction—downward through the intestines or upward onto the carpet. These large masses of fur, called bezoars, can form hard-to-budge—and life-threatening—blockages.

"If your pet's stomach swells and he frequently vomits or can't pass his stool, you need to see a veterinarian right away," says H. Ellen Whiteley, D.V.M., a veterinary consultant in Guadalupita, New Mexico, and consultant for *The Country Vet's Home Remedies for Cats.*

"Slippery elm bark (*Ulmus rubra*) can be really helpful," she says. She recommends diluting 20 drops of slippery elm tincture in an ounce of spring water and giving your pet one dropperful three times every day—20 minutes before morning and evening meals and again at bedtime. It is best to use tinctures that are alcohol-free because alcohol may be harmful for cats.

**BEST BET!** **Groom away the problem.** The most effective, if not the easiest way to prevent hair balls, especially in cats, is to brush your pet every day. This will remove loose fur before your pet has a chance to swallow it, says Dr. Carson.

# HEARING PROBLEMS

## The Signs
- Your pet doesn't perk up when you whistle or call her name.
- She doesn't hear your footsteps when you approach.
- The sound of the can opener or the rustle of a bag doesn't get her attention.

## The Cause
Dogs and cats have extraordinarily sharp hearing, which is why they can hear you opening a can of food from three rooms away. Their ears are complicated instruments with narrow canals, high levels of humidity, and plenty of fur. It doesn't take much—a buildup of earwax, a little bit of swelling, or a minor infection—to make their hearing less efficient, says Carolyn Blakey, D.V.M., a holistic veterinarian in private practice in Richmond, Indiana.

Ear and hearing problems are often treated with antibiotics or other

## Call the VET

It is not uncommon for pets to get a little deaf as they get older, and young dogs and cats may lose their hearing temporarily when they have minor problems like ear mites or infections. When hearing loss comes on suddenly, however, you need to call your vet because there is a good chance that the eardrum has been damaged, says Sandra Priest, D.V.M., a holistic veterinarian in private practice in Knoxville, Tennessee.

A ruptured eardrum will heal on its own, but using cleaning solutions or other medications in the meantime could make things worse, she warns. To be safe, it is a good idea to have your pet checked before proceeding on your own.

medications. Short-term solutions may not be efficient, however, because they don't always correct the underlying cause of the problem. In fact, some drugs used to treat ear infections occasionally cause pets to lose their hearing altogether. In the holistic view, it is often better and safer to treat hearing problems with other more-natural, less-invasive approaches.

## The Solutions FOR DOGS & CATS

**Try acupressure.** Although they aren't sure why it works, holistic veterinarians who practice traditional Chinese medicine have found that some hearing problems can be corrected with acupressure. According to Susan G. Wynn, D.V.M., a veterinarian in Atlanta and co-editor of *Comple-*

*mentary and Alternative Veterinary Medicine*, the best points to try are those near the base of the ear, specifically the following:

🐾 TH17, located just below the ear.

🐾 SI19 and GB2, both located just in front of the ear.

Press each point with your index finger once a day for 30 seconds to a minute, then release. You can follow this with a massage, which most pets love in this area, says Dr. Wynn.

**Stop the swelling with garlic.** Dogs and cats with allergies or ear infections may go a little deaf when tissue in the ear canals swells, blocking sound from reaching the eardrum. To fight the infection that is causing the swelling, heat a little aged garlic oil until it is barely warm, then put a drop or two in the ears, suggests John Limehouse, D.V.M., a holistic veterinarian in private practice in Toluca Lake, California. Some pets will get better after one or two treatments. Garlic oil may cause problems if the eardrum is ruptured, he adds, so check with your vet before doing this at home.

**Put eucalyptus to work.** It is very common for dogs and cats to lose some of their hearing when earwax or grime accumulates in their ear canals. An excellent way to clean the ears is with a product called Animal Dermatology Laboratories Foaming Ear Cleanser, which contains eucalyptus. Available from veterinarians, the cleanser's foaming action helps break up debris and float it to the surface. And eucalyptus has mild antiseptic and soothing properties, so it kills germs and reduces swelling, says Sandra Priest, D.V.M., a holistic veterinarian in private practice in Knoxville, Tennessee. This cleanser is available only through veterinarians.

**Make use of mullein.** Another way to keep the ears clear and the hearing sharp is with mullein (*Verbascum thapsus*), an herb that acts as an expectorant and helps the body keep the ears clean naturally, says Michele Yasson, D.V.M., a holistic veterinarian in private practice in New York City and Rosendale, New York. Mullein is usually taken in capsule

form. Pets under 20 pounds can take one-quarter of the human dose once a day for about a month. Dogs 20 to 50 pounds can take one-half of the human dose, and larger dogs can take the full human dose.

**BEST BET!** **Change the diet.** Some commercial pet foods, especially generic brands, may not provide all the nutrients that pets need, which can weaken immunity and increase the risk of ear infections and hearing loss. Pets with a history of hearing problems should be given natural

---

## Meet the Experts

**Carolyn Blakey, D.V.M.,** is a holistic veterinarian in private practice in Richmond, Indiana. She is certified in acupuncture.

**John Limehouse, D.V.M.,** is a holistic veterinarian in private practice in Toluca Lake, California. He is certified in acupuncture.

**Sandra Priest, D.V.M.,** is a holistic veterinarian in private practice in Knoxville, Tennessee. She is certified in chiropractic.

**Susan G. Wynn, D.V.M.,** is a veterinarian in Atlanta and co-editor of *Complementary and Alternative Veterinary Medicine.*

**Michele Yasson, D.V.M.,** is a holistic veterinarian in private practice in New York City and Rosendale, New York. She is certified in acupuncture.

foods—or at least high-quality commercial foods supplemented with meats and vegetables, says Dr. Priest. For more information on natural diets, see page 61.

**Give them spirulina.** Made from sea algae, spirulina is packed with nutrients that can help keep the ears healthy, says Dr. Priest. "I like spirulina because it is readily available and has a nice mix of trace minerals," she says. For spirulina to be effective, however, it has to be used every day.

Pets under 15 pounds can take one-quarter of the human dose listed on the label, while larger pets can take between one-half and a full dose.

Spirulina may affect the balance of blood sugars in the body, so don't give it to pets with diabetes or Cushing's disease without checking with your veterinarian first. Even in healthy pets, you shouldn't give it forever. It is best to give it for about three months, then take a month off before using it again.

# Heart Problems

## The Signs
- Your pet coughs after exercise or when she is excited.
- Breathing is rapid and irregular.
- The abdomen is puffy or swollen.
- She collapses or faints.
- Her tongue and gums are blue, gray, or purple.

## The Cause

Dogs and cats don't get artery disease like people do, but they can develop a variety of heart problems that are just as serious. When the heart doesn't beat properly, the valves get leaky. Or when the arteries are narrower than they should be, blood has trouble circulating and may accumulate in the heart or lungs, says Jeffrey Feinman, V.M.D., a holistic veterinarian in private practice in Fairfield County in Connecticut. Pets with heart disease are often weak and tired, he adds. Without quick veterinary treatment, heart problems can be extremely serious.

Puppies and kittens are sometimes born with heart defects, but pets usually develop heart problems in their golden years. Although some heart problems can't be prevented, often they are worsened by lifestyle factors, such as poor diet, dental disease, obesity, stress, or a lack of exercise, says Junia Borden Childs, D.V.M.,

# Call the VET

Heart problems are fairly common in older pets, but they don't always cause obvious symptoms—until it is too late. If you know what to look for, however, you can often detect problems in the early stages when they are easier to treat, says Jeffrey Feinman, V.M.D., a holistic veterinarian in private practice in Fairfield County in Connecticut.

It is normal for the heart to speed up and slow down with each breath. A normal heartbeat in dogs is between 80 and 160 beats a minute. In cats, it is between 120 and 180 beats per minute. (Puppies and kittens have faster heart rates.) But if your pet's heart is beating erratically—it is skipping beats, for example, or racing—you need to call your vet right away. This is especially true when the irregular heartbeat is accompanied by other symptoms like coughing or a bloated belly. These are signs of congestive heart failure, which is always an emergency, says Michelle Tilghman, D.V.M., a holistic veterinarian in private practice in Stone Mountain, Georgia.

a holistic veterinarian in private practice in Ojai, California.

"Conventional medicine can be a lifesaver for pets with heart problems, but it is much more effective when combined with natural therapies," she says. In fact, many heart problems can be prevented altogether by taking more of a holistic approach to your pet's health. Here are a few ways to keep the heart beating strong and true.

## The Solutions FOR DOGS & CATS

**Give them garlic.** This pungent herb can help prevent blood clots from forming in the arteries, Dr. Childs says. Dogs over 50 pounds can have two teaspoons of chopped garlic a day, while smaller dogs can have between one-quarter and one-half teaspoon. Cats can't tolerate too much garlic, but it is safe to give them up to one-eighth teaspoon a day for a couple of weeks at a time.

**BEST BET! Keep blood flowing with fish oil.** Fish-oil supplements contain omega-3 fatty acids, which have been shown to slow the progression of heart disease, Dr. Childs says. You can get fish-oil supplements specifically for pets in pet supply stores and from your vet. Follow the directions on the label or ask your vet what dose is right for your pet.

If you prefer a natural diet to giving pills, fresh and canned fish (especially mackerel, salmon, and sardines) contain plenty of omega-3s. Feeding your pet fish once a week will help keep her heart working well. Be sure to cook the fish before putting it in your pet's bowl because raw fish may contain parasites, says Dr. Childs.

**Strengthen the beat with hawthorn.** Hawthorn berries (*Crataegus laevigata*) help make the heart muscle stronger, says Maria H. Glinski, D.V.M., a holistic veterinarian in private practice in Glendale, Wisconsin. She recommends giving pets with heart problems a glycerin-based hawthorn berry extract. The dose for cats and dogs weighing under 15 pounds is 8 drops. Pets 15 to 50 pounds can take 16 drops, and larger dogs can take 32 drops. All doses should be given twice a day.

Pets dislike the taste of hawthorn, so you will have to disguise it in their food, she adds. If that doesn't work, you will have to put the drops directly in their mouths. They won't thank you for it, but you will be doing their hearts a lot of good.

**Get rid of excess fluids.** Pets with heart disease may develop uncomfortable (and dangerous) accumulations of fluid in their bodies, which can cause bloating in the abdomen or legs. The homeopathic remedy Apis is a mild diuretic that can help the kidneys excrete excess fluids when pets are bloating, Dr. Glinski says. She recommends giving 30C-strength pellets twice a day until the bloating goes down or for up to one week at a time. Pets weighing 15 pounds and more can take two pellets, and smaller dogs and cats can take one pellet.

**BEST BET!** **Try a protective enzyme.** In pets with heart disease, a nutritional supplement called coenzyme $Q_{10}$ may help prevent the heart muscle from weakening, says Dr. Childs. You can give dogs over 50 pounds 30 milligrams of coenzyme $Q_{10}$ a day. Pets weighing 15 to 50 pounds can take 20 milligrams, and smaller cats and dogs can take 10 milligrams.

**Soothe them with flower essences.** Pets with heart disease have a lot of physical and emotional stress, which saps their strength and makes it hard for them to recover. To help them relax, Dr. Childs uses the flower essences star-of-Bethlehem and impatiens. You can prepare the remedy ahead of time by putting 4 drops of each essence in a one-ounce brown bottle filled with spring water. Shake it well before using and give your pet 4 drops four times a day. If she fights when you put the dropper in her mouth, try putting the drops on her

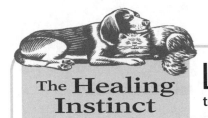

Long before there were cardiologists and EKG machines, cats were using their tongues to protect their hearts.

Veterinarians have found that cats with heart problems often spend hours licking their front legs—sometimes so vigorously that they lick away the fur, says Michelle Tilghman, D.V.M., a holistic veterinarian in private practice in Stone Mountain, Georgia. This behavior seems strange, but it makes sense from a holistic point of view. On the back of the front leg is an acupressure point called HT7, which plays a role in controlling the heart's rhythm. By licking this point, cats are instinctively performing acupressure to help the heart beat more evenly, she explains.

Licking serves another purpose as well. When dogs and cats are upset, licking calms them down, reducing the body's need for blood and oxygen. For pets with heart disease, this can help them stay relaxed and comfortable, says Dr. Tilghman.

nose or the pads of her paws, where they will be absorbed into the body. Or you can put 10 drops in her water twice a day.

**Give a calming touch.** Another way to reduce tension is with a technique called TTouch, says Dr. Childs. Massage the skin in small clockwise circles with the tips of your fingers, beginning at the six o'clock position. Complete a full circle—plus a little more—in one spot, then move to another part of the body. Doing this once or twice a day for 5 to 10 minutes will help your pet relax so that she is better able to cope with her illness.

**Restore the energy.** Holistic veterinarians believe that most physical illnesses, including heart disease, are partly caused by energy imbalances in the body. Using acupressure will help restore the proper balance, says Dr. Childs. The acupressure points to stimulate include the following:

🐾 BL13, BL14, and BL15. Stimulating these points, which are located between the third, fourth, and fifth rib spaces on either side of the spine between the shoulder blades, can help balance energy in the lungs, heart, and pericardium (the sac surrounding the heart).

🐾 HT7. Located on the outside of the front legs in a triangular depression just above the wrist, this point can help reduce heart palpitations and keep the emotions on an even keel.

**ALTERNATIVE**

## 🐾SUCCESS

### SWEET PEA'S SECOND CHANCE

Congestive heart failure is the most serious type of heart problem. Apart from giving medications, there is not a lot that mainstream veterinarians can do to treat it. So when Sweet Pea started going downhill—his vet said that he only had a few weeks to live—his owner knew that she had to try something else.

She took Sweet Pea, a 12-year-old cocker spaniel, to a holistic veterinary clinic in Stone Mountain, Georgia. After a thorough exam, Michelle Tilghman, D.V.M., gave Sweet Pea hawthorn extract (*Crataegus laevigata*) and coenzyme $Q_{10}$ to strengthen the heart muscle and vitamin E to reduce damage to the blood vessels. She used acupuncture to restore the proper balance energy in the body and encouraged Sweat Pea's owner to give him a daily massage. At the same time, she reminded her to continue with the medical treatments recommended by her veterinarian.

After a few weeks on the holistic plan, Sweet Pea had regained most of his former energy. He was breathing more easily and his heart was beating stronger. The improvement, says Dr. Tilghman, was dramatic. "His quality of life improved tremendously."

To avoid overstimulating your pet, don't hit all the acupressure points at one time, Dr. Childs adds. Stimulate one or two points a day for 30 seconds to a minute, then move on to different points later on.

**Calm her with calcium.** This essential mineral acts like a natural tranquilizer and helps the heart beat more efficiently, says Dr. Childs. A good source of calcium is bonemeal, which you can sprinkle on your pet's food. She recommends giving one-eighth teaspoon a day to cats and dogs under 15 pounds and one-half teaspoon to larger pets.

**Feed her well.** Giving your pet a top-quality diet is one of the best ways to protect her heart, says Dr. Feinman. He recommends supplementing your pet's chow with a little bit of cooked chicken or lean beef, along with fresh vegetables and maybe some fruit. (Bananas are especially good because they are rich in potassium.)

In addition, giving pets a little brown rice will help reduce fluid retention, Dr. Childs adds.

Before changing your pet's diet, ask your vet if the pet food you are using has the proper amount of sodium. Since different-size pets need different amounts of sodium, check with your vet to find out how much sodium your pet should have. Some dry dog foods contain up to 7 times the necessary amount of sodium, says Dr. Childs. Canned foods can have up to 16 times the necessary sodium for dogs and 5 times the necessary sodium for cats. This much sodium simply isn't good for pets with heart disease, she explains.

**Pump the heart with vitamins.** Vitamin C is a powerful antioxidant that can help prevent damage to the arteries in the heart, especially when it is combined with bioflavonoids, says Dr. Childs. Cats and dogs under 20 pounds can have 250 milligrams of vitamin C once or twice a day, and pets over 20 pounds can have 500 milligrams. You will know that you are giving too much if she starts having diarrhea. If that happens, reduce the amount for a few days. Keep reducing the amount until you find a dose that her bowels will tolerate.

Vitamin E is another nutrient that helps protect the heart, says Michelle Tilghman, D.V.M., a holistic veterinarian in private practice in Stone Mountain, Georgia. She recommends giving dogs and cats under 20 pounds 50 to 100 international units (IU) of vitamin E daily. Pets 20 to 50 pounds can have 200 IU. Dogs 51 to 70 pounds can have 400 IU, and larger dogs can have 600 to 800 IU a day. You don't have to force them to swallow the capsule, she adds. An easier way is to break open the capsule and squeeze the oil on their food.

**Keep them active.** "Moderate exercise is a vital factor for pets with heart problems, especially for aging pets," says Dr. Tilghman. Exercise strengthens the heart so that it beats more efficiently. It also helps keep pets trim, tones the arteries, and helps prevent fluids from accumulating in the body.

Most pets need about 20 minutes of exercise twice a day. It is easy to exercise your dog—all you have to do is put on some walking shoes and pick up the leash. Cats usually need more persuasion. Vigorous play—rolling a ball, for example, or tossing a catnip-filled mouse—is the best way to get them moving. Pets with heart problems can't always handle a lot of exercise, however, so be sure to check with your vet before starting a new exercise plan.

**Keep her teeth clean.** You wouldn't think a little dental hygiene would protect the heart, but cleaning your pet's teeth is one of the best things you can do, says Dr. Feinman. This is because pets with periodontal disease (also called gum disease) have harmful bacteria in the mouth that may get into the bloodstream, causing a dangerous inflammation in the lining of the heart or in the valves. Brushing your pet's teeth at least twice a week or, better yet, once a day with a pet toothpaste will help prevent dental problems that can lead to heart disease, he says.

## The Solutions

**FOR CATS**

**Reach for the taurine.** Cats need an essential amino acid called taurine. While there is plenty of taurine in commercial foods, cats with heart disease aren't always able to absorb enough of it. Giving your cat taurine supplements—about 500 milligrams a day—will help the heart work more efficiently, Dr. Childs says.

# HEARTWORMS

## The Signs
- Your pet is coughing or having trouble breathing.
- He is tired all the time.
- He can't tolerate exercise.

## The Cause

Mosquitoes are annoying pests, but apart from spoiling picnics and causing a little itching, they aren't a serious problem for most Americans. But for dogs—and to a lesser extent, cats—they can be life-threatening because they transmit heartworms, parasites that enter the bloodstream as larvae and migrate to the heart. Six months after reaching the heart, the larvae turn into adults, and that's when problems begin.

Full-grown heartworms remove nutrients from the body, but that is not so serious. The real threat is that heartworms eventually fill the heart like strands of spaghetti, blocking the flow of blood to the lungs and damaging the heart. "They're a silent killer," says Mona Boudreaux, D.V.M., a holistic veterinarian in private practice in Albuquerque, New Mexico. "By the time you see symptoms, they have already done damage to the heart."

Conventional and holistic veterinarians recommend giving pets medications, daily or monthly, to prevent heartworms. Once pets are infected, however, they need different medica-

tions. Unfortunately, these drugs can be dangerous for cats and, less often, for dogs. This is why holistic veterinarians supplement medical treatments with a variety of natural remedies to reduce damage to the body and help pets heal. At the same time, of course, they suggest doing everything possible to prevent pets from getting infected in the first place. Here is what they recommend.

## The Solutions FOR DOGS & CATS

**Fortify the heart.** Since heartworms and the medications used to treat them are hard on the heart,

## Call the VET

**H**eartworms are never easy to treat, and the longer your pet has been infected, the more difficult the treatments get. That is why it is so important to catch heartworms as soon as you can. The best approach is to have your dog tested for heartworms every one to three years. Dogs already infected may have symptoms such as fatigue, coughing, or rapid breathing, says Nancy Brandt, D.V.M., a holistic veterinarian in private practice in Las Vegas.

Many conditions can cause the same symptoms, she adds. But as long as you live in an area where mosquitoes thrive, it is worth getting your pet to your vet right away, even if it's the middle of winter and there aren't any mosquitoes around. It takes about six months for symptoms to appear, and your pet could have been exposed in the previous warm-weather season.

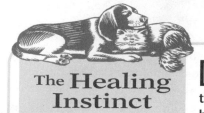

**D**ogs and cats don't like mosquitoes any more than people do, and they have their own ways of dealing with the little bloodsuckers. When mosquitoes are out in force, dogs and cats instinctively avoid the hot, muggy places where mosquitoes congregate and gravitate instead to cool, dry areas, says Michelle Tilghman, D.V.M., a holistic veterinarian in private practice in Stone Mountain, Georgia.

Dogs have an additional strategy for staying bite-free: They will roll around in dust or even in mud. This helps remove moisture from the skin and changes their scent, making them less of a target, says Dr. Tilghman.

holistic veterinarians believe it is critical to strengthen the entire cardiovascular system. One of the best ways to do this is with essential oils, says Nancy Brandt, D.V.M., a holistic veterinarian in private practice in Las Vegas. She recommends applying a drop of thyme or lavender oil behind each ear and another drop just above the pad on the back of each of the hind feet. Rub the oil into the skin, then put a drop of marjoram oil in the same places. Dilute the oils half-and-half with olive oil before applying them.

**Help him heal with noni juice.** An extract from a Tahitian plant, noni juice has antiparasitic properties. "It can help clean out the cardiovascular system as the parasites are being killed by the medicine," says Dr. Brandt. "It can also help heal the toxic effects of the drug." She recommends giving pets weighing under 15 pounds one teaspoon of noni juice once a day.

Larger dogs can take up to one tablespoon a day. Pets don't like the taste, however, so you will have to put it directly in their mouths with a needleless syringe or eyedropper.

**Strengthen the body with vitamin C.** This essential nutrient strengthens the immune system and helps the body repair tissue that has been damaged by heartworms, says Bob Ulbrich, V.M.D., a holistic veterinarian in private practice in Portland, Oregon. He recommends giving pets weighing under 15 pounds 250 milligrams of vitamin C three times a day. Dogs 15 to 50 pounds can take 500 milligrams three times daily, and larger dogs can have 1,000 milligrams three times a day. Keep giving the vitamin C until your pet is free from heartworms. Vitamin C in large amounts can cause diarrhea, so you may have to experiment a bit until you find an amount that your pet can tolerate.

**Reduce side effects with Arsenicum.** A homeopathic remedy called Arsenicum can help cleanse the body of arsenic, a key ingredient in some heartworm medications, says Dr. Ulbrich. Use a 6X to 30X potency two or three times a day for up to two weeks. Dogs and cats under 15 pounds can take one or two pellets at a time, and those over 15 pounds can take three to five pellets.

"If the pellets are too big, crush them onto a clean piece of paper and pour the powder on your pet's tongue or under his lip," he advises. Arsenicum shouldn't be given with food, he adds, so don't give it for 30 minutes before or after eating.

**Protect the liver.** Most medications are processed by the liver, so it is critical to give this organ some extra support when your pet is being treated for heartworms, says Michelle Tilghman, D.V.M., a holistic veterinarian in private practice in Stone Mountain, Georgia. She recommends using herbal supplements containing milk thistle (*Silybum marianum*), dandelion (*Taraxacum officinale*), or red clover (*Trifolium pratense*), which are known for their liver-protecting properties. Dogs over 50 pounds can take the full human dose. Pets 15 to 50 pounds can take one-half of the human dose, and those under 15 pounds can take one-quarter of the human dose. "If possible, start giving it to your pet two to three weeks be-fore treatment begins," she says. "Keep him on it during the treatment and for at least a month afterward."

Another way to protect the liver is with B vitamins, which help the body break down and detoxify the compounds in the medications, says Dr. Tilghman. She recommends giving 50 milligrams of a B-complex vitamin for every 20 pounds of weight once a day.

**BEST BET!** **Practice prevention.** Unless you live in an area with no mosquitoes, the only sure way to protect your pets is to give them preventive medications. Many holistic veterinarians are uncomfortable using these medications, but the risk of heartworms is so great, they say, that

## Meet the Experts

**Mona Boudreaux, D.V.M.,** is a holistic veterinarian in private practice in Albuquerque, New Mexico. She is certified in acupuncture and chiropractic.

**Nancy Brandt, D.V.M.,** is a holistic veterinarian in private practice in Las Vegas. She is certified in acupuncture.

**Michelle Tilghman, D.V.M.,** is a holistic veterinarian in Stone Mountain, Georgia. She is certified in acupuncture.

**Bob Ulbrich, V.M.D.,** is a holistic veterinarian in private practice in Portland, Oregon. He is certified in homeopathy.

giving preventive medicine is the only responsible alternative, especially if you live in a high-risk area. Some medications are given once a day, but most pet owners prefer longer-lasting drugs, which are given once a month.

**Strengthen his resistance with whole foods.** Dogs and cats are more likely to resist heartworms when they are given all-natural foods, which help keep the immune system strong, says Dr. Tilghman. "If you don't want to make their foods at home, use a commercial food that is free of additives and preservatives. Add fresh vegetables to the food to make sure that he gets all the nutrients he needs." For more information on natural diets, see page 61.

## The Solutions *FOR DOGS*

**Give him garlic.** This pungent herb repels mosquitoes, cleanses the blood, and strengthens the immune system, says Dr. Boudreaux. Dogs over 50 pounds can have as much as two teaspoons of garlic a day, and smaller dogs can have one-quarter to one-half teaspoon a day. Garlic can be a problem for cats, so don't give them too much. A safe limit is one-eighth teaspoon or less a day for up to two weeks at a time.

# HEAT SENSITIVITY

## The Signs
- Your pet pants a lot even when the temperature is cool.
- She appears tired during the warm months.
- Her gums are suddenly bright red.

## The Cause
Dogs and cats don't take off their coats in warm weather, and they don't sweat like people do. (An exception is the nearly hairless Sphynx cat, which sweats so much that it needs to be toweled off every day.) Pets pant in order to dispel heat, but it isn't a very efficient system; they naturally run a little on the warm side. And some pets, such as those with dark, heavy coats, are much more susceptible to heat than others.

Veterinarians worry when pets seem unusually warm, because overheating may be a symptom of underlying problems. A dog who can't walk

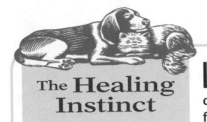

## The **Healing Instinct**

Long before there were fans, air conditioners, and comfortable backyard pools, dogs and cats developed their own strategies for beating the heat, strategies that they still use today. Besides looking for cool, shady spots, they will often dig into the ground a few inches, where the temperatures are cooler.

Another trick—one that is shared by humans—is to slow down their pace during the day when the temperatures are highest. Moving slowly and keeping the body's metabolism at idle helps prevent internal temperatures from rising.

half a block without overheating may have a heart problem or be overweight.

You will want to see your vet right away if your pet is suddenly panting much more than usual. The chances are good, however, that she just can't stand the heat. Here are a few ways to keep her a little cooler.

## The Solutions
FOR DOGS & CATS

**Mist her with essences.** A blend of five flower essences called Bach Rescue Remedy can help decrease stress when your pet is overheated, says Kimberly Henneman, D.V.M., a holistic veterinarian in private practice in Utah. You can put three to five drops of Rescue Remedy in her drinking water, but you will get quicker results if you combine five drops with a cup of spring water in a mister and give her a quick spritz whenever she seems to be getting warm.

**Stop the heat with Belladonna.** Dogs and cats that are exhausted from the heat will quickly revive when given homeopathic Belladonna, says Betsy Walker Harrison, D.V.M., a holistic veterinarian in private practice in Wimberley, Texas.

"It's also the primary homeopathic remedy for heatstroke," adds Dr. Henneman. She recommends giving pets weighing under 15 pounds one pellet of Belladonna 30C every 30 minutes until they start feeling better. Larger pets can take two pellets every 30 minutes. If your pet isn't getting better by the third dose, Belladonna probably isn't going to help, and you should call your vet, she says.

**BEST BET!** **Encourage her to drink.** Pets that are sensitive to heat need to drink a lot of water, especially during the summer months. The problem is that the body's thirst mechanism isn't always as sensitive as it should be, so pets may not drink all the water they really need. To encourage them to drink more, Dr. Harrison recommends giving them ice chips or ice cubes throughout the day. Many pets like crunching ice, and it helps get extra fluids into their systems.

Another way to get the benefits of water—at least with dogs—is to get them wet. Spritzing them with a hose or encouraging them to lie in a kiddie pool will cool them off in a hurry. Even sprinkling the grass where they play will keep them a little cooler, Dr. Harrison says.

**Replace electrolytes.** When dogs and cats lose fluids, they also lose electrolytes, essential minerals like calcium and sodium that they need to stay healthy. Giving your pets an electrolyte solution like Pedialyte or Gatorade will quickly replace these minerals, and they will probably like the taste. You can add several tablespoons of one of these drinks to your pet's water every day, says Dr. Harrison.

**BEST BET!** **Get the air moving.** Even on mild days, your pet's coat traps a lot of heat and holds it next to the skin. Putting her in front of a fan or, better yet, near an air conditioner will circulate air through the

## Call the VET

For pets that are sensitive to heat, the steamy summer months are an uncomfortable time. This is also when the risk of heatstroke is highest. The *T. rex* of overheating, heatstroke is a dangerous condition in which the body's temperature rises to over 104°F. Pets with heatstroke will have glassy-looking eyes, and they will have difficulty walking or standing up.

Heatstroke is an emergency that needs medical attention as soon as possible. Even before you take your pet to the vet, however, you need to start cooling her body down by putting her in a tub of cool water, for example, or by applying wet towels or ice packs to her body, says Susan G. Wynn, D.V.M., a veterinarian in Atlanta and co-editor of *Complementary and Alternative Veterinary Medicine*. When you are in the car, turn the air conditioner on high and get to the vet as quickly as you can.

## Meet the Experts

**Betsy Walker Harrison, D.V.M.,** is a holistic veterinarian in private practice in Wimberley, Texas. She is certified in homeopathy.

**Kimberly Henneman, D.V.M.,** is a holistic veterinarian in private practice in Utah. She is certified in acupuncture and chiropractic.

**Susan G. Wynn, D.V.M.,** is a veterinarian in Atlanta and co-editor of *Complementary and Alternative Veterinary Medicine*.

fur and help keep her cool, says Dr. Harrison.

**Check for dehydration.** Since pets that are sensitive to heat may run low on fluids, you need to watch for dehydration, says Dr. Harrison. A quick test is to gently pinch the area between the shoulder blades. The skin should snap back into its usual position when you let go. Skin that stays in the pinched position for three to five seconds is a sign that your pet is dehydrated, and you will need to call your vet right away.

# HIP DYSPLASIA

## The Signs
- Your pet has trouble getting up or climbing stairs.
- She limps or sways unevenly when she walks.
- She cries or winces when you touch her hips.

## The Cause

The ball-shaped upper end of the thighbone is designed to fit snugly into the socket of the hipbone. But in dogs with hip dysplasia, the hip socket may be too shallow to firmly cradle the thighbone, or the surrounding muscles and tendons may be too weak to hold the bones together. In either case, hip dysplasia puts a lot of stress on one or both hip joints, causing pain and inflammation as well as difficulty walking or getting up.

Hip dysplasia can strike any dog (cats rarely get it), although large breeds like German shepherds and Saint Bernards have the highest risk. Since hip dysplasia is usually an inherited condition, there is no easy way to prevent it, although keeping your dog trim and active will help reduce her risks. Once a dog has it, the usual treatment is to give anti-inflammatory painkilling medications like cortisone or aspirin-like drugs during flare-ups.

These drugs can stop the symptoms, but they can cause uncomfortable and sometimes dangerous side effects. That is why holistic veterinarians prefer natural alternatives that may be just as effective as drugs for relieving pain and increasing mobility.

## The Solutions FOR DOGS

**BEST BET!** **Press away pain.** There are three acupressure points—BL54, GB29, and GB30—surrounding the bony hipbone that can be stimulated for quick pain relief, says Albert J. Simpson, D.V.M., a holistic veterinarian in private practice in Oregon City, Oregon. "Make a three-finger tripod with your thumb and index and middle fingers and surround the bone," he says. Place your index finger at the top of the bone and your thumb and middle finger on each side, then press for about 60 seconds.

**Supplement the joints.** Hip dysplasia puts uneven pressure on the joints, which can wear away the protective cartilage and possibly cause a painful form of arthritis, says Nancy Scanlan, D.V.M., a holistic veterinarian in private practice in Sherman Oaks, California. Glucosamine supplements, available in health food stores, help the body repair cartilage and increase lubrication in the joints, she says. Dogs weighing under 50 pounds can take 250 milligrams of glucosamine once a day, while larger dogs need about 500 milligrams.

Some veterinarians recommend giving Cosequin, a combination of glucosamine and another supplement called chondroitin sulfate, which can help repair damaged cartilage in the hip. You can give pets 10 milligrams per pound of body weight twice a day, says Susan G. Wynn, D.V.M., a veterinarian in Atlanta and co-editor of *Complementary and Alternative Veterinary Medicine*. Cosequin is available from veterinarians and shouldn't be used in pets with liver problems or clotting disorders, she adds.

**Stop the swelling.** Much of the pain of hip dysplasia is caused by inflammation inside and surrounding the joint. Vitamins E and C have been shown to reduce inflammation as well as cartilage damage, says Dr. Simpson. Dogs weighing under 15 pounds need about 10 international units (IU) of vitamin E a day. Dogs between 15 and 50 pounds need 20 IU, and larger dogs can take 30 IU.

For vitamin C, Dr. Simpson recommends using the powdered ester form, which is easier to digest than the ascorbic acid form that people use. He recommends giving dogs over 50 pounds one-quarter teaspoon (about 1,000 milligrams) of ester vitamin C a day. Dogs between 15 and 50 pounds can take one-eighth teaspoon, and smaller dogs need just a sprinkling. The easiest way to give vitamin C is to sprinkle it on your pet's food, he says. Vitamin C can cause diarrhea, so you may have to reduce the dose until you find an amount your pet will tolerate.

**BEST BET!** **Massage away the pain.** Giving dogs a daily massage relaxes tight muscles and relieves pain by increasing circulation, says Patricia Whalen-Shaw, a registered massage therapist and owner of Optissage, an animal massage school in Circleville, Ohio. She recommends starting with slow, firm strokes to warm up the muscles, followed by fingertip pressure on the muscles along either side of the spine in the lower back and then down the back legs. Don't press on the bones, she adds. Just rub the muscles that lie alongside them.

**Give herbal relief.** A popular Indian remedy for joint pain is the herb boswellia (*Boswellia serrata*), says Dr. Simpson. The herb is available from some holistic veterinarians and pet supply catalogs. You will probably need to give your dog between 150 and 200 milligrams twice a day, although you will want to check with your vet to get the precise dose, he advises.

**Put heat on the hips.** One of the quickest remedies for hip dysplasia is to apply a little warmth to the area, which increases circulation and reduces pain in the joint, says Randy Caviness, D.V.M., clinical instructor of small animal acupuncture at Tufts University School of Veterinary Medicine in North Grafton, Massachusetts, and a holistic veterinarian in Concord. He recommends wrapping a hot-water bottle or heating pad in a thick towel and applying it to achy hips for about 10 minutes once or twice a day.

**BEST BET!** **Keep her trim.** Nothing is cuter than a chubby puppy, but research has shown that young dogs that are fed too much grow too quickly, which can cause hip problems later on, says Dr. Scanlan. If your dog is already showing too much padding, talk to your vet about putting her on a weight-loss plan.

## Meet the Experts

**Randy Caviness, D.V.M.,** is a clinical instructor of small animal acupuncture at Tufts University School of Veterinary Medicine in North Grafton, Massachusetts, and a holistic veterinarian in Concord. He is certified in acupuncture and chiropractic.

**Nancy Scanlan, D.V.M.,** is a holistic veterinarian in private practice in Sherman Oaks, California. She is certified in acupuncture and chiropractic.

**Albert J. Simpson, D.V.M.,** is a holistic veterinarian in private practice in Oregon City, Oregon. He is certified in acupuncture and chiropractic.

**Patricia Whalen-Shaw** is a registered massage therapist and owner of Optissage, an animal massage school in Circleville, Ohio.

**Susan G. Wynn, D.V.M.,** is a veterinarian in Atlanta and co-editor of *Complementary and Alternative Veterinary Medicine*.

**BEST BET!** **Exercise often.** Dogs that stay active develop strong muscles that help support the hip joints, says Dr. Simpson. Even if your dog already has hip dysplasia, regular exercise can reduce pain and stiffness, he says. Walking is great exercise (running may be too hard on sore hips). Swimming is even better because the water helps support your dog's weight, taking pressure off her hips. Vigorous exercise isn't always good for dogs with hip problems, so be sure to check with your veterinarian before starting a new program.

# HIVES

## The Signs
- Your pet has red welts and is unusually itchy.
- The skin on his face is swelling.

## The Cause

Even though it is protected by fur, your pet's skin can be pretty sensitive at times. When dogs and cats brush against something that they are allergic to, they may break out in hives—ugly, itchy welts that can appear within minutes. Hives usually go away within 24 hours, but, like unwelcome guests, they sometimes come right back.

Hives can be triggered by many different things, states Stephanie Chalmers, D.V.M., a veterinary dermatologist and holistic veterinarian in private practice in Santa Rosa, California. Insect stings, pollen, and ingredients in food may cause hives. In some cases, even sunlight may trigger an outbreak.

Mainstream veterinarians sometimes give pets antihistamines to quell the allergic reaction and, in severe cases, steroids to control inflammation. Since hives go away fairly quickly, it usually isn't necessary to use powerful drugs, Dr. Chalmers says. A better approach is to use natural remedies to ease the discomfort—and to figure out why your pet is having reactions in the first place.

## The Solutions FOR DOGS & CATS

**Give an oatmeal bath.** A time-tested remedy to ease the itching of hives is to give pets an oatmeal bath. Dr. Chalmers recommends filling the bathtub—or, for large dogs, a kiddie pool—with cool water and adding half a packet of colloidal oatmeal (like Aveeno). Encourage your pet to soak

## Call the VET

Hives usually aren't serious and disappear almost as quickly as they show up, but sometimes they keep coming back. This may be a sign that your pet has a weak or damaged immune system, and you are going to need a veterinarian's help—both to solve the underlying problem and to figure out what your pet is sensitive to.

It doesn't happen often, but sometimes hives are the first sign of a more serious allergic reaction. If your pet breaks out in hives and seems weak or is having trouble breathing, it is an emergency, and you should get him to a vet right away.

in the water for about 10 minutes. If the water doesn't cover the itchy areas, you can use a pitcher of water to pour water over his body until his fur and skin are soaked. Keep giving baths once a day until he is feeling better.

Of course, cats (and some dogs) hate baths and won't get in without a fight. An alternative is to use a colloidal oatmeal compress. "Mix some oatmeal powder with cool water in a bowl until you get a milky solution. Then saturate a washcloth in the mixture, squeeze it out, and gently hold it over the irritated skin for 5 to 10 minutes," Dr. Chalmers advises.

**Lather up some relief.** Pet supply stores sell a variety of oatmeal shampoos, which can help relieve itchy skin. Dr. Chalmers recommends using an oatmeal shampoo that also contains aloe vera, an herb that is soothing for the skin. After working

up a lather, let it soak into the fur for a few minutes, then rinse your pet well, she advises.

**Brew some tea.** Black and green teas contain compounds called tannins, which can help stop itching, says Dr. Chalmers. Brew a cup of tea, allow it to cool, and pour it into bathwater. Or you can soak a cloth in room-temperature tea and apply it as a compress.

**Soothe with flower essences.** Holistic veterinarians often use flower essences to relieve itchy skin. A good combination of essences is agrimony, beech, cherry plum, crab apple, olive, and walnut, says Wanda Vockeroth, D.V.M., a holistic veterinarian in private practice in Calgary, Alberta, Canada. To prepare the mixture, put two or three drops of each essence in a one-ounce dropper bottle filled with spring or purified water. Give your pet a dropperful of the mixture twice a day. "You can also put it in a spray bottle and spritz the itchy spots or dab some on a cloth and wipe it on," she adds.

**BEST BET!** **Beat the bees.** When hives are caused by insect stings, you can ease the discomfort with homeopathic Ledum or Urtica urens, says Dr. Chalmers. She recommends using the 30C potency, giving cats one to three pellets and dogs three to five pellets once a day. If necessary, you can repeat the treatment 24 hours later, she says. Use these remedies one at a time. If your pet doesn't improve in two to three hours, try another remedy.

**Block the poison.** Some dogs and cats are sensitive to poison ivy and will break out in hives at the slightest contact. Homeopathic Rhus tox., given every 15 to 30 minutes for up to two hours, will often ease the

---

**Meet the Experts**

**Stephanie Chalmers, D.V.M.,** is a veterinary dermatologist and holistic veterinarian in private practice in Santa Rosa, California. She is certified in homeopathy.

**Jeanne Olson, D.V.M.,** is a holistic veterinarian in private practice in North Pole, Alaska.

**Wanda Vockeroth, D.V.M.,** is a holistic veterinarian in private practice in Calgary, Alberta, Canada. She is certified in acupuncture.

---

discomfort, says Jeanne Olson, D.V.M., a holistic veterinarian in private practice in North Pole, Alaska. She recommends using the 30C or 30X potencies. Pets under 50 pounds can take one pellet. Dogs 50 pounds and over can take two or three pellets.

# HOT SPOTS

## The Signs
- Your dog has one or more circular sores that are red, swollen, and oozing.
- The sores get larger within hours.
- The sores are painful, smelly, and hot to the touch.

## The Cause
During the warm months especially, the combination of bug bites, allergy flare-ups, and even hair mats can make dogs perpetually itchy. They react by scratching and biting their skin—sometimes for hours. "Eventually, all that scratching does some damage," states Lowell Ackerman,

## Call the VET

The amazing thing about hot spots is how quickly they spread. Your dog might have a thumb-size sore on his flank in the morning and a palm-size sore by nightfall. The sores look ugly but are rarely serious. "They heal so quickly that you almost never need to give your dog antibiotics," says Lowell Ackerman, D.V.M., a veterinary dermatologist in Mesa, Arizona, and author of the *Guide to Skin and Haircoat Problems in Dogs*.

Sometimes, however, hot spots get so sore and tender that your dog won't let you near them. Less often, the infection that is causing the sore travels deep inside, rather than spreading across the surface of the skin. This usually occurs when the hot spot has been covered by a thick ointment, Dr. Ackerman explains. "The infection can't get through the ointment, so it turns around and goes the other way."

Hot spots that are extremely tender or don't get better within a day or two need to be treated by your vet. He may need to give the sores a deep cleaning and possibly use medications such as steroids to reduce the inflammation.

---

D.V.M., a veterinary dermatologist in Mesa, Arizona, and author of the *Guide to Skin and Haircoat Problems in Dogs*.

Once the skin is damaged, bacteria move in and quickly spread among the hair follicles. This can cause painful, rapidly spreading sores known as hot spots. Cats rarely get hot spots, but they are quite common in dogs, especially breeds like Chow Chows, which have heavy double coats that often get matted. The sores can appear anywhere but usually crop up in areas dogs are able to reach, like on the tail, flanks, back, and rump.

Hot spots look scary, but in most cases they only involve the top layer of skin. You don't need to use powerful drugs or lotions, says Dr. Ackerman. Most hot spots are easy to treat with natural home remedies. Here is what veterinarians advise.

## The Solutions

**BEST BET!** **Dry the sore with Burow's.** A traditional remedy called Burow's solution, available in some drugstores and grocery stores, dries the sores and helps them heal more quickly, says Dr. Ackerman. He recommends spraying the hot spots with Burow's solution two or three times a day until they heal.

**Coat it with boric acid.** It sounds like powerful stuff from a laboratory, but boric acid is a natural element that acts as a mild antiseptic. Applied to sores, it kills bacteria and helps speed healing, says Steven A. Melman, V.M.D., a veterinarian in private practice in Potomac, Maryland, and Palm Springs, California, and author of *Skin Diseases of Dogs and Cats*. He recommends dabbing a solution containing acetic and boric acids (like DermaPet Ear and Skin Cleanser), available from veterinarians, on hot spots once or twice a day.

**BEST BET!** **Soothe pain with calendula (*Calendula officinalis*).** Made from marigolds, calendula tincture is very soothing and helps ease the pain of hot spots, says Michelle Tilghman, D.V.M., a holistic veterinarian in private practice in Stone Mountain, Georgia. Dilute the tincture half-and-half with water and place the bottle into steaming (not boiling) water for seven minutes to remove the alcohol. Apply it with a cotton ball two or three times a day.

**BEST BET!** **Cool the heat with witch hazel.** As the name suggests, hot spots can literally be warm to the touch. You can cool things down a bit by applying a little witch hazel. Made from a plant called hamamelis, witch

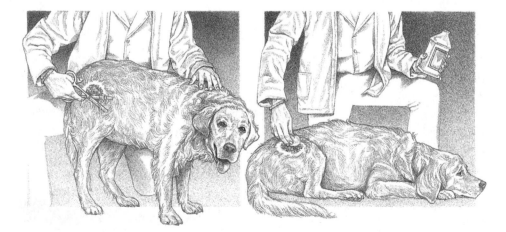

Hot spots will heal quickly as long as they get plenty of air and stay dry and clean. To help air circulate, use electric clippers or a pair of blunt-nosed scissors to trim a one-inch border around the hot spot so that the fur is about one-eighth inch high.

Rinse the area thoroughly with warm water. Using a cotton ball, dab the spot with witch hazel, then gently pat it dry.

hazel evaporates almost instantly, making hot spots feel more comfortable. You can use witch hazel two or three times a day, says Dr. Ackerman.

**BEST BET!** **Brew some tea.** Another natural remedy for hot spots is black tea. It contains tannic acid, which acts as an astringent—meaning that it dries the sores and helps them heal more quickly, says Dr. Ackerman. All you have to do is soak a tea bag in hot water, let it cool, and apply the bag directly to the sore for five minutes. Do this three or four times a day.

**Stop the itch cycle.** To stop the itching that causes hot spots, try a homeopathic remedy, such as Homeo-Pet Hot Spot Dermatitis, says Carolyn Blakey, D.V.M., a holistic veterinarian in private practice in Richmond, Indiana. Dogs can take 10 drops and cats 3 drops, both three times a day. If the problem doesn't go away in a few days or if it clears up and then returns, you will want to call your vet, she adds.

**Stop the scratching from the inside out.** Holistic veterinarians sometimes give dogs with hot spots a Chinese medicine called Armadillo Counter-Poison Pill. It contains a combination of herbs that can help relieve itchy skin. "I use it in place of antihistamines," says Dr. Tilghman. You can find Armadillo Counter-Poison Pill in health food stores and natural apothecaries. Give pets weighing under 15 pounds one pill a day. Pets 15 to 50 pounds can take two pills a day, and larger dogs can take three pills a day, she advises.

**Stop the fleas.** Hot spots often occur when dogs have an allergic reaction to flea bites, so it is essential to get rid of fleas as well as ticks, says Alexander Werner, V.M.D., a veterinary dermatologist in private practice in Studio City, California. For more information on getting rid of fleas, see page 259.

**Comb out the mats.** Hair mats

---

## Meet the Experts

**Lowell Ackerman, D.V.M.,** is a veterinary dermatologist in Mesa, Arizona, and the author of the *Guide to Skin and Haircoat Problems in Dogs*.

**Carolyn Blakey, D.V.M.,** is a holistic veterinarian in private practice in Richmond, Indiana. She is certified in acupuncture.

**Steven A. Melman, V.M.D.,** is a veterinarian with practices in Potomac, Maryland, and Palm Springs, California, and the author of *Skin Diseases of Dogs and Cats*.

**Michelle Tilghman, D.V.M.,** is a holistic veterinarian in private practice in Stone Mountain, Georgia. She is certified in acupuncture.

**Alexander Werner, V.M.D.,** is a veterinary dermatologist in private practice in Studio City, California.

**Susan G. Wynn, D.V.M.,** is a veterinarian in Atlanta and co-editor of *Complementary and Alternative Veterinary Medicine*.

that lie against the skin are another common cause of hot spots. "They are a great hiding place for fleas and ticks," says Dr. Ackerman. "And when moisture and heat collect, bacteria can grow like crazy."

Hair mats can be difficult (and painful) to remove because they lie so close to the skin. Preventing them is easy, however. All you have to do is brush your dog at least twice a week, preferably once each day. Regular grooming also helps the skin breathe, which makes it harder for infections to get started, says Dr. Ackerman.

**Discourage the licking.** A dog's idea of first-aid is to lick whatever hurts. It is not a bad approach—some experts believe saliva helps some wounds heal—but dogs can take a good thing a little too far. They will sometimes lick hot spots so long and so vigorously that they never heal. A good way to stop the licking is to use a distraction, says Susan G. Wynn, D.V.M., a veterinarian in Atlanta and co-editor of *Complementary and Alternative Veterinary Medicine*. A treat or a walk around the block can help your dog focus on something other than the hot spot. A game of catch or a quick training session can also help.

# House Soiling

## The Signs
- Your pet has recently started having accidents.
- Your cat is missing the litter box.
- Your dog urinates when she is excited or nervous.
- You are finding deposits on your possessions.
- Your dog leaves wet spots where she has been sleeping.

## The Cause

Bathroom etiquette can have a significant impact on your relationship with your pets. After all, it is hard to feel loving and affectionate when you are always discovering piles or puddles in the house.

Cats and dogs have an instinctive need to perform potty duty away from their "den." This is what makes it easy to train dogs to use the yard and cats to use a litter box. But all pets occasionally have accidents, especially puppies and kittens, which sometimes aren't fully reliable until they are about six months old. Even adult dogs can hold it for only 8 to 10 hours and

## Call the VET

Even though occasional accidents are nearly inevitable, most pets quickly learn the house-training basics. Dogs and cats that have always been reliable but are suddenly starting to make messes in the house probably have a health problem, says George Carley, D.V.M., a holistic veterinarian in private practice in Tulsa, Oklahoma.

Bladder infections, parasites, and diabetes are just a few of the conditions that can make it difficult for pets to control themselves, Dr. Carley explains. So you should consider house soiling to be a valuable warning sign and call your vet right away.

will give up trying when they have been left alone too long.

Accidents are understandable, but some pets are much more accident-prone than others. Dogs and cats that are upset or under stress, for example, may forget their training. "In some cases, older pets develop a kind of senility in which they just don't remember their house training anymore," adds George Carley, D.V.M., a holistic veterinarian in private practice in Tulsa, Oklahoma.

House soiling is often caused by physical problems such as urinary tract infections or conditions such as arthritis, which make it hard for pets to move quickly enough to get outside. It is also common in spayed females because they don't produce a lot of estrogen, a hormone that adds tension to the muscle that controls urination.

Veterinarians sometimes use med-

ications to reduce stress, add holding power to the urinary muscles, or improve behavior problems. The problem with medications is that they may cause side effects. As long as your pet is generally healthy, you can often control house soiling by combining natural treatments with simple training procedures, in which you encourage your pet to go in the right place, then praise her lavishly when she does. Even if your pet does need medications for a physical condition, approaching house soiling from a whole-life perspective may take care of the symptom as well as the underlying problems.

## The Solutions FOR DOGS & CATS

**Refresh their memories with supplements.** Older pets sometimes have trouble absorbing all the nutrients from their food, and this can lead to memory lapses and accidents, says Dr. Carley. He recommends giving them a combination supplement called Missing Link, which contains important nutrients along with digestive enzymes that will help them digest their food more thoroughly. You can get Missing Link at pet supply stores. Cats need one-half teaspoon once a day. Dogs under 15 pounds can take a teaspoon. Those weighing 15 to 50 pounds need two teaspoons, and larger dogs can take one tablespoon once a day.

**Improve control with acupressure.** There are a number of acupressure points that can help direct healing energy to the parts of the body that play a role in house soiling, says Joanne Stefanatos, D.V.M., a holistic veterinarian in private practice in Las Vegas. For example:

🐾 Pressing the points LI4, LI11, and ST25 can help stop diarrhea and other bowel-control problems.

🐾 The acupressure points BL67, BL1, SP6, and SP10 can be stimulated to stop urinating in the house.

Use your index finger to apply even pressure to each of the points.

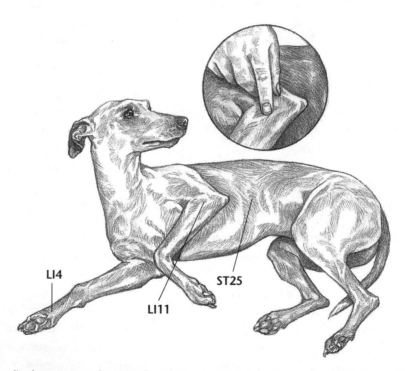

To stop diarrhea, you need to stimulate three acupressure points: LI4, located between the dewclaw and the first long toe of the paw in the front leg; LI11, located on the outside of the front legs at the elbow creases; and ST25, located on the abdomen.

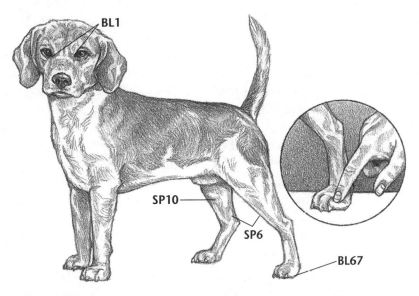

There are four points for stopping inappropriate urination: BL67, located on the outside edge of the outside toe on the rear foot; BL1, located on the inside corner of each eye; SP6, located on the inside of the rear legs, just above the hocks (the ankles); and SP10, located above the knee on the inside of the rear leg.

Press each point for about 30 seconds twice a day until your pet has gained more control, says Dr. Stefanatos.

**Reduce stress with lavender.** The scent of the essential oil of lavender acts as a natural sedative that helps calm pets that are upset or anxious, says Donna M. Starita, D.V.M., a holistic veterinarian in private practice in Boring, Oregon. She recommends dabbing a little bit of the oil, diluted half-and-half with vegetable oil, on the fur on your pet's throat. This keeps the scent near her face but in a place where she can't lick it off. You can apply the oil every day for up to a month after the problem is under control.

**Reduce stress with essences.** Another way to keep pets calm is to give them the flower essence mimulus, says Thomas Van Cise, D.V.M., a holistic veterinarian in private practice in Norco, California. It works fairly quickly, and you should start seeing an improvement within a week. He recommends putting a dropperful of the essence in your pet's water once a day.

**BEST BET! Lower your voice.** Dogs and cats crave our approval almost more than we can imagine, and yelling at them when they have made a mess can rattle them so much that they are more likely to do it again, says H. Ellen Whiteley, D.V.M., a veterinary consultant in Guadalupita, New Mexico, and consultant for *The Country Vet's Home Remedies for Cats*. What's more, unless you actually catch them in the act, they won't have the foggiest idea why you are yelling, she explains.

A better approach is to clean the area thoroughly so that your pet won't be attracted to the scent later on. And take advantage of those times when you see a "mistake" in progress, Dr. Whiteley adds. That's your chance to quickly hustle your pet outside or to her box and praise her for doing her thing. This positive reinforcement works better than yelling to help her understand which places make you happy, she says.

## The Solutions FOR DOGS

**BEST BET!** **Give her a smaller space.** Unless your dog has a medical problem, one of the easiest ways to stop house soiling is to confine her in a crate when you aren't going to be around, says Dr. Whiteley. Dogs that are trained to stay in a crate will do everything possible to control themselves, and they will be more likely to let you know when they need to go out.

Puppies take naturally to crates, but older dogs may be a bit resistant at first. Ask your vet for advice on the best way to crate-train your dog, she advises.

**Build her confidence.** Dogs that live in the wild will sometimes show deference to other dogs by urinating. Vets call this submissive urination, and some dogs do it whenever they are anxious or excited, says Dr. Stefanatos. The flower essences centaury or larch will help make dogs more confident and secure so that they are less likely to feel the need for submissive displays, she says. You can squirt a dropperful of either essence in your dog's water for her to sip throughout the day.

Another way to stop submissive urination is simply to walk away and ignore the behavior, says Wayne Hunthausen, D.V.M., a veterinary behaviorist in Westwood, Kansas, and author of the *Handbook of Behaviour Problems in Dogs and Cats*. Dogs urinate submissively because they want you to acknowledge their subordinate status. If you simply ignore it, your dog will learn that the message isn't having an impact, and she will be more likely to find other more acceptable ways to communicate, he explains.

## The Solutions FOR CATS

**BEST BET!** **Keep the box clean.** Cats hate a messy litter box and will sometimes take their business elsewhere rather than use it, says Pam Johnson Bennett, a feline behavior consultant in Nashville and author of

*Twisted Whiskers*. Cleaning the box daily is the best way to ensure that it gets used, she says. It is also important to have a different litter box for each cat in the family and to find a litter that your cat likes. Your best bet is to use unscented litter. The scented kind may smell good to you, but cats often dislike the smell and won't go near it.

**Find a cat-friendly location.** Just as cats are particular about what goes in their litter box, they are also fussy about where it goes. When your cat starts missing, it could be a sign that you need to find another place for the box—preferably in an area where there is some privacy and not too much foot traffic, such as the laundry room, Bennett says.

**Stop territorial spraying.** Some cats, usually unneutered males, will spray urine as a way of marking their territory. The urine contains chemical scents called pheromones that tell other cats to stay away. You can use their instincts against them by using a product such as Feliway, available from vets, which contains feline pheromones. By spraying it in the same places where your cat sprays, he will think another cat has already claimed the area and will be less likely to spray, says Dr. Carley.

**BEST BET!** **Use an odor neutralizer.** Just as cats are repelled by the pheromones from other cats, they are attracted to their own, which means they will often return to the same place. The only way to stop the cycle is to clean the area thoroughly, then treat it with a urine neutralizer such as Simple Solution Stain and Odor Remover. Available in pet supply stores and catalogs, it contains natural enzymes that break down and eliminate the scents in urine. A good

## Meet the Experts

**Pam Johnson Bennett** is a feline behavior consultant in Nashville and the author of *Twisted Whiskers* and *Psycho Kitty*.

**George Carley, D.V.M.,** is a holistic veterinarian in private practice in Tulsa, Oklahoma. He is certified in acupuncture.

**Wayne Hunthausen, D.V.M.,** is a veterinary behaviorist in Westwood, Kansas, and the author of the *Handbook of Behaviour Problems in Dogs and Cats*.

**Donna M. Starita, D.V.M.,** is a holistic veterinarian in private practice in Boring, Oregon.

**Joanne Stefanatos, D.V.M.,** is a holistic veterinarian in private practice in Las Vegas. She is certified in acupuncture and chiropractic.

**Thomas Van Cise, D.V.M.,** is a holistic veterinarian in private practice in Norco, California. He is certified in acupuncture.

**H. Ellen Whiteley, D.V.M.,** is a veterinary consultant in Guadalupita, New Mexico, and consultant for *The Country Vet's Home Remedies for Cats*.

follow-up treatment is to clean the area with a lemon-scented cleaner. Cats dislike the smell of lemon and will be reluctant to return to the scene of the crime.

One problem with cat urine is that even when you can smell that there is a problem, you can't always tell where it is coming from. A handy way to find out is to dim the lights and walk around with a portable black light, which causes cat urine to glow.

# Hyperactivity

## The Signs
- Your pet is always pacing or following you around.
- He constantly races around, chases his tail, or spins in circles.
- His eyes looked unfocused, and you can't get his attention.

## The Cause

It is normal for puppies and kittens to zoom around and always be underfoot. They have tons of energy and will start calming down within the first year or two. But some pets, usually dogs, are hyperactive and never get past this high-energy stage. "It's as if they don't have an Off switch," says Mary Lee Nitschke, Ph.D., professor of psychology at Linfield College in Portland, Oregon, and an animal behaviorist in Beaverton.

Hyperactivity, caused by an imbalance of chemicals in the brain, is fairly rare. Mainstream veterinarians sometimes use mood-altering drugs like fluoxetine (Prozac) to make hyperactive pets a little bit calmer. But holistic veterinarians have found that there are simpler—and safer—approaches. Here is what they recommend.

## The Solutions  FOR DOGS

**Calm them with scents.** Holistic veterinarians often use aromatherapy to make dogs calmer and easier to be around. "Oil of bergamot works for very wild, hyperactive pets," says Donna M. Starita, D.V.M., a holistic veterinarian in private practice in Boring, Oregon. She recommends using oil of bergamot only when your pet is seriously wound up. The rest of time, you can use oil of lavender just to take the edge off. Dilute the oil half-and-half with vegetable oil and apply it to the fur on the back of your pet's neck. Or you can soak a cotton ball in the oil and hang it from a small pouch on his collar. The scent will stay active for 4 to 12 hours, and one treatment a day is enough, she says.

**Stop impatience with impatiens.** Impatiens is a flower remedy that can help dogs relax, says Dr. Starita. She recommends putting two to four drops of impatiens in your pet's mouth several times a day. You also can put a few drops into each fresh bowl of water. It is just as effective as putting the drops in his mouth, and he will be able to sip the benefits all day long.

**Calm him with music.** Some pets are indifferent to music, but others seem to listen and be affected by it, says Dr. Starita. "Choose music that is calming for you. It likely will affect your pet the same way." The best music for hyperactive dogs has a slow, even tempo. Soft jazz is good, she says. So are New Age and country music.

**BEST BET! Exercise his energy.** Dogs that are hyperactive have more energy than they know what to do with. One way to slow them down is to burn off some of the excess, says Dr. Nitschke. A walk or two each day is enough exercise for most dogs, but not for those that are hyperactive. They need a lot of exercise—a mile-long run, for example, or a few hours playing agility sports like Frisbee. You can also give them a tough workout without leaving your yard. "Tie a fuzzy little toy to the end of a stick and run your dog in circles to wear him out," she suggests. Vigorous exercise can sometimes be hard on young puppies, however, so ask your vet how much exercise he needs.

**Use a natural sedative.** Milk contains a chemical called tryptophan that plays a role in promoting sleep, says Dr. Nitschke. Giving your dog one-quarter cup of warm milk once or twice a day will help take the edge off his energy, she says.

**Calm him with color.** Research has shown that colors affect how pets (and people) feel. Some colors—

## Meet the Experts

**Nicholas Dodman, B.V.M.S.,** is professor of behavioral pharmacology and director of the behavior clinic at Tufts University School of Veterinary Medicine in North Grafton, Massachusetts. He is the author of *The Dog Who Loved Too Much* and *The Cat Who Cried for Help.*

**Mary Lee Nitschke, Ph.D.,** is a professor of psychology at Linfield College in Portland, Oregon, and an animal behaviorist in Beaverton.

**Donna M. Starita, D.V.M.,** is a holistic veterinarian in private practice in Boring, Oregon.

**Joanne Stefanatos, D.V.M.,** is a holistic veterinarian in private practice in Las Vegas. She is certified in acupuncture and chiropractic.

red, for example—are stimulating, while others are calming. To keep your dog calm, try using a blue light-bulb in the room where he sleeps. Blue can stimulate the pituitary gland to produce calming hormones, says Joanne Stefanatos, D.V.M., a holistic veterinarian in private practice in Las Vegas.

**Relax him with herbs.** An herbal combination called Calm Pet, available from veterinarians, contains kava kava, chamomile, St. John's wort, and valerian root, all of which may help dogs be a little calmer, says Nicholas Dodman, B.V.M.S. (bachelor of medicine and surgery, a British equivalent of D.V.M.), professor of behavioral pharmacology and director of the behavior clinic at Tufts University School of Veterinary Medicine in North Grafton, Massachusetts. Every pet will need different amounts, so ask your vet for the proper dose.

# INFLAMMATORY BOWEL DISEASE

## The Signs
- Your cat is vomiting a lot.
- Your dog or cat has chronic diarrhea.
- There is blood in his stools.
- Your pet is losing weight, has diarrhea, and is vomiting.

## The Cause

Dogs and cats are always eating things they shouldn't, which is why vomiting and diarrhea are so common in pets. But when they are getting sick for weeks or months instead of days, they could have a more serious digestive problem called inflammatory bowel disease.

Veterinarians aren't sure what causes inflammatory bowel disease, although they suspect it occurs when the immune system mistakenly attacks tissues in the digestive tract. Food allergies or problems with the pancreas may play a role in causing it. Even hair balls, which irritate the intestines, may be involved, says Kathleen Carson, D.V.M., a holistic veterinarian in private practice in Hermosa Beach, California.

The conventional therapy for inflammatory bowel disease is to give medications to stop the symptoms: steroids to suppress the immune system and sometimes antibiotics to control bacteria in the gut. Holistic veterinarians, on the other hand, believe it is possible to cure inflammatory bowel disease by strengthening the body's organs—especially digestive and regulatory organs like the pancreas and liver—and by helping the immune system work the way it is supposed to. Here is what they recommend.

## The Solutions FOR DOGS & CATS

**Give digestive enzymes.** Some veterinarians believe that inflammatory bowel disease occurs when the pancreas is working harder than it should to produce enzymes. Giving your dog or cat digestive enzymes made for pets, such as Prozyme, allows the pancreas to work more efficiently, says Joanne Stefanatos, D.V.M., a holistic veterinarian in private practice in Las Vegas. She recommends giving one-quarter teaspoon of Prozyme twice a day to cats and dogs under 15 pounds. Pets 15 to 50 pounds can take one-half teaspoon twice a day. Dogs up to 80 pounds can take one teaspoon twice a day, and larger dogs can have one tablespoon twice a day. Available from veterinarians and some pet supply stores and catalogs, this enzyme should be given with food, she says.

**BEST BET!** **Ask your vet about a change of diet.** Some pets with inflammatory bowel disease are sensitive to ingredients in commercial foods, says Dr. Carson. Switching to a high-quality food or, better still, to a homemade diet will often help prevent the diarrhea and vomiting that accompany inflammatory bowel disease, she says. For more information on natural diets, see page 61.

**Control bacteria with yogurt.** The normal acid balance in the intestines can change when the pancreas is overactive, allowing harmful bacteria to flourish. This, in turn, can cause painful inflammation. Giving your pet between one and three teaspoons a day of live-culture yogurt will help replenish the supply of beneficial bacteria and get the intestines back into balance, says H. Ellen Whiteley, D.V.M., a veterinary consultant in Guadalupita, New Mexico, and consultant for *The Country Vet's Home Remedies for Cats*.

Instead, you can give supplements containing *Lactobacillus acidophilus*, the same organism that is in yogurt. Make the following adjustments to the human dosage listed on the label: For pets weighing under 20 pounds, use one-fourth of the human dose; for pets 21 to 50 pounds, use one-half of the human dose; and for pets over 50 pounds, use the full human dose.

**Switch to spring water.** Municipal water supplies often contain chlorine, which can kill helpful bacteria in the intestines, says Dr. Carson. Giving your pet bottled water, which doesn't contain chlorine, will help these bacteria thrive.

**Strengthen the liver with milk thistle.** The liver produces large amounts of metabolic enzymes. You can help it work more efficiently by giving your pet milk thistle (*Silybum marianum*) once a day, says Dr. Carson. Available in health food stores, milk thistle may help the liver generate new cells. Ask your veterinarian what dose will be right for your pet.

**Give glutamine supplements.** Inflammatory bowel disease can damage cells in the intestine, causing scarring. Supplements containing glutamine can help rebuild the intestinal lining so that it functions better, says Susan G. Wynn, D.V.M., a veterinarian in Atlanta and co-editor of *Complementary and Alternative Veterinary Medicine*. She recommends giving pets with inflammatory bowel disease 500 milligrams of L-glutamine, available at health food stores, twice a day.

**Absorb toxins with clay.** Harmful bacteria in the intestines, including bacteria that come from eating rotten food, give off toxins that irritate the gut. You may be able to stop the vomiting and diarrhea by giving pets bentonite or montmorillonite clays. Available at health food stores and some pet supply catalogs, the clays can absorb up to 2,000 times their weight in toxins, says Dr. Stefanatos.

She recommends a clay called Gastrex, which contains bentonite and other ingredients. Give pets under 20 pounds half a capsule twice a day. Pets 20 to 50 pounds can take one capsule twice a day, and larger dogs can take two to three capsules twice a day. A product that may be easier to find is Cholacol II, says Dr. Stefanatos. Give pets the same doses as you would with

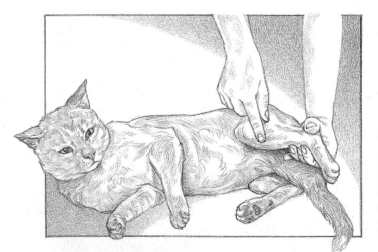

The acupressure point ST36, located just below the knees on the hind legs, can be used to ease a variety of intestinal complaints, including inflammatory bowel disease.

Gastrex. The easiest way to give Gastrex or Cholacol II is to mix it in your pet's food, she adds.

**Improve digestion with homeopathy.** The homeopathic remedies Nux vomica and Arsenicum are very effective at stopping both diarrhea and vomiting, says Dr. Stefanatos. Mix 20 drops of the 6X potency of Nux vomica in an ounce of spring water and give your pet half a dropperful. When using Arsenicum, give pets weighing less than 15 pounds one to two of the 6X-potency pellets. Larger pets can take three to five 6X pellets. If your pet seems better in a few hours, give him another dose. If he isn't getting better, you will want to call your vet.

**Cleanse the intestines with acupressure.** An acupressure point called ST36, located just below the knee on the outside of the hind legs, is the master point for the entire gastrointestinal tract. Pressing this point for 30 seconds once a day will help stimulate the intestines so that they work more efficiently and with less discomfort, Dr. Carson says.

**Boost immunity with herbs.** Echinecea (*Echinacea purpurea* or *Echinacea angustifolia*) has been shown to strengthen the immune system by increasing the number of specialized cells called T-lymphocytes. Another herb, goldenseal (*Hydrastis canadensis*), is a natural antibiotic that

helps control harmful bacteria in the gut, giving mucous membranes a chance to heal, says Dr. Carson.

**Surround him with red.** "The color red stabilizes the immune system," says Dr. Stefanatos. She recommends surrounding your pet with red-colored bedding or put a red lightbulb in the room where he sleeps.

**Stop spasms with essential oils.** Pets with inflammatory bowel disease often have painful intestinal spasms. "Oil of basil, oil of chamomile, and thyme and peppermint oils all have wonderful antispasmodic properties," says Dr. Stefanatos. She recommends putting one or all of these oils in a nebulizer (a small heating unit that va-

---

## Meet the Experts

**Kathleen Carson, D.V.M.,** is a holistic veterinarian in private practice in Hermosa Beach, California.

**Joanne Stefanatos, D.V.M.,** is a holistic veterinarian in private practice in Las Vegas. She is certified in acupuncture and chiropractic.

**H. Ellen Whiteley, D.V.M.,** is a veterinary consultant in Guadalupita, New Mexico, and consultant for *The Country Vet's Home Remedies for Cats*.

**Susan G. Wynn, D.V.M.,** is a veterinarian in Atlanta and co-editor of *Complementary and Alternative Veterinary Medicine*.

porizes the oil) and letting your pet breathe the scent for a few hours a day. Nebulizers are available by mail order.

**Soothe him with slippery elm.** Long-term intestinal problems are often helped by giving pets slippery elm (*Ulmus rubra*) tincture, says Dr. Carson. She recommends diluting 20 drops of the tincture in a one-ounce bottle filled with spring water. Give cats and dogs under 15 pounds a dropperful three times a day. Pets 15 to 50 pounds can have two droppersful, and larger dogs can take three droppersful. It is best to give slippery elm about 20 minutes before meals and again at bedtime. It is best to use tinctures that are alcohol-free because alcohol may be harmful for cats.

# Insect Bites and Stings

## The Signs
- Your pet has one or more raised, itchy bumps on his skin.
- The area around the sting is red and swollen.

## The Cause

Humans would just as soon avoid bees and other stinging insects. But to dogs and cats, they are endlessly fascinating things to chase, paw, or swallow. The reward for all their efforts, of course, is likely to be a painful sting.

Most stings aren't too serious, but even small amounts of toxin can raise a painful, itchy bump. Veterinarians often recommend treating stings by applying hydrocortisone ointment, which reduces inflammation. Although hydrocortisone is safe for pets, many veterinarians prefer a more natural approach.

## The Solutions **FOR DOGS & CATS**

**Remove the stinger.** Before you can treat a sting, you have to remove the stinger. "If the stinger stays in your pet's skin, there will be a stronger reaction and more likelihood of an allergic response," says Nancy Brandt, D.V.M., a holistic veterinarian in private practice in Las Vegas. To remove the stinger, put your fingers at the base of the bump and squeeze upward. This will push the stinger up so that it is easier to remove with your fingers or tweezers. Don't push down on the bump, or

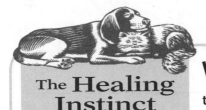

## The **Healing Instinct**

**W**hen dogs and cats get stung or bitten by insects, their immediate response is to start licking. A wet tongue is more than just soothing. "The enzymes in saliva help to neutralize poisons," says Patricia Cooper, D.V.M., a holistic veterinarian in private practice in Houston. When they are bitten in a place where they can't lick, they will often rub the area on grass or in the dirt in an attempt to eliminate the venom, she adds.

you will push more of the venom into the skin, she says.

**Apply a mud poultice.** Mud acts like a sponge and will pull venom out of a sting. It also helps reduce inflammation, says Beatrice Ehrsam, D.V.M., a holistic veterinarian in private practice in New Paltz, New York. You can leave the mud on the sting until it dries out, she adds.

**Apply chamomile tea.** One problem with stings is that the area

often gets infected, says Dr. Brandt. You can reduce the irritation by soaking a cotton ball or a piece of gauze in room-temperature chamomile tea and applying it to the sting. Leave the compress in place for 15 to 30 minutes and repeat three times on the first day. For the next two days, apply a fresh compress for a few minutes three times a day.

**Cover it with a tea bag.** Black tea contains compounds that act as astrin-

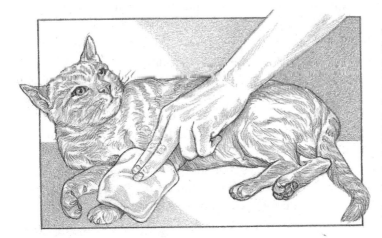

You can stop swelling fast by applying a chamomile compress. Soak a cotton ball in room-temperature chamomile tea, squeeze it out, and put it on the bite. Cover the cotton ball with a square of cotton gauze and hold the wet compress in place with your fingers for 15 to 30 minutes.

## Call the VET

For pets with allergies, a single sting can be deadly. "If your pet has an allergic reaction, with severe swelling around his head or neck, difficulty breathing, persistent pain, or drowsiness, go to the vet right away," says Beatrice Ehrsam, D.V.M., a holistic veterinarian in private practice in New Paltz, New York. He may need a shot of epinephrine, a medication that blocks serious allergic reactions called anaphylaxis. You should also call your vet if your dog or cat has been bitten by a black widow or brown recluse spider.

If you can't get to a vet immediately, try the homeopathic remedy Apis, giving two or three 200C pills, says Gerald Buchoff, B.V.Sc.A.H. (bachelor of veterinary science and animal husbandry, the Indian equivalent of D.V.M.), a holistic veterinarian in private practice in North Bergen, New Jersey. "It works immediately," he says. Apis will help get your pet past the danger, but you will still have to get him to a vet as quickly as possible, he says.

gents, which help draw toxins out of a sting, says Mona Boudreaux, D.V.M., a holistic veterinarian in private practice in Albuquerque, New Mexico. Moisten a tea bag in warm water, squeeze it out, then hold it on the sting for 10 to 15 minutes, she advises.

**Treat it with Ledum.** The homeopathic remedy Ledum helps puncture wounds heal and prevents swelling as long as you give it quickly after the sting occurs, says Patricia Cooper, D.V.M., a holistic veterinarian in private practice in Houston. She recommends giving two or three tablets of Ledum 30C, either by putting them in your pet's mouth or by dissolving them in a few teaspoons of water and then putting the water in your pet's mouth. Repeat the treatment every 30 minutes for two to three hours, she advises.

**Ease the irritation.** For small bites from gnats, the essential oils lavender or thyme will quickly relieve irritation and itching, says Dr. Brandt. Mix three drops of either oil in a teaspoon of apple cider vinegar and dab the solution on the bites, she advises. Vinegar by itself is also effective.

**Apply some ammonia.** Another way to ease the pain of insect bites and stings is to apply ammonia, says Susan G. Wynn, D.V.M., a veterinarian in Atlanta and co-editor of *Complementary and Alternative Veterinary Medicine*. A number of commercial products, like After Bite, use ammonia as the active ingredient.

 **Give an oatmeal bath.** A single bite isn't too bad, but sometimes pets—usually puppies or kittens—will lie down on a pile of ants and wind up with a rash of itchy bites on their bellies. You can stop the itching fast by soaking them in cool water spiked with oatmeal, says Dr. Boudreaux. Put about a cup of oatmeal in a cloth and tie it up with a piece of string. Put the bag in a cool-water bath and soak your pet for about 20 minutes. You can repeat the treatment once a day until the rash and itching improve, she says.

**Reduce inflammation with an Indian herb.** An herbal supplement called ashwagandha (*Withania somnifera*), available in health food stores, will reduce inflammation caused by stings, says Tejinder Sodhi, D.V.M., a holistic veterinarian in private practice in Bellevue and Lynnwood, Washington. You can add ashwagandha powder to your pet's food. Pets under 15 pounds can take one-quarter teaspoon of the powder two or three times a day. Those weighing 15 to 50

## Meet the Experts

**Mona Boudreaux, D.V.M.,** is a holistic veterinarian in private practice in Albuquerque, New Mexico. She is certified in acupuncture and chiropractic.

**Nancy Brandt, D.V.M.,** is a holistic veterinarian in private practice in Las Vegas. She is certified in acupuncture.

**Gerald Buchoff, B.V.Sc.A.H.,** a holistic veterinarian in private practice in North Bergen, New Jersey. He is certified in chiropractic.

**Patricia Cooper, D.V.M.,** is a holistic veterinarian in private practice in Houston.

**Beatrice Ehrsam, D.V.M.,** is a holistic veterinarian in private practice in New Paltz, New York. She is certified in acupuncture.

**Tejinder Sodhi, D.V.M.,** is a holistic veterinarian in private practice in Bellevue and Lynnwood, Washington. He is certified in acupuncture, chiropractic, and homeopathy.

**Susan G. Wynn, D.V.M.,** is a veterinarian in Atlanta and co-editor of *Complementary and Alternative Veterinary Medicine*.

pounds can take one-half teaspoon two or three times a day, and dogs over 50 pounds can take as much as a teaspoon two or three times a day.

**Stop swelling with spice.** Another Indian remedy for inflammation is the spice turmeric (*Curcuma longa*). Dr. Sodhi recommends mixing powdered turmeric with a little chicken broth and slipping it in your pet's food. "It's relatively bland, despite its bright yellow color," he adds.

Pets under 15 pounds can take about one-half teaspoon of turmeric twice a day. Those that weigh 15 to 50 pounds can take a teaspoon twice a day, and larger pets can have two teaspoons twice a day.

# INSOMNIA

## The Signs
- Your pet is unusually restless when the lights go out.
- He wakes up very early in the morning.
- He gets anxious at night.

## The Cause

When it comes to getting a good night's sleep, dogs and cats are the undisputed champs. They have the enviable ability to curl up and enjoy what Shakespeare called "Nature's soft nurse" on a moment's notice.

Pets don't get insomnia very often. When they do, you need to pay attention because there is almost certainly something wrong. Pain from such things as arthritis or a pinched nerve can make them a little wakeful. A lack of exercise will sometimes keep pets awake. So will anxiety or other kinds of stress, says Wanda Vockeroth, D.V.M., a holistic veterinarian in pri-

vate practice in Calgary, Alberta, Canada. "Things that cause them stress during the day can bother them at night, too," she says. Insomnia can also be caused by serious conditions, like an overactive thyroid gland, diabetes, or problems in the brain.

Of course, pets don't necessarily keep the same hours that people do. Cats, for example, are nocturnal creatures who get their sleep in installments; what may seem like insomnia to you may be perfectly normal for them. But when your pet's usual sleep patterns have suddenly changed, and the all-night scratching, pacing, and collar-jingling is keeping *you* awake, you will need a few natural remedies to help your pet sleep more soundly.

## The Solutions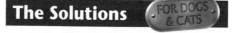

**Move the bed.** Pets sometimes get restless at night when their beds are in an "unfriendly" place—close to a chilly outside wall, for example, or near sources of electricity, says Deborah C. Mallu, D.V.M., a holistic veterinarian in private practice in Sedona, Arizona. "Appliances emit frequencies that may disturb your pet's sleeping patterns," she explains. "It is important not to place their beds near appliances or a wall outlet."

**BEST BET!** **Calm them with herbs.** The herbs valerian (*Valeriana officinalis*) and kava kava (*Piper methysticum*) can soothe anxiety and help pets sleep more comfortably, says Greig Howie, D.V.M., a holistic veterinarian in private practice in Dover, Delaware. He recommends mixing equal parts of valerian and kava kava tinctures. "For all cats or for dogs weighing less than 15 pounds, use three or four drops of the mixed tincture," he says. "For dogs weighing 15 pounds or more, you can give up to two dropperfuls." You can put the drops directly in their mouths or in their food or water once a day, about an hour before bedtime, he says. You can continue this treatment for up to two weeks. It is best to use tinctures that are alcohol-free because alcohol may be harmful for cats.

**Rescue their rest.** Flower essences can help pets sleep more soundly. A drop or two of an essence called Bach Rescue Remedy, rubbed on the gums periodically, relieves anxiety and nighttime agitation, says Pat Bradley, D.V.M., a holistic veterinarian in private practice in Conway, Arkansas. "If it's an acute situation, like you have moved to a new house, I would use it three or four times a day,"

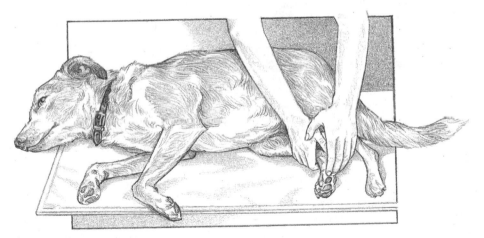

To massage your pet to sleep, stroke the insides of the hind paws, moving downward from the ankles to the tips of the toes. Some pets don't like having their feet touched, so don't try to force things if your pet won't hold still.

ALTERNATIVE

## ❧ SUCCESS

### AFRAID NO MORE

Chops developed a very strange habit that had his family very worried: The 14-year-old cat would wake up every night between 2:00 and 4:00 and start screaming at full throttle. He seemed unusually nervous during the day and was easily startled.

Chops's owners, puzzled by his strange behavior and feeling a little sleepless themselves, took him to Deborah C. Mallu, D.V.M., a holistic veterinarian in private practice in Sedona, Arizona.

Dr. Mallu quickly discovered that Chops, like many older pets, had lost some of his sight and hearing. She suspected that this was making him afraid of the dark. "I suggested that they give him a moist snack at bedtime, put Rescue Remedy flower essence in his water, and keep a night-light on," she recalls.

During her exam, she also discovered something else: Chops had an overactive thyroid gland, which was speeding his metabolism, and a kidney problem. Chops didn't need drugs, but he did need a comprehensive plan to restore his health—physically and emotionally.

"With acupuncture, herbs, and changes in his diet, he is doing much better," Dr. Mallu says. "He sleeps through the night at least four times a week, and that is a big improvement."

she says. "If it's ongoing anxiety, I would use it perhaps once or twice a day for several weeks."

**Feed your pet late.** Like Dagwood in the comic strip *Blondie*, dogs and cats occasionally wake up at night simply because they are hungry. If you want your pet to sleep through the night, try feeding him right before he goes to sleep and make sure that there is plenty of fat in the food. Fat causes food to stay in the stomach longer, so he will be less likely to wake up hungry later on. Try adding one-half teaspoon of butter or a raw egg to your pet's nighttime meal for a few nights to see if it helps. Some pets can develop pancreatitis when they are given high-fat diets, however, so check with your vet before doing this on a regular basis.

**BEST BET!** **Give him a workout.** Young pets sometimes have too much pent-up energy to sleep well, says Dr. Vockeroth. Regular exercise in the evening may be just the outlet they need to calm down.

Adding another pet to the family is a sure way to help your pet sleep more soundly, Frazier adds. "Nobody can exercise an animal like another animal."

**Rub them to sleep.** Dogs and cats sometimes have trouble sleeping because their circulation isn't as good as it could be, says Cheryl Schwartz, D.V.M., a holistic veterinarian in San Francisco and author of *Four Paws, Five Directions: A Guide to Chinese Medicine for Cats and Dogs*. They become agitated because there is not enough circulatory pressure in their muscles to provide the oxygen and nutrients they need to stay calm, she explains. Giving your pet a bedtime massage will boost circulation and help him sleep more soundly. She recommends stroking the insides of his hind paws, moving downward from

## Meet the Experts

**Pat Bradley, D.V.M.,** is a holistic veterinarian in private practice in Conway, Arkansas. She is certified in homeopathy.

**Greig Howie, D.V.M.,** is a holistic veterinarian in private practice in Dover, Delaware. He is certified in acupuncture and homeopathy.

**Deborah C. Mallu, D.V.M.,** is a holistic veterinarian in private practice in Sedona, Arizona. She is certified in acupuncture.

**Cheryl Schwartz, D.V.M.,** is a holistic veterinarian in San Francisco and the author of *Four Paws, Five Directions: A Guide to Chinese Medicine for Cats and Dogs*. She is certified in acupuncture.

**Wanda Vockeroth, D.V.M.,** is a holistic veterinarian in private practice in Calgary, Alberta, Canada. She is certified in acupuncture.

the tops of the ankles to the tips of the toes.

**Give magnesium.** Available in capsules and pills, magnesium supplements have a calming effect, says Dr. Vockeroth. Every dog and cat needs different amounts of magnesium, so be sure to ask your vet for the correct dose.

# ITCHING

## The Signs
- Your pet is scratching or biting his skin.
- His coat looks patchy.
- The skin is raw and inflamed.
- He chews on his paws.
- He scratches his ears or shakes his head.

## The Cause

Few things make dogs and cats more uncomfortable than itchy skin. And since the skin is the body's largest organ, there are plenty of places for trouble to begin.

Itching is usually caused by allergies to pollen, molds, fleas, or even food. Some pets handle allergies just fine, while others go into a veritable scratching frenzy. Itching is most likely to be a problem when your pet's overall health isn't what it should be. "Itching is just one symptom of your pet's whole-health picture, but it is the symptom that screams the loudest," says Jordan A. Kocen, D.V.M., a holistic veterinarian in private practice in Springfield, Virginia.

Mainstream veterinarians usually treat the itching itself by giving antihistamines, for example, while holistic vets focus more on the underlying problems, which can range from emotional stress to problems with the immune system. "The holistic approach is not magic, and it takes time to work," Dr. Kocen says. It can, however, give long-lasting benefits. Here is what holistic veterinarians recommend.

## The Solutions FOR DOGS & CATS

**Stop fleas with neem.** An Indian herb called neem (*Azadiracta indica*) repels fleas and soothes sore skin, says Michael W. Lemmon, D.V.M., a holistic veterinarian in Renton, Washington, and past president of the American Holistic Veterinary Medical Association. Neem can be applied to the skin as an oil or lotion. One popular brand available from veterinarians is PhytoGel, which contains neem along with other essential oils. Neem has a bitter taste that fleas dislike. Dogs and cats dislike it, too, which means that they are less inclined to bite and chew at their skin, he says.

Neem is also available in capsule form, Dr. Lemmon adds. Ask your vet what dose is right for your pet.

**Cool the skin.** The herb calendula (*Calendula officinalis*), also known as marigold flowers, will quickly soothe hot, irritated areas on

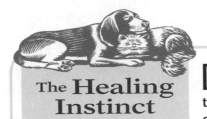

## The **Healing Instinct**

**D**ogs that live in the wild are nomadic. They will stay in one place for a while, then move on. This peripatetic lifestyle has one big advantage: Every time they leave a place, they also leave behind the eggs of parasites that otherwise could cause problems within the pack, says Jordan A. Kocen, D.V.M., a holistic veterinarian in private practice in Springfield, Virginia.

What works in the wild, of course, isn't an option for today's one-house pets, which is one reason fleas and other parasites are so common. "Even the healthiest dog is likely to be affected," says Dr. Kocen. Since dogs can't heed their instincts and wander off, it is up to us to treat the house and yard to keep parasites under control.

your pet's skin, says Charles E. Loops, D.V.M., a veterinarian in private practice in Pittsboro, North Carolina. He recommends adding 10 to 15 drops of calendula tincture to four ounces of distilled or spring water and putting the mixture in a spray bottle. You can spray the area as often as needed to help stop your pet from scratching. It is best to use tinctures that are alcohol-free because alcohol may be harmful for cats.

The herbs chickweed (*Stelleria media*) and plantain (*Plantago*, various species) are also good for skin problems, says Dr. Lemmon. You can buy both herbs as a lotion, or you can use bulk leaves to brew a tea. Boil a pint of water, remove it from the heat, and pour it over two tablespoons of dried herbs or a handful of fresh herbs. Cover and steep for 10 to 20 minutes. Let the tea cool to room temperature,

strain if you have used loose leaves, dip a cloth in the solution, and apply it to your pet's sore spots for 5 to 10 minutes a few times a day.

**Throw him a bone.** Raw, meaty bones, like chicken and turkey necks, are filled with nutrients that strengthen the immune system and help control allergy-related itching, Dr. Lemmon says. Chicken and turkey necks that are not free-range or organically grown may be contaminated with salmonella bacteria. So don't let them sit around unrefrigerated for more than a half-hour. "Some dogs get so excited to be given something so good that they will gulp the bones down without chewing and may vomit them back up," he adds. Cats love raw bones, too, although you may want to help them out by first chopping the bones with a cleaver.

**Give him extra zinc.** Research

has shown that zinc supplements can help relieve a variety of skin problems, including itching. Veterinarians usually recommend chelated zinc. Ask your vet what dose is right for your pet.

**BEST BET!** **Give him extra fatty acids.** Two common fatty acids, omega-3s and omega-6s, can help reduce itching and inflammation, says Susan G. Wynn, D.V.M., a veterinarian in Atlanta and co-editor of *Complementary and Alternative Veterinary Medicine*. You can buy supplements that contain both of these fatty acids in health food and pet supply stores, and many dogs and cats will gobble them like treats. Ask your vet which supplement and dose are right for your pet.

**BEST BET!** **Improve his diet.** Giving your pet a balanced, top-quality diet can build up the immune system so that he is better able to fight itching from the inside out. Some commercial pet foods may be a problem because they often contain chemical additives and poor-quality ingredients that contribute to skin problems, says Dr. Lemmon. A better choice is an all-natural food like Flint River Ranch, Solid Gold, or PetGuard Premium that doesn't contain artificial ingredients. Natural foods are available at some pet supply stores or from mail-order companies. Or you can make a homemade diet that includes plenty of raw meat. For more tips on homemade diets, see page 61.

## A Modern Problem

For years, veterinarians have assumed that pets are simply itchier than people. But there is some evidence that continual itching isn't normal.

Holistic veterinarians suspect that yearly vaccinations, such as corona, may be involved. They have found that pets given natural diets and fewer vaccines tend to be a lot less itchy than their counterparts who are given traditional foods and yearly shots. Annual vaccines can contain up to seven viruses (in an altered, non-disease-causing form) in one shot. The vaccines immediately go into the lymphatic system, bypassing the immune system's first line of defenses, such as the mouth, nose, and skin. This can weaken the immune system, causing more allergies and itching, says Charles E. Loops, D.V.M., a veterinarian in private practice in Pittsboro, North Carolina.

The immune system is further weakened by the chemicals in many commercial pet foods as well as by their processed ingredients, Dr. Loops explains.

Switching pets to an all-natural diet and giving them only the essential vaccines that your vet recommends can help the immune system recover. Not only will your pet be healthier, says Dr. Loops, but you will probably see a decrease in "normal" scratching as well.

**Slip some vegetables in his bowl.** An easy way to increase the amounts of immune-boosting nutrients in your pet's diet is to give him raw vegetables like carrots and green beans, Dr. Kocen says. Many pets don't like raw vegetables, however, so you may find it is best to chop and lightly steam them, then mix them in his food.

**Give him vitamin supplements.** The vitamins A, C, and E have been shown to strengthen the immune system and may help reduce itching, Dr. Lemmon says. Each nutrient works in a different way, he adds.

🐾 Vitamin A helps irritated skin heal and strengthens the immune system. This nutrient can be harmful in large amounts, however, so check with your vet for the correct dose before giving it at home.

🐾 Vitamin C also strengthens the immune system and may help relieve allergies as well. Give cats and dogs weighing under 15 pounds 250 milligrams of vitamin C a day. Pets 15 to 50 pounds can take 500 milligrams, and larger dogs can take 1,000 milligrams. Vitamin C may cause diarrhea, so be prepared to reduce the dose until you find an amount that your pet will tolerate.

🐾 Vitamin E reduces inflammation in the skin and is an essential nutrient for healthy immunity. Give cats and dogs under 15 pounds 100 international units (IU) of vitamin E a day. Dogs 15 to 40 pounds can take 200 IU. Those 41 to 70 pounds can have 400 IU, and dogs over 70 pounds can take 800 IU, says Dr. Lemmon.

**Stop itching with homeopathy.** Holistic veterinarians often treat itchy

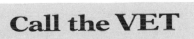

## Call the VET

Even the healthiest pets will scratch occasionally, sometimes for the pure pleasure of it. Itchy skin is normal, as long as it is not too serious and doesn't last too long. Dogs and cats that are constantly scratching, however, probably have an underlying problem that needs looking into.

"Your pet needs to see a veterinarian if he doesn't get relief from the itching within a few days," says Michael W. Lemmon, D.V.M., a holistic veterinarian in Renton, Washington, and past president of the American Holistic Veterinary Medical Association.

pets with homeopathic Sulfur, Petroleum, or Graphites, Dr. Lemmon says. Each of the remedies can be effective, but pets react to them differently, so you will need to check with your vet before using them at home, he adds.

**BEST BET!** **Soothe him with an oatmeal bath.** A classic remedy for itchy skin is to lather pets with an oatmeal shampoo or to soak them in cool water to which you have added colloidal oatmeal (like Aveeno), says Dr. Loops. Many vets prefer colloidal oatmeal to shampoo because it doesn't contain soaps that may irritate itchy skin. Give your pet a bath every day for two or three days. After that, if it doesn't seem to be working, find another way to soothe the skin.

# JEALOUSY

## The Signs
- Your pet gets upset when you are near other people or pets.
- She periodically disappears or seems withdrawn.
- She is aggressive toward family members.

## The Cause

You often hear about a "one-person dog" or a cat who "only eats when *I* feed her." Dogs and cats are intensely loyal; it is one of their most endearing traits. Sometimes, however, their emotional attachments get too intense and turn into jealousy.

A little bit of jealousy usually isn't a problem. Maybe your cat disappears when you pay attention to another pet, or your dog misbehaves when you turn your attention elsewhere. But jealousy has a way of escalating, and small signs of displeasure may give way to more aggressive displays like growling, scratching, or even biting.

"Jealousy is about fear," explains Jean Hofve, D.V.M., a holistic veterinarian in private practice in Denver. "It's often a fear of losing your love."

Some veterinarians have begun treating jealousy with mood-altering drugs such as fluoxetine (Prozac). Medications can control the signs of jealousy, but they won't help solve the underlying problems, says Dr. Hofve. That is why holistic veterinarians prefer a wider-ranging approach. Here is what they advise.

## The Solutions FOR DOGS & CATS

**Help her with holly.** Holistic veterinarians recommend giving jealous pets flower essences because they can make them calmer, more content, and less prone to jealous feelings, says Dr. Hofve. Holly is the essence usually recommended for jealousy, although beech, agrimony, heather, chicory, elm, and aspen may be helpful as well. You can use the remedies separately, but they are usually more effective in combination, she says. Your vet will help you choose essences that are best for your pet's personality.

To prepare a "jealousy remedy," put four drops each of one or more of the essences that your vet recommends in a one-ounce brown glass bottle filled with spring water, says Junia Borden Childs, D.V.M., a holistic veterinarian in private practice in Ojai, California. Give your pet four

## Call the VET

**M**ost dogs and cats get jealous from time to time, and usually they get over it fairly quickly. When a little jealousy turns into aggression, however, you need to call your vet right away. If you don't get help, the bad behavior is only going to get worse, says Greig Howie, D.V.M., a holistic veterinarian in private practice in Dover, Delaware.

Your veterinarian will probably recommend that you see a professional trainer or behavior specialist, who will teach you ways to reduce or even eliminate the jealous behavior, says Dr. Howie. He will also want to give your pet a thorough exam to make sure that there is nothing physically wrong that could be causing the problem.

drops of the remedy four times a day—either by putting them straight in her mouth or by putting the drops on her nose or foot pads, where they will be absorbed into the body.

**Switch to a natural diet.** Commercial pet foods may contain chemical preservatives such as ethoxyquin that can make pets cranky. When they are already prone to jealousy, the additional emotional and physical turmoil can make them even more upset, says Dr. Hofve. She recommends giving pets natural, chemical-free foods such as Precise, Natural Life, or PetGuard Premium, available from some pet supply stores and mail-order catalogs.

**BEST BET!** **Respect the hierarchy.** Dogs and cats can get very emotional about their food, and they attach a lot of meaning to who gets fed first, says Dr. Hofve. If you have more than one pet and jealousy has been a problem, feed the jealous one first. "She should know that she's the one being favored," she states. Feeding pets separately may be helpful as well.

**Give her some pampering.** Jealousy usually occurs when pets are feeling insecure about your affections. "Go off by yourselves every day and give her extra-special attention," suggests Dr. Hofve. You don't have to do anything fancy—maybe take a longer walk than usual or give her an extra petting session. The more special she feels, the less threatened she

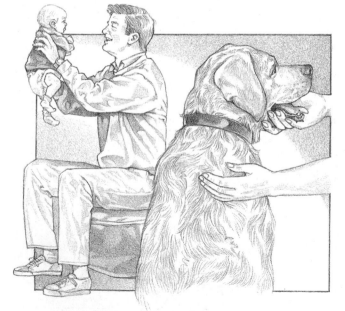

To perform the healing touch known as Clouded Leopard, cup your hand slightly and use the index and two middle fingers to push the skin clockwise in a small circle. It is best to start at the head and move downward to the tail. You can repeat the touch several times a day to reduce jealous feelings.

is likely to be when you spend time with others.

**Touch her fears.** One of the best ways to calm jealous pets is with a technique called TTouch, says Dr. Hofve. "It's very supporting and comforting to animals," she says. "It helps connect pets with themselves and makes them feel more whole."

She recommends using a touch called Clouded Leopard. Cup your hand slightly with the index and two middle fingers together. Rest your hand lightly on your pet's body and, using the tips of your fingers, gently push the skin clockwise in a small circle. After completing one circle—plus a little more—move to another part of her body. You can do this once or twice a day, starting at the head and working all the way down to the tail and feet, Dr. Hofve says.

**Focus on the physical.** It is common for pets to get cranky when they are ill, so what appears to be jealousy may be a medical problem, says Michelle Tilghman, D.V.M., a holistic veterinarian in private practice in Stone Mountain, Georgia. "A lot of pets appear to be jealous when they are actually hurting," she says. Check with your vet just to be sure, she advises.

## The Solutions

**BEST BET!** **Take control.** Dogs will occasionally show signs of jeal-ousy when they think they are not getting their just deserts—it is their way of pushing you around. "You have to get better control of the situation," says Dr. Tilghman. "You are the leader of the pack."

The next time your dog starts acting jealous, tell him, "No!," she suggests. Make it clear that you are in charge and her behavior isn't acceptable. You may want to start practicing basic obedience drills as well. Once your dog remembers who is "top dog," she will learn to keep her grumbling to herself.

**Cut back on protein.** Veterinarians have found that dogs that get too much protein in their diets sometimes get jealous or aggressive. Your vet may recommend switching her to a lower-protein food—preferably one con-

## Meet the Experts

**Junia Borden Childs, D.V.M.,** is a holistic veterinarian in private practice in Ojai, California.

**Jean Hofve, D.V.M.,** is a holistic veterinarian in private practice in Denver.

**Greig Howie, D.V.M.,** a holistic veterinarian in private practice in Dover, Delaware. He is certified in acupuncture and homeopathy.

**Michelle Tilghman, D.V.M.,** is a holistic veterinarian in private practice in Stone Mountain, Georgia. She is certified in acupuncture.

taining no more than 22 to 23 percent protein, says Dr. Tilghman.

## The Solutions
**FOR CATS**

**BEST BET!** **Give them their space.** "Cats are solitary animals, so if you put several of them in a small house, it can be really hard on them," says Dr. Tilghman. The next time your cats are feuding or vying for your attention, try giving them plenty of space by putting them in separate rooms, for example. Giving each cat a separate litter box can also help ease the tension.

# JUMPING UP

## The Signs
- Your dog jumps up whenever he is excited.
- He jumps on visitors or strangers.

## The Cause

No matter how much you love your dog's perky energy and exuberant displays of affection, it is hard to love washing paw prints off your skirt or watching guests get bowled over when they walk in the door.

In the world of dogs, it is natural to jump up and lick their friends' faces, says Deborah C. Mallu, D.V.M., a holistic veterinarian in private practice in Sedona, Arizona. What's appropriate among dogs, however, isn't always welcome in the human clan. Jumping on people can be annoying or even dangerous. That's why it is important to find ways to keep your dog grounded, no matter how much he wants to leap up and say "hi."

Dogs that jump on people need to be trained to keep their feet on the floor, says Pat Bradley, D.V.M., a holistic veterinarian in private practice in Conway, Arkansas. They also may need some help keeping all that extra energy under control. Here are a few tips that you may want to try.

## The Solutions
**FOR DOGS**

**Take the edge off of his excitement.** "If your dog gets really excited and is jumping up, you may want to try giving Phosphorus," says Michael

W. Lemmon, D.V.M., a holistic veterinarian in Renton, Washington, and past president of the American Holistic Veterinary Medical Association. He recommends giving one homeopathic dose of Phosphorus 30C once a day for a week. If it is going to work at all, you should see results within a week, he adds.

**Try some yeast.** Veterinarians have found that natural forms of B vitamins can help keep dogs calmer. "Nutritional yeast is a very good source of B vitamins," states Dr. Lemmon. He recommends giving dogs under 15 pounds one-half teaspoon of yeast a day. Dogs 15 to 50 pounds can take one teaspoon, and larger dogs can take a tablespoon. Some dogs are allergic to yeast, so it is a good idea to check with your vet before using it at home.

**Manage him with magnesium.** This essential mineral may have a calming effect. Dr. Lemmon recommends giving dogs chelated magnesium, available in capsule form in health food stores. Dogs under 15 pounds can take 100 milligrams a day. Dogs weighing 15 to 50 pounds can take 300 milligrams, and larger dogs can take up to 600 milligrams

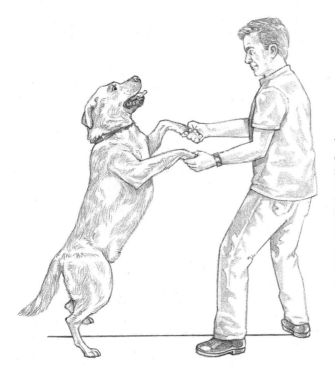

The traditional way to teach dogs not to jump up is to swiftly raise your knee so that it smacks them in the chest. A gentler technique is to lightly squeeze your dog's front paws while they are in the air, but *before* they make contact with you. Dogs don't like having their feet touched, and this also throws off their timing. If you do this every time he tries to jump, he will learn to give other less enthusiastic greetings.

## ALTERNATIVE

# ✷ SUCCESS

## TAKING THE JUMP OUT OF JEHOSHAPHAT

Jehoshaphat was unusually energetic even for an eight-month-old Labrador retriever. In his owner's words, he was a "maniac" who was perpetually airborne. He would leap on family members or even strangers at the slightest excuse.

Jehoshaphat's owner, concerned that he might hurt the children, took him to the veterinarian, who recommended giving him barbiturates. But before resorting to powerful drugs, she wanted to try a more natural approach. So she took Jehoshaphat to Karen Komisar, D.V.M., a holistic veterinarian in private practice in Lynn, Massachusetts.

"We treated him with the homeopathic remedy Silicea," says Dr. Komisar. There are a number of homeopathic remedies that can calm excitable dogs, she adds, but for Jehoshaphat, Silicea was the right choice. "After five days, Jehoshaphat's owner called and said he was much calmer," she says. "He would eat his food and go lie down, and he wasn't jumping on people anymore."

a day. You can either pop the capsule right down his throat or open it up and mix the contents in his food, he says.

**Calm him with St. John's wort.** This popular herbal remedy appears to work as well for pets as it does for people. "St. John's wort is a good herb to use for behavioral problems," says Robin Cannizzaro, D.V.M., a holistic veterinarian in private practice in St. Petersburg, Florida. Different dogs will need different amounts, and in some cases St. John's wort may cause side effects. So talk to your vet before using it at home.

**BEST BET! Teach them the ropes.** Dogs aren't always sure what is expected of them, so you need to make it very clear that jumping up is always a problem, says Susan G. Wynn, D.V.M., a veterinarian in Atlanta and co-editor of *Complementary and Alternative Veterinary Medicine*. To help them get the message, use simple commands like "Off" or "No."

## Meet the Experts

**Pat Bradley, D.V.M.,** is a holistic veterinarian in private practice in Conway, Arkansas. She is certified in homeopathy.

**Robin Cannizzaro, D.V.M.,** is a holistic veterinarian in private practice in St. Petersburg, Florida. She is certified in acupuncture and homeopathy.

**Anitra Frazier** is an animal behavior consultant in New York City and the author of *The New Natural Cat* and *It's a Cat's Life*.

**Karen Komisar, D.V.M.,** is a holistic veterinarian in private practice in Lynn, Massachusetts. She is certified in homeopathy.

**Michael W. Lemmon, D.V.M.,** is a holistic veterinarian in Renton, Washington, and past president of the American Holistic Veterinary Medical Association.

**Deborah C. Mallu, D.V.M.,** is a holistic veterinarian in private practice in Sedona, Arizona. She is certified in acupuncture.

**Susan G. Wynn, D.V.M.,** is a veterinarian in Atlanta and co-editor of *Complementary and Alternative Veterinary Medicine*.

When you are teaching your dog to stay down, it is important for all family members to be consistent, says Dr. Wynn. It is confusing if one person tells him to stay down one day, and someone else permits him to jump up the next. Dogs need very clear directions in order to learn, and giving mixed messages will undermine the entire training process.

Of course, there may be times—while playing in the yard, for instance—when it is perfectly acceptable for your dog to jump up. Just make sure that he knows the difference. "You can have different word or hand signals for when he can jump and when he can't," says Anitra Frazier, an animal behavior consultant in New York City and author of *The New Natural Cat*.

**Give a hand signal.** Dogs don't like it when hands move quickly toward their faces. You can often discourage jumping up by moving the palm of your hand quickly toward your dog's nose just as he leaps. "You don't hit him," Frazier says. "You just move your hand toward the nose."

# KENNEL COUGH

## The Signs
- Your dog has a dry, gagging, or hacking cough.

## The Cause

You thought you were doing the right thing by boarding your dog in a nice, comfortable kennel when you went on vacation. But now he is coughing up a storm, and you are starting to think that his canine companions away from home gave him more than just company.

"Kennel cough is caused by different viral and bacterial infections that spread from dog to dog, usually in kennels," says Allen M. Schoen, D.V.M., director of the Veterinary Institute for Therapeutic Alternatives in Sherman, Connecticut, and author of *Love, Miracles, and Animal Healing.*

Depending on the cause of the infection and the severity of the symptoms, kennel cough may be treated with antibiotics or cough suppressants, and mainstream veterinarians often recommend vaccinations to prevent it. These are pretty serious treatments for a condition that usually goes away on its own in a few weeks, says Adriana Sagrera, D.V.M., a holistic veterinarian in private practice in New Orleans. Veterinarians who practice alternative medicine usually favor a more natural—and drug-free—strategy for keeping kennel cough under control. Here is what they advise.

## The Solutions FOR DOGS

**BEST BET!** **Stop it with loquat.** A Chinese herbal liquid called loquat will soothe your dog's irritated throat and help him heal more quickly, says Dr. Schoen. "It's very sweet," he says. "Your dog will lick it right off the spoon." He recommends giving dogs under 15 pounds one-eighth teaspoon of loquat a day. Dogs 15 to 50 pounds can take one-half teaspoon, and larger dogs can take one-half to three-quarters tablespoon. You can get loquat from mail-order companies.

Since loquat is very sweet, Dr. Schoen adds, you don't want to give it to dogs that have diabetes without first checking with your veterinarian.

**Battle the infection.** The herbs echinacea (*Echinacea purpurea* or *Echinacea angustifolia*) and goldenseal (*Hydrastis canadensis*) have antiviral and antibacterial properties and can strengthen the immune system, says

Dr. Schoen. He recommends giving dogs with kennel cough an extract that combines both of these herbs. Dogs under 15 pounds can take 7 drops twice a day, and larger dogs can take 15 drops twice a day. The taste is very bitter, he adds, so you will need to disguise the drops by mixing them in your dog's food.

**Use a natural cough syrup.** Most homeopathic remedies come in liquid or tablet form, but those used for kennel cough are available as a soothing syrup, says Christina Chambreau, D.V.M., a holistic veterinarian in Sparks, Maryland, and education chairperson for the Academy of Veterinary Homeopathy. Two popular brands are Hyland's Cough Syrup and B and T Homeopathic Cough and Bronchial Syrup.

"Some dogs will lick the syrup, but for others, you will need to squirt it down their throats with a needleless dosing syringe," she says. She recommends giving dogs under 15 pounds one-quarter of the human dose. Dogs 15 to 50 pounds can take one-half of the human dose, and larger dogs can take the full human dose.

**Try lemon and honey.** For centuries, natural healers have used honey and lemon juice to soothe coughs and sore throats in humans. The combination is equally effective for dogs with kennel cough, says Dr. Chambreau. She recommends mixing

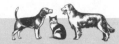

## Questionable Protection

Many veterinarians recommend (and most kennels require) that dogs be vaccinated against kennel cough before being boarded. But some vets specializing in natural healing feel the vaccinations aren't necessary and may cause problems.

"Vaccinations of any sort can compromise the immune system and weaken an animal overall, even though they provide some specific protection," says Christina Chambreau, D.V.M., a holistic veterinarian in Sparks, Maryland, and education chairperson for the Academy of Veterinary Homeopathy. "Giving repeated vaccinations for diseases that aren't life-threatening is not good for the health of the animal."

The problem, of course, is that unless your dog gets the vaccination, you may have trouble finding a kennel that will board him. Even if you do find a high-quality kennel that doesn't require the shots, you may be asked to sign a release saying that you won't hold the owners responsible should your dog get infected.

If you decide to get your dog vaccinated, keep in mind that the shot provides protection for less than six months.

two tablespoons of honey and a teaspoon of lemon juice in one-half cup of water and giving the solution to your dog a few times a day.

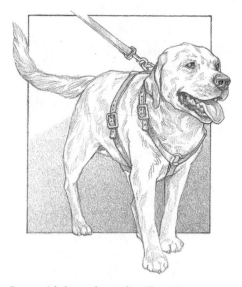

Dogs with kennel cough will go into a coughing frenzy at the slightest pressure from a collar and leash. While your dog recovers, it is a good idea to swap his usual collar for a harness that buckles around the chest. This will keep him under control without putting pressure where it hurts.

"Honey and lemon are very safe, so you can give more or less of it depending on how your dog responds," she says.

**Ease congestion with mullein.** The herb mullein (*Verbascum thapsus*), available in capsule form, is very effective at breaking up the congestion that often accompanies kennel cough, says Beatrice Ehrsam, D.V.M., a holistic veterinarian in private practice in New Paltz, New York. "You can empty the capsule into hot water to make a tea, then cool it down and squirt it in his mouth with a syringe," she says. Or you can empty the cap-

sule into his food. She recommends giving mullein twice a day until your dog's cough is getting better. Give dogs under 15 pounds one-quarter of the human dose. Dogs 15 to 35 pounds can take one-half of the human dose, and dogs 36 to 60 pounds can take three-quarters of the human dose. Larger dogs can take the full dose.

**Help the body heal itself.** The vitamins E, C, and A strengthen the immune system and can help dogs with kennel cough heal more quickly, says Dr. Ehrsam. Dogs under 15 pounds can take 30 to 100 international units (IU) of vitamin E, 250 to

## Meet the Experts

**Christina Chambreau, D.V.M.,** is a holistic veterinarian in Sparks, Maryland, and education chairperson for the Academy of Veterinary Homeopathy.

**Beatrice Ehrsam, D.V.M.,** is a holistic veterinarian in private in New Paltz, New York. She is certified in acupuncture.

**Adriana Sagrera, D.V.M.,** is a holistic veterinarian in private practice in New Orleans.

**Allen M. Schoen, D.V.M.,** is director of the Veterinary Institute for Therapeutic Alternatives in Sherman, Connecticut, and the author of *Love, Miracles, and Animal Healing.* He is certified in acupuncture and chiropractic.

500 milligrams of vitamin C, and 500 IU of vitamin A a day. Dogs 15 to 40 pounds can take 200 to 300 IU of vitamin E, 500 milligrams of vitamin C, and 1,000 IU of vitamin A a day. Larger dogs can take 400 IU of vitamin E, up to 1,000 milligrams of vitamin C, and 5,000 IU of vitamin A a day. Since vitamin C can cause diarrhea, you may have to cut back the dose until you find an amount your pet will tolerate.

# LAMENESS

## The Signs
- Your pet is limping or walking with one leg off the ground.
- He is reluctant to move, and he cries when he does.

## The Cause

Almost anything can cause lameness, from jumping and landing wrong to having a broken bone or a "trick" knee. It can also be caused by long-term problems like arthritis or hip dysplasia, says Albert J. Simpson, D.V.M., a holistic veterinarian in private practice in Oregon City, Oregon.

Most lameness is temporary, he adds. Your dog or cat may limp for a few days, then gradually get better. You will need to call your vet when the pain seems to be severe or the lameness lasts longer than about three days. In most cases, however, natural home remedies will help your pet walk comfortably and recover more quickly. Here is what veterinarians advise.

## The Solutions FOR DOGS & CATS

**Stop the soreness.** Pets sometimes limp a bit when they have pushed their muscles too much during a hard run, for example, or from an extra-long swim. "A homeopathic remedy called Arnica can help relieve soreness," says Greig Howie, D.V.M., a holistic veterinarian in private practice in Dover, Delaware. "For really deep bruising, Bellis perennis can help." You will want to use 30C-potency pills, he advises. Give two or three pills every few hours until the lameness starts to improve. Only use one remedy at a time, he adds. If Arnica doesn't work, try Bellis perennis instead. Both remedies are available in some health food stores and mail-order catalogs. If your pet isn't better

## Call the VET

Lameness is usually caused by minor injuries and will clear up on its own within a few days. But sometimes it is caused by more serious problems, like a broken bone, a tumor, or the onset of arthritis, which will get worse if you don't get treatment right away. So if your pet is crying when he tries to walk or he doesn't improve within two to three days, you will want to call your vet, says Randy Caviness, D.V.M., a clinical instructor of small animal acupuncture at Tufts University School of Veterinary Medicine in North Grafton, Massachusetts, and a holistic veterinarian in Concord.

within two to three days, ask your vet for advice.

**Add some ankle pressure.** There is an acupressure point called BL60, which is on the outside of the back leg in the depression midway between the tendon and the anklebone. Stimulating this can temporarily ease pain, says Dr. Simpson. This spot is also known as the aspirin point because it relieves pain anywhere in the body. Press gently but firmly on the point for about 60 seconds, he advises. There should be a slight improvement right away. You can stimulate this point several times a day or as often as necessary to help control the pain.

**Treat the knees.** When lameness is caused by a sore knee, press the acupressure points known as Eyes of the Knee, located in the hollows on either side of the knees on the rear legs. These are very powerful points for easing knee pain, says Dr. Simpson. Press them for about 60 seconds several times a day as needed.

**Reverse the pain cycle.** When a pet pulls or sprains a muscle, the body floods the area with pain-causing chemicals that can cause swelling and inflammation, says Randy Caviness, D.V.M., clinical instructor of small animal acupuncture at Tufts University School of Veterinary Medicine in North Grafton, Massachusetts, and a holistic veterinarian in Concord. Applying cold for 15 to 20 minutes—either by using a commercial cold pack or a plastic bag filled with ice and wrapped in a thin towel—will constrict blood vessels and help reduce painful swelling. You can repeat this treatment three times a day for up to two days, he says. Only use cold when an injury is recent. After a day or two, veterinarians usually recommend using heat instead.

**Add some warmth.** When lameness isn't accompanied by swelling or when the swelling has begun to go down, it is a good idea to heat the sore spot with a hot pack, hot-water bottle, or a heating pad, says Dr. Caviness. Applying heat improves circulation to the area, which will help loosen muscles and flush out pain-causing chemicals. You don't want your pet to get too hot, he adds. To be safe, insulate the heat source by wrapping it in a blanket or towel. Keep the heat in place for 15 to 20 minutes, or until your pet lets you know he has had enough.

**BEST BET! Rub away the aches.** Overexertion often causes muscles to contract and tighten into painful little bands. Massaging the sore spot will improve circulation and speed healing, says Patricia Whalen-Shaw, a registered massage therapist and owner of Optissage, an animal massage school in Circleville, Ohio. Massage the shoulders for front-end lameness and around the hipbones for problems at the back end. Don't press on the bones, which can be painful, she adds. Just massage the muscles that lie alongside the bones.

**BEST BET! Try a healing cream.** "A homeopathic combination remedy called Traumeel cream is won-

## Meet the Experts

**Randy Caviness, D.V.M.,** is a clinical instructor of small animal acupuncture at Tufts University School of Veterinary Medicine in North Grafton, Massachusetts, and a holistic veterinarian in Concord. He is certified in acupuncture and chiropractic.

**Greig Howie, D.V.M.,** is a holistic veterinarian in private practice in Dover, Delaware. He is certified in acupuncture and homeopathy.

**Albert J. Simpson, D.V.M.,** is a holistic veterinarian in private practice in Oregon City, Oregon. He is certified in acupuncture and chiropractic.

**Michelle Tilghman, D.V.M.,** is a holistic veterinarian in private practice in Stone Mountain, Georgia. She is certified in acupuncture.

**Patricia Whalen-Shaw** is a registered massage therapist and owner of Optissage, an animal massage school in Circleville, Ohio.

derful for treating bruises, sprains, and strains," says Michelle Tilghman, D.V.M., a holistic veterinarian in private practice in Stone Mountain, Georgia. Gently rub the cream onto the injured area several times a day, she advises, making sure to get it beneath the fur and onto the skin. You can get Traumeel from veterinarians or, under the name Traumed, at some health food stores.

# LETHARGY

## The Signs

- Your pet tires easily or has lost his spunk.
- He is staying out of sight.
- He is not playing or eating as much as usual.
- Nothing seems to excite him.

## The Cause

It doesn't take much to get dogs and cats excited. A jiggle of the leash, a rolling ball of yarn, or, when all else fails, rattling a box of food is sure to fire up some enthusiasm. When it becomes obvious that your pet's get-up-and-go has got up and gone, you need to take a closer look.

"A loss of vim and vigor is an indication that something is up," says Beatrice Ehrsam, D.V.M., a holistic veterinarian in private practice in New Paltz, New York. Sometimes it is just a temporary thing. In summer, for example, dogs and cats naturally slow down a little. Pets that are getting older or have gained some weight will also lose some of their pep. But lethargy that doesn't go away may also be a sign of nutritional deficiencies, a hormone imbalance, or even serious illnesses like cancer or heart disease.

Holistic veterinarians believe that everything in your pet's life, from the food he eats to his emotional health, plays a direct role in how energetic he feels. Here are a few ways to help him shake off the cobwebs and start feeling excited again.

## The Solutions FOR DOGS & CATS

**Lift your pet's spirits.** Boredom, loneliness, or a lack of stimulation can make pets lethargic, says John F. Sangiorgio, D.V.M., a holistic veterinarian in private practice in Staten Island, New York. "Give him more to do, more contact with humans, more meaningful activity," he advises.

**Help him sleep with chamomile.** Most dogs and cats don't have any trouble falling asleep, but some have the human equivalent of insomnia, which can make them tired and poopy during the day. If your pet seems restless at night, give him some chamomile tea, an ancient herbal remedy for insomnia and jangled nerves, says Dr. Sangiorgio. In the evening, steep two tablespoons of dried chamomile in a pint of hot water for 10 to 20 minutes. Strain and let it cool to room temperature, then pour one-quarter to one-half cup into a bowl and see if he will drink it. Don't put it in his water bowl because some pets don't care for the taste of chamomile and will stop drinking altogether, he adds.

**Provide a ginseng jolt.** The herb ginseng is renowned for giving people and pets a quick boost of energy, says Dr. Sangiorgio. He recommends using ginseng capsules, giving cats about one-tenth of the human dose once a day. Dogs can take a little more. Dogs weighing 15 to 50 pounds, for example, can take one-quarter to one-third of the human dose. Ginseng can have side effects, so don't use it longer than two weeks.

**Give him a rise with yeast.** Yeast is an excellent source of B vitamins, which are vital for producing energy. Use nutritional yeast instead of brewer's yeast because it is less likely to cause allergic reactions, says Tejinder Sodhi, D.V.M., a holistic veterinarian in private practice in Bellevue and Lynnwood, Washington. Most pets like the taste, and you can sprinkle it on their food. Pets weighing under 15 pounds can take one-half teaspoon of yeast with every meal. Pets 15 to 50 pounds can take a teaspoon, and larger dogs can have two teaspoons with every meal. Some pets are allergic to yeast, so it is a good idea to check with your vet before using it at home.

## Call the VET

It isn't normal for pets to be droopy all the time. If you aren't able to give your pet some extra pep in three to five days using home remedies, you will want to play it safe and call your vet. It is probably nothing more than temporary fatigue, but some serious conditions, including heart disease and cancer, can make pets crushingly tired, says Bob Ulbrich, V.M.D., a holistic veterinarian in private practice in Portland, Oregon.

As soon as you notice lingering signs of lethargy, take your pet's temperature, Dr. Ulbrich adds. The normal temperature range for a dog is 100° to 102.5°F; for cats, it is 101° to 102.5°. If the temperature is low, your pet could be dehydrated, which may be a sign of kidney or liver disease. If it is 103.5° or higher, he should see the vet.

**BEST BET!** **Improve his diet.** One of the main causes of lethargy in dogs and cats is poor nutrition, says Katherine Evans, D.V.M., a holistic veterinarian in private practice in Concord, New Hampshire. Even though commercial pet foods contain all the essential vitamins and minerals, they don't always use the best-quality ingredients. She recommends giving pets an all-natural diet, preferably one that is made from scratch. "Home-cooked whole foods can increase a pet's energy dramatically," she says. For more information on making natural diets at home, see page 61.

**Improve his digestion with enzymes.** To help ensure that your pet absorbs all the nutrients in his food, supplement his meals with digestive enzymes, says Patricia Cooper, D.V.M., a holistic veterinarian in private practice in Houston. She recommends giving pets Zymex wafer enzymes, available from veterinarians. Pets under 15 pounds can have half a wafer with every meal. Those weighing 15 to 50 pounds can have one wafer, and larger dogs can have two. Some cats dislike the taste, she adds, so you may need to dissolve it in water and mix it in their food.

**Reduce stress with flower essences.** Dogs and cats may experience a physical slump when they are disturbed emotionally, says Bob Ulbrich, V.M.D., a holistic veterinarian in private practice in Portland,

---

## Meet the Experts

**Nancy Brandt, D.V.M.,** is a holistic veterinarian in private practice in Las Vegas. She is certified in acupuncture.

**Patricia Cooper, D.V.M.,** is a holistic veterinarian in private practice in Houston.

**Beatrice Ehrsam, D.V.M.,** is a holistic veterinarian in private practice in New Paltz, New York. She is certified in acupuncture.

**Katherine Evans, D.V.M.,** is a holistic veterinarian in private practice in Concord, New Hampshire. She is certified in acupuncture.

**John F. Sangiorgio, D.V.M.,** is a holistic veterinarian in private practice in Staten Island, New York.

**Tejinder Sodhi, D.V.M.,** is a holistic veterinarian in private practice in Bellevue and Lynnwood, Washington. He is certified in acupuncture, chiropractic, and homeopathy.

**Bob Ulbrich, V.M.D.,** is a holistic veterinarian in private practice in Portland, Oregon. He is certified in homeopathy.

---

Oregon. The flower essence walnut, for example, is helpful for pets that are having trouble adjusting to a new environment, while the essences pine and chestnut are recommended for pets that are grieving. There are many flower essences, so you will want to ask your vet which is the best choice.

Mix about 10 drops of the essence in a cup of spring water, then put three or four drops of the diluted essence on your pet's tongue three or four times a day. Or add one-half dropperful of the full-strength essence to his water once a day.

**Give a natural sleep aid.** A Tahitian herbal remedy called noni juice can be very helpful for pets that are having trouble getting enough sleep, says Nancy Brandt, D.V.M., a holistic veterinarian in private practice in Las Vegas. "It stimulates the pineal gland to make more melatonin, which regulates sleep patterns, and serotonin, which is a nerve regulator," she says. "Noni juice jump-starts the cells so that they clear out toxins and work better."

She recommends giving a teaspoon of the juice once a day to cats and dogs under 15 pounds. Larger pets can take between one and three teaspoons a day. Noni juice isn't always easy to find, so you may want to ask your veterinarian to recommend a supplier.

**Mix vegetables in his food.** Fresh vegetables such as carrots, squash, zucchini, pumpkin, and greens are an excellent source of trace minerals and soluble fiber. "They are very good for the intestinal tract, which, if not working properly, can make animals sluggish," says Dr. Sodhi. "If you are not feeding your pet home-cooked meals, try adding grated, lightly steamed vegetables to your pet's food, he suggests. You don't have to give a lot to get the benefits, he adds. Pets under 15 pounds only need about a teaspoon of vegetables with every meal. Those weighing 15 pounds or more can have as much as a tablespoon. It is fine to give a little more, he adds, although pets that eat too much vegetables will often get soft stools.

# LICKING

## The Signs
- Your pet has licked away fur, or the skin is getting irritated.
- She is concentrating on certain parts of her body.

## The Cause

It doesn't take dogs and cats long to learn the art of licking. Their mothers lick them all over as soon as they are born, and they quickly discover that it feels good and is comforting. As they mature, they continue to lick for comfort, to remove dead hair and skin cells, to scratch itches, and to relieve pain.

The problem is that some pets can't get enough of a good thing. They will lick themselves so often and so vigorously that they will rub away fur and irritate the skin underneath. Pets with allergies are especially likely to indulge in nonstop licking. So are those that are bored or experiencing stress. "It's similar to a person who bites his nails," says Thomas Van Cise, D.V.M., a holistic veterinarian in private practice in Norco, California.

No matter what is causing the licking, the only way to reduce it is to treat all parts of your pet's life—her emotions along with her body. Here is what holistic veterinarians advise.

## The Solutions
FOR DOGS & CATS

**Give comfort with chamomile.** The herb chamomile is renowned for reducing stress and imparting feelings of calm. It is especially good for pets that have recently had a stressful experience, like a quarrel with another pet, says Susan G. Wynn, D.V.M., a veterinarian in Atlanta and co-editor of *Complementary and Alternative Veterinary Medicine*. Brew a cup of chamomile tea and let it cool to room temperature, then mix the tea in your pet's food. You can give a teaspoon of tea to pets under 15 pounds, one tablespoon to pets 15 to 50 pounds, and

## Call the VET

The ceaseless "slurp, slurp" of inveterate lickers is usually more annoying for owners than it is harmful to pets. But dogs and cats that lick too long and too often may develop serious sores called lick granulomas.

Lick granulomas resemble an irritated callus and can lead to painful, hard-to-heal infections, says Thomas Van Cise, D.V.M., a holistic veterinarian in private practice in Norco, California. They rarely go away with home treatments and invariably get worse over time, he adds. Any sore that is slow to heal, especially one that occurs on the lower legs, could be a lick granuloma, and you should ask your vet to take a look.

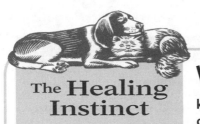

## The Healing Instinct

With our flexible hands and opposable thumbs, it just seems natural to rub or knead itchy spots on the skin. Rubbing increases circulation and reduces both pain and itching.

Dogs and cats don't have hands, but they do have tongues, and licking the skin is nature's way of boosting blood flow and relieving discomfort, says Maria Chelaru-Williams, D.V.M., a veterinarian in private practice in Boulder, Colorado. In addition, licking creates moisture, which produces a form of topical anesthesia when it evaporates, she adds.

two tablespoons to pets over 50 pounds.

An easier way to give chamomile is to mix crushed leaves in your pet's food, Dr. Wynn suggests. Give one-quarter teaspoon of leaves to pets under 15 pounds, one-half teaspoon to those 15 to 40 pounds, three-quarters teaspoon to those 41 to 70 pounds, and a full teaspoon to dogs over 70 pounds. Or you can buy a glycerin-based chamomile tincture and add a few drops to her food.

**BEST BET!** **Serve extra fatty acids.** Veterinarians have discovered that fatty acids, especially omega-3 and omega-6 fatty acids, help recondition dry skin and relieve irritation, says Dr. Van Cise. Health food stores stock a wide variety of fatty acids, but you will want to ask your vet to recommend one that contains the proper mix of omega-3s and omega-6s. One product you may want to try is Eskimo Oil. Available in drugstores and

from veterinarians, it comes in a liquid form, and dogs and cats love the taste. You can give cats and dogs under 15 pounds one-quarter teaspoon of the oil with every meal, while larger pets can take one-half teaspoon.

**Stop pain and itching.** Dogs and cats often lick when they are in pain—because of arthritis, for example, or even a pulled muscle. An herb called neem (*Azadiracta indica*) reduces joint and muscle pain and soothes the skin, says Michael W. Lemmon, D.V.M., a holistic veterinarian in Renton, Washington, and past president of the American Holistic Veterinary Medical Association. He recommends applying neem oil or neem hand-and-body lotion to the affected area once or twice a day. It has a bitter taste, so most pets won't lick it off, he adds.

**Stop licking with homeopathy.** Given in tandem, the homeopathic remedies Ignatia and Gelsemium can reduce the urge to lick, says Maria

Chelaru-Williams, D.V.M., a veterinarian in private practice in Boulder, Colorado. She recommends giving dogs four pellets of Ignatia 30X in the morning and four pellets of Gelsemium 30X in the afternoon. Cats can take two pellets of each remedy. Repeat the treatments every day for a week, then once a month for three months, she advises.

**Reduce the urge with essences.** Used for a variety of emotional problems, flower and other essences can help curtail stress-related or compulsive licking, says Dr. Van Cise. He recommends giving the essences in combination, either camellia and forsythia or barnacle and urchin. Both combinations are available in mail-order catalogs. Mix three drops of each essence in an ounce of spring or distilled water, then put three drops on your pet's tongue or gums three times a day for four to six months.

**Add some entertainment to her life.** Just as humans will sometimes crack their knuckles or twirl a strand of hair when they are bored, dogs and cats lick, sometimes for hours. Keeping your pet entertained is a great way to give her tongue a rest. Take a 15-minute walk instead of the usual 5-minute stroll. Throw a ball or a ball of string for half an hour in the morning. Or just get down on the floor and roll around with her. Pets that are active have a lot less nervous energy than those that lie around all day, says

## Meet the Experts

**Pam Johnson Bennett** is a feline behavior consultant in Nashville and the author of *Twisted Whiskers* and *Psycho Kitty*.

**Maria Chelaru-Williams, D.V.M.,** is a veterinarian in private practice in Boulder, Colorado.

**Michael W. Lemmon, D.V.M.,** is a holistic veterinarian in Renton, Washington, and past president of the American Holistic Veterinary Medical Association.

**Thomas Van Cise, D.V.M.,** is a holistic veterinarian in private practice in Norco, California. He is certified in acupuncture.

**Susan G. Wynn, D.V.M.,** is a veterinarian in Atlanta and co-editor of *Complementary and Alternative Veterinary Medicine*.

Pam Johnson Bennett, a feline behavior consultant in Nashville and author of *Twisted Whiskers*.

**Switch to a simple diet.** Pets usually take up licking because they are sensitive to something in their diets, says Susan G. Wynn, D.V.M., a veterinarian in Atlanta and co-editor of *Complementary and Alternative Veterinary Medicine*. Switching them to a natural diet, which won't contain the artificial additives found in many commercial foods, can help calm the immune system and reduce the need to lick, she says. For more information on natural diets, see page 61.

# Liver Problems

## The Signs

- Your pet isn't eating as much as usual.
- He is vomiting repeatedly or has had diarrhea for more than a few days.
- He seems tired and run-down.
- The eyes or insides of the ears are slightly yellow.
- His abdomen is swollen.

## The Cause

As the largest organ in the body, the liver performs more than 500 different tasks. It is a food processor, a storehouse for nutrients, and a factory that makes hormones and other substances. It is also a filter that removes toxins, such as drugs or the chemical additives in foods, from the blood. "It is the best detoxification organ there is," says Roger L. DeHaan, D.V.M, a holistic veterinarian in private practice in Frazee, Minnesota.

The liver is designed to withstand most things that the body throws at it. But when it is exposed to large amounts of toxins or to viruses or bacteria, it can literally shut down. "Unfortunately, pets don't often show signs of liver problems until the damage is severe," says Dr. DeHaan.

And except for using antibiotics for bacterial infections, there aren't a lot of drugs for treating liver problems. "But if you nourish the organ with natural medicines, a lot of times it will regenerate, and your pet can live a normal life," he says.

## The Solutions FOR DOGS & CATS

**Pull away poisons.** Applying magnets to your pet's feet can redirect the energy flowing through his body and help remove toxins from the liver, says Joanne Stefanatos, D.V.M., a holistic veterinarian in private practice in Las Vegas. She recommends applying one magnet (with a strength of about 550 gauss) underneath the right front foot and another one under the left rear foot. The magnets are quite large, and you can simply rest your pet's feet on them as long as he will hold still. Make sure that the "north pole" of the magnet is facing the foot on the right side, and the "south pole" is facing the foot on the left. Hold the magnets in place for 20 to 30 minutes twice a day, she advises.

**Use a dandelion purifier.** The ubiquitous dandelion (*Taraxacum officinale*) is an extremely powerful herb

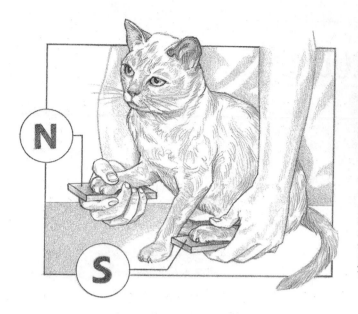

Many veterinarians are using magnets to help detoxify the liver and other parts of the body. Position your cat's right front paw pad on top of the "north pole" side of a magnet and the left rear paw pad on the "south pole" side of another magnet. For healing, the magnets must be in contact with the cat's paw pads. Hold the magnets against the paw pads for about 20 minutes, giving the magnets time to adjust energy fields throughout the body.

that can also help remove toxins from the liver, says Dr. DeHaan. Although you can use fresh dandelion, it is easier to give dandelion capsules, available in health food stores. He recommends giving cats with liver problems half a capsule of dandelion once a day. Dogs weighing less than 15 pounds can take a whole capsule. Those weighing 15 to 50 pounds can take two capsules, and larger dogs can take three capsules a day.

**BEST BET!** **Strengthen the liver with milk thistle.** The liver is susceptible to damage from toxins and infection. Available at health food stores, milk thistle (*Silybum marianum*) has been shown to help the liver generate new cells and protect it from toxins, says Susan G. Wynn, D.V.M., a veterinarian in Atlanta and co-editor of *Complementary and Alternative Veterinary Medicine*. Give cats and dogs weighing under 15 pounds one-quarter of the human dose. Pets 15 to 30 pounds can take one-half of the human dose, and those 31 to 50 pounds can take three-quarters of the human dose. Larger dogs can take the full human dose.

Other herbal supplements that can help cleanse the liver or even rejuvenate damaged cells include wheat grass, barley greens, and green chlorella. Chlorophyll tablets are also good, says Dr. Stefanatos. Wheat grass is especially helpful because it helps remove heavy metals like lead, mercury, and aluminum from the body, she adds. Your vet can advise you as to which supplements and doses will be best for your pet.

**Get the drop on toxins.** Giving your pet a dropperful of homeopathic medicine, either Liver Liquescence or Detoxification, can remove toxins in the body that may put excessive strain on the liver. You can use either one twice a day for up to four weeks, says Dr. DeHaan. Both homeopathic medicines are available from veterinarians.

**Feed them naturally.** The artificial flavors, additives, and preservatives in many commercial pet foods can overburden the liver, says Dr. DeHaan. He recommends giving pets with liver problems a homemade diet or a commercial food, such as Wysong, which don't contain artificial

ingredients. You can buy Wysong and similar all-natural foods in some pet supply stores and through mail order. For more information on natural diets, see page 61.

**Help his body clean house.** The lymphatic system is responsible for capturing toxins throughout the body and carting them to the liver for removal. To help this system work more efficiently, Dr. DeHaan recommends vigorously rubbing your pet's right side, just over the last three ribs. Doing this for 10 to 15 seconds once a day will stimulate the flow of lymph and help remove harmful compounds from the bloodstream.

**Put beets in his bowl.** Raw beets contain natural chemicals that can

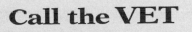

## Call the VET

It's no big deal when dogs skip a few meals, but a lost appetite can lead to serious problems for cats. Cats that don't eat for a day or two can develop a life-threatening condition called hepatic lipidosis, or fatty liver disease, in which fat deposits move into the liver and clog up the cells, says Pat Zook, D.V.M., a holistic veterinarian in private practice in Stone Mountain, Georgia.

Symptoms of hepatic lipidosis include a swollen abdomen, loss of appetite, and yellowish eyes and ears—signs that bile from the liver is accumulating in the body. This condition is always an emergency, says Dr. Zook, and you will need to see your vet immediately.

**ALTERNATIVE**

## 🐾 SUCCESS

### HEALING FROM THE HEART

Opie always had a big appetite, so his owner, Betsy Stowe of Slippery Rock, Pennsylvania, wasn't too surprised when she noticed that his orange-and-white tummy growing a little rounder. But she started getting worried when her seven-year-old cat starting acting tired and depressed, and his nose and gums suddenly turned white.

Her veterinarian had bad news: Opie had liver cancer. Betsy took him home, fussed over him, and cried. "But that seemed to make him worse," she says. "He didn't want to be reminded that he was sick."

A friend suggested that Opie might feel better if Betsy were more positive and upbeat. "She said to talk to him about the things that he liked to do, call him by his special nicknames—Chief and Boss—sing him silly songs, and just treat him normally." Betsy took the advice—and the change was amazing. Within a week, the swelling in the abdomen went down, and Opie's appetite came back. When Betsy returned to the vet, she got some incredible news: The cancer was in remission.

"When you are close to a cat, you can look in his eyes and communicate," Betsy says. "Opie just wanted to hear the same old stuff, to be king of the manor, and to strut around. That is his job, and he thrived on it. You just have to listen with your heart."

---

help remove toxins from the liver and make it stronger. Dr. DeHaan recommends giving pets weighing under 15 pounds about one-quarter teaspoon of grated raw beets a day. Pets 15 to 50 pounds can have one-half teaspoon, and larger dogs can have one to two teaspoons. Cats shouldn't have more than a few slivers. "It's quite powerful, so don't give too much," he says. Dr. DeHaan advises giving beets once a day for five days, then letting the body rest for two.

**Treat the liver with liver.** Sheep and beef livers contain enzymes that can help repair liver damage in dogs and cats, says Dr. DeHaan. He recommends giving cats and dogs under 15 pounds about one teaspoon of raw liver a day. Larger dogs can take up to two tablespoons. Talk to your vet before giving liver because it contains a lot of copper, which may cause problems for pets with certain liver conditions.

**Add enzymes to his diet.** Giving your pet digestive enzymes, such as Prozyme or FloraZyme LP, which are available from veterinarians and at some pet supply stores, will cause food to be digested more completely, putting less strain on the liver, says Dr. DeHaan. Check the label for the proper doses.

**Restore energy with aromatherapy.** Dogs and cats that are recovering from liver problems are invariably weak and tired. They will often feel energized if you apply a little essential oil of basil to the inside tips of their ears once a day, says Dr. Stefanatos. The oil is too strong to use directly, so dilute it half-and-half with vegetable oil and only use it for a few days, she adds.

**Push their appetites into motion.** Pets with liver problems often lose their appetites, and the less they eat, the weaker they get. A quick way to restore lost appetite is to press the GV7 acupressure point, located on each side of the spine seven vertebrae back from the shoulder blades, for a minute or two each day, suggests Dr. DeHaan.

## Meet the Experts

**Roger L. DeHaan, D.V.M.,** is a holistic veterinarian in private practice in Frazee, Minnesota. He is certified in chiropractic.

**Joanne Stefanatos, D.V.M.,** is a holistic veterinarian in private practice in Las Vegas. She is certified in acupuncture and chiropractic.

**Susan G. Wynn, D.V.M.,** is a veterinarian in Atlanta and co-editor of *Complementary and Alternative Veterinary Medicine.*

**Pat Zook, D.V.M.,** is a holistic veterinarian in private practice in Stone Mountain, Georgia. She is certified in acupuncture.

## The Solutions — FOR CATS

**Give a high-powered snack.** When your cat won't eat anything else, try giving him a raw liver formula, says Dr. DeHaan. In a blender combine a raw egg yolk, a tablespoon of raw sheep or beef liver, a teaspoon of honey, two tablespoons of plain yogurt, and a cup of water, and mix it well. "Give your cat one teaspoon—or as much as he will eat—every hour or two," says Dr. DeHaan. "You can use this for a week or two when he is refusing to eat regular food."

# MANGE

## The Signs

- Your pet is scratching furiously.
- Her skin looks red and irritated, or there are bumps or sores.
- She is losing patches of hair or has a bad smell.

## The Cause

Mange has a reputation for being the scourge of junkyard dogs, but any dog can get it, and sometimes cats get it, too.

There are two kinds of mange. One kind, called scabies, occurs when sarcoptic mites tunnel under the skin and trigger an allergic reaction. Scabies is highly contagious to pets as well as people, which is why it is important to treat all the pets in your family even when only one is infected, says Susan G. Wynn, D.V.M., a veterinarian in Atlanta and co-editor of *Complementary and Alternative Veterinary Medicine*.

The second kind of mange, called demodectic mange, occurs when demodex mites that normally live on the skin suddenly multiply to enormous numbers. Demodectic mange usually occurs in puppies because their immune systems are changing constantly and aren't able to control the mites, says Dr. Wynn.

Both types of mange can cause ferocious itching, which is why holistic and mainstream veterinarians sometimes recommend killing the mites quickly with a medication called ivermectin (Stromectol). Other vets use a toxic dip. But drugs may not be necessary as long as you keep your pet's natural immunity strong and use home remedies to control the itching, says Jane Laura Doyle, D.V.M., a holistic veterinarian in private practice in Berkeley Springs, West Virginia.

## The Solutions FOR DOGS & CATS

**BEST BET!** **Kill mites with a natural dip.** One of the quickest ways to eliminate mange mites and stop itching is to douse your pet with a lime-sulfur solution, says Steven A. Melman, V.M.D., a veterinarian with practices in Potomac, Maryland, and Palm Springs, California, and author of *Skin Diseases of Dogs and Cats*. Available from vets, products such as Lymdyp are safe and very effective, although you will probably have to repeat the treatment about once a week until your pet is feeling better.

**Soothe the skin with an oatmeal bath.** "Shampoos containing oatmeal are soothing and can be helpful in relieving the itch caused by mange," says Dr. Doyle. Be sure to use an oatmeal shampoo made specifically for pets, she adds. Shampoos meant for humans may be harmful for dogs and cats.

**BEST BET!** **Use natural medicines to strengthen immunity.** Since mange thrives when the immune system is weaker than it should be, it is critical to boost immunity. Holistic veterinarians sometimes recommend giving pets reishi mushroom (*Ganoderma lucidum*) supplements, available in pet supply and health food stores, says Dr. Wynn. She recommends giving pets under 20 pounds one-quarter of the human dose. Those weighing 20 to 50 pounds can take half the human dose. Dogs 51 to 80 pounds can take three-quarters of the human dose, and larger dogs can take the full human dose.

Another herb that strengthens immunity is astragalus (*Astragalus membranaceus*), which is given in the same amounts as reishi mushrooms. Charlene Kickbush, D.V.M., a dog breeder and holistic veterinarian in private practice in Watkinsville, Georgia, advises giving astragalus along with echinacea (*Echinacea angustifolia* or *Echinacea purpurea*). The dosage recommendations for astragalus and echinacea are the same as those given above for reishi mushroom.

## Call the VET

Mange usually isn't that hard to treat with a combination of medications, dips, or natural treatments to relieve itching and strengthen the immune system. But sometimes a small patch of mange spreads to other parts of the body. Vets call this condition generalized demodectic mange, and it can be quite serious, if only because it usually occurs when another, underlying problem, like genetic immune-deficiency, a hormonal imbalance, diabetes, or cancer, has weakened the immune system and allowed the mites to thrive.

It is fine to treat small patches of mange at home, but you will need to call your vet if it seems to be spreading.

**BEST BET!** **Switch to a natural diet.** Dogs and cats are most likely to get mange and other skin problems when they aren't getting all the nutrients they need from their diets. Even though most commercial pet foods are nutritionally balanced, they may contain low-quality ingredients, along with chemical preservatives and additives that can weaken the immune system. "A good diet is crucial in fighting mange," says Dr. Wynn.

The best diets are those that are homemade and consist of fresh, natural foods, Dr. Kickbush says. For more information on making natural diets at home, see page 61.

**Give a vitamin supplement.** Many veterinarians believe that all pets, especially those with mange, will benefit from getting extra antioxidant vitamins in their diets. Nutrients such as vitamins C and E help strengthen immunity and block the release of histamine, a chemical in the body that causes itching, says Nancy Scanlan, D.V.M., a holistic veterinarian in private practice in Sherman Oaks, California. Pets under 15 pounds can be given about 100 international units (IU) of vitamin E a day, along with 250 milligrams of vitamin C. Those weighing 15 to 40 pounds can take 200 IU of vitamin E and between 500 and 1,000 milligrams of vitamin C. Dogs 41 to 80 pounds can take 400 IU of vitamin E and 1,000 milligrams of vi-

tamin C, and dogs over 80 pounds can take 600 IU of vitamin E and between 1,000 and 2,000 milligrams of vitamin C. Every pet needs different amounts of these nutrients, so ask your vet for the precise dose.

**Keep things calm.** Pets with demodectic mange tend to have flare-ups whenever they are feeling stressed, such as when you have out-of-town guests or even during spring cleaning when their usual routines are

---

## Meet the Experts

**Jane Laura Doyle, D.V.M.,** is a holistic veterinarian in private practice in Berkeley Springs, West Virginia. She is certified in acupuncture and homeopathy.

**Charlene Kickbush, D.V.M.,** is a dog breeder and holistic veterinarian in private practice in Watkinsville, Georgia. She is certified in acupuncture and chiropractic.

**Steven A. Melman, V.M.D.,** is a veterinarian with practices in Potomac, Maryland, and Palm Springs, California, and the author of *Skin Diseases of Dogs and Cats*.

**Nancy Scanlan, D.V.M.,** is a holistic veterinarian in private practice in Sherman Oaks, California. She is certified in acupuncture and chiropractic.

**Susan G. Wynn, D.V.M.,** is a veterinarian in Atlanta and co-editor of *Complementary and Alternative Veterinary Medicine*.

disrupted. It is worth doing everything you can to keep your pet calm and comfortable until the mange clears up, says Dr. Kickbush.

**Give the house a thorough cleaning.** The mites that cause scabies can survive for several days even when they are off your pet. To prevent a reinfestation, it is important to vacuum rugs, sweep and mop floors, and wash your pet's bedding, crate, collar, and any grooming tools that you happen to use.

# NOISE ANXIETY

## The Signs
- Your pet trembles, cries, hides, or gets destructive when she hears loud noises.

## The Cause

The sounds of storms—such as thunder, lightning, blowing winds, and drumming rain—make some pets go berserk with terror. Other pets cower at the sounds of fireworks or truck doors slamming. Some even quiver when they hear paper rustling, says Nicholas Dodman, B.V.M.S. (bachelor of veterinary medicine and surgery, a British equivalent of D.V.M.), professor of behavioral pharmacology and director of the behavior clinic at Tufts University School of Veterinary Medicine in North Grafton, Massachusetts.

Vets aren't sure why so many pets are terrified of loud sounds. In some cases, it is probably due to bad experiences. A puppy swatted with the sports section of the newspaper may grow up to be afraid of all paper sounds. Some pets are simply afraid of things that they don't understand, like the crash of thunder.

"Sedatives are commonly used to treat severe noise anxiety," says Wayne Hunthausen, D.V.M., a veterinary behaviorist in Westwood, Kansas, and author of the *Handbook of Behaviour Problems in Dogs and Cats*. The problem with drugs, of course, is that they often have side effects. And they are only effective when your pet is actually taking them. If she hears a loud noise when she is not taking the drug, she will get terrified all over again.

Holistic veterinarians have a lot of experience treating noise anxiety. They have found that it is possible to retrain pets to change their reactions to certain sounds. In addition, there are a number of natural remedies that can relieve anxiety and make pets less likely to react to the sounds they fear.

## The Solutions · FOR DOGS & CATS ·

**Comfort them with music.** When you know that noise is imminent—on the Fourth of July, for example—you may want to turn up the stereo and leave it on. "Pets have very acute hearing, but music may screen out some sounds," says Pam Johnson Bennett, a feline behavior consultant in Nashville and author of *Twisted Whiskers*. It doesn't matter what you play, although music with a slow, even rhythm is probably the most soothing, she says. Leaving the TV on can also help mask outside sounds.

**Give them a natural sedative.** Milk contains a natural chemical called tryptophan that tells the brain when to relax and sleep. "Pets with anxiety calm down when given warm milk," says Mary Lee Nitschke, Ph.D., professor of psychology at Linfield College in Portland, Oregon, and an animal behaviorist in Beaverton. You can give pets between one-quarter and one-half cup of milk, along with a little bread, she adds.

**Soothe them with color.** Veterinarians have found that different colors affect the brain and body in different ways. Some colors, such as red, are stimulating, while others have a calming effect. To keep your pet calm during noisy times, you may want to get a blue lightbulb and put it in the room with her bed. Blue can stimulate the pituitary gland to produce calming hormones, says Joanne Stefanatos, D.V.M., a holistic veterinarian in private practice in Las Vegas.

**BEST BET!** **Give a soothing supplement.** "Given the choice between terror and sleep, sometimes it is kinder for pets to sleep," says Dr. Dodman. One way to help them nod off is with melatonin, a supplement that is similar to a natural chemical in the brain that helps regulate sleep. Pets may react in different ways to melatonin, so be sure to ask your vet for the correct dose, he advises.

"Another home treatment is a product called Calm Pet," he says. "It contains melatonin, kava kava, chamomile, St. John's wort, and valerian root, and it will help relax your pet." Follow the directions on the label.

**Reduce panic with flower essences.** Dogs and cats in the throes of noise anxiety can suffer extreme panic. You can quickly calm them with a combination of the flower essences aspen, mimulus, and Rescue Remedy, says Jeanne Olson, D.V.M., a holistic veterinarian in private practice in North Pole, Alaska. Mix eight drops of each in an ounce of distilled water, she says.

One way to use flower remedies is to put the two to four drops between your pet's lip and gums several times a day, ideally, just before things get a little noisy. Or put a dropperful in her water so that she can sip it all day.

**Relax her with magnets.** It sounds like something out of science fiction, but you can literally readjust the body's electromagnetic field to help relieve anxiety attacks, says Dr. Stefanatos. She recommends holding a magnet, available from holistic veterinarians and some pet supply catalogs, on your pet's forehead right between the eyes for about 20 minutes or until she is calm. The "north pole" of the magnet should face her forehead.

**BEST BET!** **Be kind—but not too kind.** It is fine to give your dog or cat a little reassurance when she is scared, but you don't want to give too much. Pampering pets when they are frightened rewards the behavior and teaches them to be more fearful in the future, says Dr. Hunthausen. The next time she is startled by noise, give her a quick pat and a kind word, then go about your business, he advises. When she realizes that you aren't concerned, she will get the idea that there is nothing to be concerned about and will gradually learn to be a little calmer.

**BEST BET!** **Give her a distraction.** "When your pet starts acting a little bit nervous, make an unusual noise—toss a key chain, squeak a toy, or slap the side of your chair," suggests Dr. Hunthausen. Once her attention is focused on you, she will forget to be fearful for a few moments. Take advantage of this opportunity to distract her even more with some sort of physical game or—dear to every pet's heart—with food. "This is a technique called counter-conditioning, in which you are teaching your pet to associate noise with play and food instead of fear," he explains.

## Meet the Experts

**Pam Johnson Bennett** is a feline behavior consultant in Nashville and the author of *Twisted Whiskers* and *Psycho Kitty*.

**Nicholas Dodman, B.V.M.S.,** is professor of behavioral pharmacology and director of the behavior clinic at Tufts University School of Veterinary Medicine in North Grafton, Massachusetts. He is the author of *The Dog Who Loved Too Much* and *The Cat Who Cried for Help*.

**Wayne Hunthausen, D.V.M.,** is a veterinary behaviorist in Westwood, Kansas, and the author of the *Handbook of Behaviour Problems in Dogs and Cats*.

**Mary Lee Nitschke, Ph.D.,** is a professor of psychology at Linfield College in Portland, Oregon, and animal behaviorist in Beaverton.

**Jeanne Olson, D.V.M.,** is a holistic veterinarian in private practice in North Pole, Alaska.

**Joanne Stefanatos, D.V.M.,** is a holistic veterinarian in private practice in Las Vegas. She is certified in acupuncture and chiropractic.

# Nose Fading

## The Signs
- Your pet's nose changes from black to light brown, gray, or pink.
- His nose is pale all the time, or it fades in winter and darkens in summer.

## The Cause

The skin on your pet's nose, like the skin on his paws, is usually dark brown or black, possibly with a little pink thrown in. When a nose that is normally dark fades to light, there is usually a problem, says John Limehouse, D.V.M., a holistic veterinarian in private practice in Toluca Lake, California. The problem isn't always serious, he adds. When dogs bury bones, for example, they use their noses as scoops and can actually wear away the color.

More often, nose fading is caused by internal problems such as allergies,

## Call the VET

Nose-color changes are fairly common in dogs because they will shove their snouts into just about anything, from ice-covered ponds to thorny thickets. In cats, however, nose-color changes tend to be more serious. "I just don't see a lot of faded-nosed cats unless they have a problem," says Steven A. Melman, V.M.D., a veterinarian with practices in Potomac, Maryland, and Palm Springs, California, and author of *Skin Diseases of Dogs and Cats*. If your cat's nose is suddenly fading, you need to call your vet right away, he says.

For dogs and cats, you should call your vet when nose-color changes are accompanied by other symptoms, such as scabs or bleeding, which may be symptoms of cancer. Be especially alert if you have a golden retriever, since changes in this breed's nose color are often an early sign of thyroid disease, says Dr. Melman.

thyroid disease, or nutritional imbalances, says Carvel Tiekert, D.V.M., executive director of the American Holistic Veterinary Medical Association and a holistic veterinarian in Bel Air, Maryland.

Alternative veterinarians believe that changes on the outside of the body are valuable warning signs of problems within, and you may need to act quickly to keep things from getting worse. Here are a few things to try.

## The Solutions FOR DOGS & CATS

**Nourish the nose.** Zinc and vitamin E are two nutrients that are essential for healthy skin, including skin on the nose, says Steven A. Melman, V.M.D., a veterinarian with practices in Potomac, Maryland, and Palm Springs, California, and author of the *Skin Diseases of Dogs and Cats*. If your pet is running low on either of these nutrients, his nose may pay the price. Dr. Melman recommends giving five milligrams of zinc per pound of pet once a day. For vitamin E, he suggests giving one international unit (IU) per pound of pet twice a day. Stop giving your pet the nutrients once his nose color has returned.

**BEST BET!** **Stick with natural foods.** Many commercial pet foods contain artificial flavors and preservatives that may cause nose-color changes. "Pick a food that is balanced and has no artificial chemicals or preservatives," advises Dr. Tiekert. "I often recommend Natural Life and Precise brands." You can buy natural foods in some pet supply stores and through mail order.

**Give them fatty acids.** Supplements containing omega-3 and omega-6 fatty acids will help keep the nose looking bright and healthy, says Dr. Tiekert. He recommends giving 180 milligrams for every 20 pounds of dog or every 10 pounds of cat. You can pop the pills right down the hatch. Since pets like the fishy taste of fatty acids, however, it is usually easier to cut open the capsule and squeeze the oil on their food.

**Put some fish on the menu.** Another way to supply your pet with more fatty acids is to add a little bit of

## Meet the Experts

**John Limehouse, D.V.M.,** is a holistic veterinarian in private practice in Toluca Lake, California. He is certified in acupuncture.

**Steven A. Melman, V.M.D.,** is a veterinarian with practices in Potomac, Maryland, and Palm Springs, California, and the author of *Skin Diseases of Dogs and Cats*.

**Carvel Tiekert, D.V.M.,** is executive director of the American Holistic Veterinary Medical Association and a holistic veterinarian in Bel Air, Maryland. He is certified in acupuncture and chiropractic.

fish—especially salmon, mackerel, and sardines—to his diet, says Dr. Tiekert. He recommends using about 90 percent of your pet's usual food and adding 10 percent cooked fish. Don't use raw fish, he adds, because it may contain harmful parasites.

**BEST BET!** **Try a dish switch.** Some dogs and cats are sensitive to plastic, aluminum, and some kinds of stainless steel. "I suggest changing water and food bowls to Pyrex," says Dr. Limehouse. "Just changing dishes will help a lot of pets."

# Oily Coat

## The Signs
- Your pet's fur looks dull or dirty, or it sticks together.
- His skin looks greasy.
- There are greasy flakes in the fur, or the fur smells bad.

## The Cause

Dogs and cats secrete a natural oil called sebum that lubricates the skin and puts shine in the coat. Sebum is usually invisible. When pets produce too much of it, however, the coat may look greasy and dull, says Steven A. Melman, V.M.D., a veterinarian in private practice in Potomac, Maryland, and Palm Springs, California, and author of *Skin Diseases of Dogs and Cats*.

Some breeds, such as Yorkshire terriers, naturally secrete too much sebum and need frequent baths to keep their coats clean. In fact, any pet with an oily coat will benefit from more frequent washings, says Dr. Melman. But according to holistic veterinarians, an oily coat is more than skin-deep. What's happening on the inside of your pet's body is probably affecting how he looks on the outside. Here is what they recommend.

## The Solutions *FOR DOGS & CATS*

**Give them algae.** Pets with oily coats may not be getting all the minerals they need. One way to supplement their diets is to give them kelp. "Kelp is a really good source of trace minerals," says Nancy Scanlan, D.V.M., a holistic veterinarian in private practice in Sherman Oaks, California. Cats and dogs weighing under 15 pounds can take one-eighth teaspoon of powdered kelp, and larger dogs can have up to one teaspoon. "Give it every day," she says. "It is fine to divide it into two or three feedings."

**Clear out the toxins.** Many harmful substances in the body are excreted through the skin, which can cause the coat to get a little oily. "The way to help get gunk out of the body is to put pets on a modified fast for a day," says Dr. Scanlan. She recommends giving dogs plain white rice cooked in chicken broth, plus a heaping tablespoon or two of cooked ground meat. For cats, give them cream of rice cereal cooked in chicken broth and mix it half-and-half with their regular food. This diet will allow your pet's body to cleanse itself, and the amount of oil on the skin should return to normal, she says.

For two days after this modified fast, continuing adding a little bit of rice to your pet's usual food. After three days, he should be back on his regular food, preferably one that is all-natural, which will help keep his coat clean.

**Give a tonic.** Another way to cleanse the body is with a product called Hokamix, from veterinarians and pet supply catalogs. "It is an herbal supplement specifically for pets that acts like a body tonic," says Dr. Scanlan. "It helps build the body up." When using Hokamix, follow the directions on the label.

**BEST BET!** **Feed them naturally.** Many commercial pet foods contain chemical preservatives and artificial flavors and dyes that can disrupt the normal balance of the skin, causing an oily coat, says Carolyn Blakey, D.V.M., a holistic veterinarian

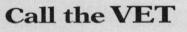

## Call the VET

Giving your pet a good shampooing is the easiest way to clean the skin and coat, but it won't stop whatever is causing the extra oil in the first place. It is worth looking into because some internal conditions, such as a hormonal imbalance, can cause the coat to look dull and greasy, says Steven A. Melman, V.M.D., a veterinarian with practices in Potomac, Maryland, and Palm Springs, California, and author of *Skin Diseases of Dogs and Cats*.

Your pet's coat should stay clean for at least a week or two after a bath, says Dr. Melman. If it gets oily within just a few days, you should ask your vet to take a look, he advises.

in private practice in Richmond, Indiana. She recommends giving pets an all-natural diet, either one made from scratch or one of the healthful commercial foods like Innova or Wysong, available at pet supply stores and through mail-order companies. Another brand that she recommends is Sojourner Farms. "They have prepared the grain, herbal, vitamin, and mineral base—it looks like dry oatmeal," she says. "You just add the fresh meat, vegetables, and water." For more on preparing natural diets for your pets, see page 61.

**BEST BET!** **Restore the balance.** To stay healthy, the skin requires the right balance of fatty acids, especially omega-3 and omega-6 fatty acids, says Joanne Stefanatos, D.V.M., a holistic veterinarian in private practice in Las Vegas. She recommends giving pets a product called Omega-derm Oil, which has a healthful mix of these fatty acids. Give pets under 25 pounds one teaspoon twice a day. Larger pets can take one tablespoon twice a day. Fatty acids smell like fish, and most pets will lap them up.

**Give some homeopathic skin relief.** Health food stores stock a variety of homeopathic remedies for skin, including HomeoPet Skin and Seborrhea and HomeoPet Hot Spot Dermatitis. Dogs can take 10 drops and cats 3 drops, both three times a day, says Dr. Blakey. If the problem doesn't go away in a few days or clears

## Meet the Experts

**Carolyn Blakey, D.V.M.,** is a holistic veterinarian in private practice in Richmond, Indiana. She is certified in acupuncture.

**Steven A. Melman, V.M.D.,** is a veterinarian with practices in Potomac, Maryland, and Palm Springs, California, and the author of *Skin Diseases of Dogs and Cats*.

**Nancy Scanlan, D.V.M.,** is a holistic veterinarian in private practice in Sherman Oaks, California. She is certified in acupuncture and chiropractic.

**Joanne Stefanatos, D.V.M.,** is a holistic veterinarian in private practice in Las Vegas. She is certified in acupuncture and chiropractic.

up and then returns, you will want to call your vet.

**Get the shampoo ready.** Regardless of what's causing the "wet look," giving your pet a bath every week or two will reduce the odor and help his fur shine. Pet supply stores sell a number of degreasing shampoos, some of which contain strong chemicals like benzoyl peroxide. You can get the same results by using an all-natural shampoo, which may contain ingredients such as oatmeal, tea tree oil, or natural salicylic acid that is derived from willow bark. Professional groomers often use a natural product called D'Grease Shampoo, which helps to dissolve the skin oil.

# OVERWEIGHT

## The Signs

- Your cat has a potbelly.
- Your dog doesn't have a waist.
- You can't feel your pet's ribs.
- He snores or is having trouble breathing.

## The Cause

Like people, some pets have an inherited tendency to gain weight. But most of the time, also like people, pets get heavy because they eat too much rich food and don't get enough exercise. "People are plugged into the TV, and pets are plugged into their owners," says Ihor Basko, D.V.M., a holistic veterinarian in private practice in Honolulu and Kilauea, Hawaii. "Poor diet and no exercise create fat pets." About one in three pets in this country is overweight.

Part of the problem is that commercial pet foods have been spiked with artificial flavors to make them more appealing. They taste so good, in fact, that many pets keep eating even when they are no longer hungry. In addition, dogs and cats don't have to hunt for a living anymore. Their bodies are designed for motion, but their modern lifestyles aren't, so they take in a lot more calories than they burn.

Holistic and mainstream veterinarians agree that the best way to help pets lose weight is to reduce the amount of calories they take in and encourage them to exercise more. Traditionally, veterinarians have recommended that overweight pets be switched to "lite" diets. While low-calorie foods can help, they don't work for all pets. And because these foods are low in certain fatty acids, they have a tendency to cause dry, flaky skin and a dull coat, says Susan G. Wynn, D.V.M., a veterinarian in Atlanta and co-editor of *Complementary and Alternative Veterinary Medicine*. "Some of the fattest animals I see are on these diets," she adds. Another problem with low-calorie diets, which are typically very low in fat, is that some pets become intolerant to fat in the future. This means that they could develop pancreatitis if they are ever switched back to a regular food, she says.

When you are helping your pet lose weight, you need to make changes in all parts of his life—not only what goes in the food bowl but also how he spends his days. Here is what holistic veterinarians advise.

# The Solutions

FOR DOGS & CATS

**Try a fat-burning herb.** Holistic veterinarians sometimes recommend giving overweight pets a Chinese herbal formula called Coptis Purge, which helps the body burn more fat, says Dr. Basko. Unlike many diet aids, which are intended for long-term use, you only have to give Coptis Purge for three to five days. "It doesn't take much to work really well," he says. You can buy Coptis Purge in health food stores. Every pet will need a different amount, so check with your vet before giving it at home, he advises. Another herb that can reduce body fat is hawthorn berry (*Crataegus laevigata*). It improves liver function, which helps reduce the amounts of fat and cholesterol in the blood, says Dr. Basko. He recommends giving 10 milligrams of hawthorn berry three times a day for every 10 pounds of weight. Hawthorn berry can be dangerous for pets with heart disease, however.

**BEST BET!** **Switch to a natural diet.** Most commercial pet foods contain way too much fat and not enough fiber, says Dr. Basko. They are also highly flavored, so dogs and cats tend to eat more than they really need. The best way to control your pet's weight is to switch to an all-natural pet food, one that more closely duplicates the balance of nutrients that nature intended. You can buy natural foods such as Innova, PetGuard Premium, Wysong, and Solid Gold in some pet supply stores and from mail-order companies.

Natural pet foods are more wholesome than many of their commercial counterparts, but holistic veterinarians believe that homemade diets are a better choice. "At least half of the protein in a cat's diet should be raw meat," says Dr. Basko. "Cats that are fed raw meat rarely get fat."

If you decide to start making your pet's meals at home, you will need to follow a few basic guidelines to help him lose weight. For cats, the diet should be 50 to 60 percent raw meat, 20 to 30 percent grains, such as rice or millet, with the rest coming from cooked vegetables. For dogs, the diet should be 35 percent protein from meat, 30 percent grains, and 35 percent raw or cooked vegetables. To kill harmful organisms such as salmonella, you can lightly steam meat before adding it to your pet's food. Your vet may also advise giving your pet nutritional supplements. For more information on natural diets, see page 61.

Dogs and cats don't always take kindly to changes in their diet. It is not uncommon for them to refuse to eat—or, in some cases, to get diarrhea—when you switch them to a new food, says Anne Lampru, D.V.M., a holistic veterinarian in private practice in Tampa, Florida. She recommends making the change gradually by mixing the new and old foods together, gradually increasing the percentage of new food over a few weeks. Dogs adjust fairly quickly, but cats may take as long as a month before they are entirely comfortable with the new diet, she says.

**Control the food flow.** Many pets that are overweight have food available all the time. This buffet style of eating—vets call it free-choice feeding—is convenient for owners, but it makes it easy for pets to overindulge. A better strategy is to feed your pet twice a day, once in the morning and again in the afternoon. This allows you to better control how much he is eating, says Dr. Wynn.

**BEST BET!** **Round out his meals with vegetables.** "Most pets can lose weight if you cut back on how much they eat," says Donn W. Griffith, D.V.M., a holistic veterinarian in private practice in Dublin, Ohio. Try giving your pet about 25 percent less of his regular food and replacing it with chopped raw or cooked vegetables. (Don't use onions, which can be dangerous for cats.)

Vegetables have fewer calories than grains or meats, and they won't cause him to gain weight, says Dr. Wynn. And because they are high in fiber, they will help him feel full even when he is getting fewer calories.

If your pet hasn't lost any weight in four weeks, reduce the pet food by

## Call the VET

Crash diets aren't particularly healthful for people, and they can be life-threatening for cats. Cats that don't eat for a day or two have a high risk of developing a condition called fatty liver disease, or hepatic lipidosis. Going without food may prompt body fat to migrate into the liver, overloading it, and possibly shutting it down. There is nothing wrong with reducing the amount of calories your cat consumes or giving him a different food, adds Anne Lampru, D.V.M., a holistic veterinarian in private practice in Tampa, Florida. Just be sure to make the change slowly because cats sometimes refuse to eat when the menu changes. If your cat does stop eating, don't wait more than a day or two before calling your vet, she says.

another 25 percent. If you still don't see any changes, you will need to talk to your vet about finding a more efficient weight-loss plan, says Dr. Wynn.

**Stimulate his metabolism with massage.** Giving your pet a vigorous, whole-body rubdown stimulates everything from digestion to circulation to the activity of the adrenal glands. The faster your pet's "motor" runs, the more calories he will burn, says Dr. Basko, who recommends giving overweight pets a 20- to 30-minute massage once a day.

**Rebalance his body with glandular supplements.** Some pets gain weight after being spayed or neutered because the hormonal balance affecting metabolism has been altered, says Dr. Lampru. You can help restore their normal metabolism by giving them glandular supplements, available in health food stores. Cats and dogs weighing less than 15 pounds can take about one-sixth of the human dose once a day. Pets between 15 and 50 pounds can take one-third of the human dose, and dogs over 50 pounds can have about one-half of the human dose, she says.

**BEST BET!** **Burn off fat with exercise.** Dogs and cats that lie around all day are going to gain weight no matter how little they eat. The only way to help them shed weight is to increase their metabolism

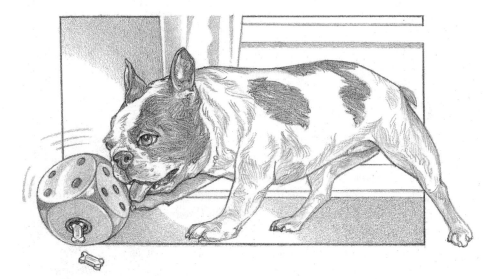

Pets are less likely to overeat when there is a lot of excitement in their lives. And few things are more exciting than the opportunity to get more food. Interactive toys like the Buster Cube have hidden compartments that contain tasty morsels. In order to get a bite, however, your pet will have to nudge, shove, and push the toy around, causing him to burn a lot more calories than he will take in.

with regular exercise. Start with 5 minutes of exercise three to five times a week, then, as your pet can tolerate it, increase the duration to 20 to 60 minutes a day, says Dr. Wynn. Too much exercise can be harmful for pets that are elderly or have heart problems, so talk to your vet before starting an exercise routine.

**Entertain their brains along with their stomachs.** Many dogs and cats become overweight because they depend on food to keep them entertained, says Dr. Lampru. Keeping their minds busy with interactive toys will make them less likely to depend on food for amusement. Many vets recommend toys such as the Buster Cube or the Goody Ship.

Of course, some of the best interactive toys, including the Buster Cube, use food as a way of getting their attention. But because the food is concealed inside the toy, they aren't able to eat much, and the fun of trying to get it out will keep them entertained for hours.

## The Solutions
### FOR CATS

**Get them moving with catnip.** Some cats are content to be doorstops,

---

## Meet the Experts

**Ihor Basko, D.V.M.,** is a holistic veterinarian in private practice in Honolulu and Kilauea, Hawaii, and the creator of the video *The Healing Touch for Your Dogs*. He is certified in acupuncture.

**Donn W. Griffith, D.V.M.,** is a holistic veterinarian in private practice in Dublin, Ohio. He is certified in acupuncture and chiropractic.

**Anne Lampru, D.V.M.,** is a holistic veterinarian in private practice in Tampa, Florida. She is certified in acupuncture and homeopathy.

**Susan G. Wynn, D.V.M.,** is a veterinarian in Atlanta and co-editor of *Complementary and Alternative Veterinary Medicine*.

---

and it can be a real challenge to entice them to exercise, says Dr. Basko. "If they are really lethargic, you may have to get them stimulated with catnip first." Catnip, both fresh and dried, lowers their inhibitions, he explains. "They will be more willing to play games and exercise when they have had some catnip first," he says.

Give cats one-quarter to one-half teaspoon of dried catnip, recommends Dr. Wynn.

# Pad Cracks

## The Signs
- Your pet's paw pads are rough, crusty, cracked, or swollen.
- She is limping on one or more paws.

## The Cause
The paw pads are shock-absorbing cushions covered with thick, durable skin. They can easily withstand the wear and tear of normal ramblings. But dogs and cats often push the pads to their limits by scrambling down gravel paths, running on hot cement, or navigating icy sidewalks. The skin on the pads sometimes cracks or bleeds, making it painful to walk. Cats occasionally have pad cracks, but they are much more likely to occur in dogs.

Veterinarians usually treat cracked paw pads with lotions or oils, and that is the best way to help them heal. But treating the cracks doesn't go far enough, says Donna M. Starita, D.V.M., a holistic veterinarian in private practice in Boring, Oregon. "Hitting the pavement a lot might make pad cracks worse, but the problem begins inside," she says. Here are a few ways to treat pad cracks, starting on the inside and working your way out.

## The Solutions  FOR DOGS & CATS

**Heal them with minerals.** "Many of the cracked pads I see are caused by a zinc or selenium deficiency in the diet," says Dr. Starita. Zinc strengthens the skin and helps it heal more quickly, while selenium boosts immunity so that the body is better able to heal itself. She recommends giving pets weighing under 30 pounds 2½ to 5 milligrams of zinc and 50 micrograms of selenium a day. Larger pets can take 5 to 10 milligrams of zinc and 100 micrograms of selenium a day. You can give your pet these supplements for two weeks at a time.

**Speed healing with vitamin E.** An important nutrient, vitamin E improves blood circulation so that cracked pads heal more quickly, says Dr. Starita. It also strengthens immunity and helps prevent parasites or infections from causing cracking. You can give pets under 15 pounds 50 international units (IU) of vitamin E a day. Those weighing 15 to 50 pounds can take 100 IU, and larger dogs can have 200 IU of vitamin E a day. She recommends opening a vitamin E gel capsule and squeezing the oil into your pet's food.

**BEST BET!** **Soften the pads with oil.** You don't want to moisturize the paw pads too much because they need to be tough to maintain their strength. But when the pads are cracked, applying a little sesame or olive oil will help them heal, and the oils are safe if your pet decides to lick them off, says Kathleen Carson, D.V.M., a holistic veterinarian in private practice in Hermosa Beach, California.

Lotions containing vitamin E are also good, although you will need to keep your pet distracted for a few minutes while the lotion soaks into the skin. It is best to use all-natural lotions, available at health food stores.

**Increase internal moisture.** Dogs and cats with internal problems like infections can lose tremendous amounts of water from their bodies, causing the pads to crack, says George Carley, D.V.M., a holistic veterinarian in private practice in Tulsa, Oklahoma. Chinese medicines containing rehmannia root can strengthen the organs and help prevent moisture loss, he says.

Rehmannia root is used in many different formulas, he adds. When cracked pads are caused by kidney problems, for example, your vet may recommend using Rehmannia 6. If lung problems are to blame, your pet may need Rehmannia Schizandra Formula. You would need to check with a veterinarian who practices traditional Chinese medicine to get the right formula and dose for your pet.

**BEST BET!** **Strengthen the skin with fatty acids.** The body needs essential fatty acids to build and maintain the membranes of skin cells. It also needs fatty acids to reduce inflammation that may accompany pad cracks. Dr. Starita recommends giving pets a fatty-acid supplement called Eskimo Oil, available from veterinarians or in drugstores. Pets love the taste, so you can put it in their mouths or mix it in their food. Cats and dogs under 15 pounds can take an one-eighth teaspoon of Eskimo Oil twice a day. Pets weighing 15 to 50 pounds can take one-quarter teaspoon twice a day, and larger dogs can take one-half teaspoon twice a day.

**Strengthen the immune system with acupressure.** Infections or infestations with parasites can cause the pads to thicken, crack, or bleed. You can use acupressure to boost immunity and help the body resist the organisms that are causing the cracks, says Dr. Carley. Three important points for immunity are the following:

🐾 SP6, located on the inside rear of the back legs just above the hock (the ankle)

🐾 BL20, located beside the spine directly between the last two ribs

🐾 LI11, located on the outside of the front legs at the elbow crease

## Meet the Experts

**George Carley, D.V.M.,** is a holistic veterinarian in private practice in Tulsa, Oklahoma. He is certified in acupuncture.

**Kathleen Carson, D.V.M.,** is a holistic veterinarian in private practice in Hermosa Beach, California.

**Donna M. Starita, D.V.M.,** is a holistic veterinarian in private practice in Boring, Oregon.

**Joanne Stefanatos, D.V.M.,** is a holistic veterinarian in private practice in Las Vegas. She is certified in acupuncture and chiropractic.

Press each of the points for 60 seconds several times a day until the cracks heal, Dr. Carley advises.

Another natural remedy for stopping infections is the herb pau d'arco (*Tabebuia impetiginosa*). It contains a natural substance called quechua that kills fungi, bacteria, and some viruses, says Joanne Stefanatos, D.V.M., a holistic veterinarian in private practice in Las Vegas. She recommends combining equal parts pau d'arco tincture and mineral oil and applying this mixture to the pads once a day until the cracks start to heal.

# PANCREATITIS

## The Signs
- Your pet refuses to eat.
- He is vomiting or having diarrhea.
- He is extremely lethargic and may have a fever.
- Because he is crying or hunching his back, you suspect his abdomen hurts.

## The Cause

The pancreas is an organ that manufactures hormones and enzymes needed to digest proteins and fats. For reasons that aren't clear, sometimes the pancreas gets swollen and inflamed and begins producing huge amounts of enzymes. It produces so much, in fact, that the highly corrosive enzymes may spill into the abdominal cavity and begin damaging internal organs. This condition, called pancreatitis, can be quite painful and often makes pets—especially dogs—very ill.

"Cats tend to have milder symptoms than dogs," says Jory Olsen, D.V.M., a veterinary internal-medicine specialist in private practice in Marietta, Georgia. "They won't eat for a day and may vomit, and then they will be fine for a while. This can go on for years and never be diagnosed." In dogs, pancreatitis may also cause vomiting as well as diarrhea and abdominal pain. "They may even collapse," says Susan G. Wynn, a veterinarian in Atlanta and co-editor of *Complementary and Alternative Veterinary Medicine*.

Although veterinarians aren't sure what causes pancreatitis, they have found that pets given rich diets are more likely to get it than those given leaner foods, says Roger L. DeHaan, D.V.M., a holistic veterinarian in private practice in Frazee, Minnesota. And once they have had it, they will often get it again. Serious flare-ups are usually treated by giving pets intravenous fluids. The rest of the time, you can protect your pets at home with a combination of supplements and easy dietary changes. Here is what holistic veterinarians advise.

## The Solutions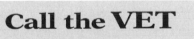

**Turn off the enzymes.** When your pet first gets sick, you can reduce the flood of digestive enzymes by putting him on a fast for 24 hours. "Any stretching of the stomach can stimulate the pancreas to keep spilling out enzymes," Dr. Olsen explains. A short-term fast will also slow the diarrhea that often accompanies pancreatitis, he adds.

**Give extra fluids.** Pets that are having an attack of pancreatitis become dehydrated very quickly because of diarrhea and vomiting. "Give them

## Call the VET

Even though pancreatitis can be a life-threatening condition, most pets recover just fine, although they can get quite sick during flare-ups.

You can manage most flare-ups of pancreatitis at home, but severe attacks can be very painful, says Roger L. DeHaan, D.V.M., a holistic veterinarian in private practice in Frazee, Minnesota. If your pet refuses to move, is acting depressed, or is having severe vomiting or diarrhea, you are going to need some help—fast. "These acute symptoms mean that it is an emergency, and you need to see your vet right away," he says.

small amounts of water frequently," suggests Dr. Wynn. Or give them a re-hydration solution such as Pedialyte, which is loaded with essential minerals called electrolytes. "Fluids improve circulation, which may help get them over the attack," she says.

Don't give too much fluid at one time because this will stretch the stomach and stimulate enzyme production. Keep the servings small: Every hour give one to two teaspoons to pets under 15 pounds, one to two tablespoons to pets 15 to 35 pounds, one to three ounces to dogs 36 to 50 pounds, and three to five ounces of fluid to dogs over 50 pounds. Once your pet is feeling better, usually within a day or two, you can slowly increase the amount, says Dr. Wynn.

**Keep the diet bland.** The fat and protein in foods stimulate the pancreas to release digestive enzymes. To help your pet recover, it is a good idea to give him simple meals, such as boiled chicken with rice or potato. "You want protein that is very digestible but bland like no-fat cottage cheese, chicken, or turkey baby food," Dr. Olsen says.

As with water, you don't want to give a lot of food all at once. Give your pet small amounts throughout the day. Even when he is better, you may want to keep feeding him a homemade diet consisting of low-fat, high-digestibility foods. Chicken and turkey, for ex-ample, are easier to digest than beef and will put less strain on the pancreas, says Dr. Olsen. Your vet will help you plan a diet that is right for your pet.

**Switch to a natural diet.** "Years and years of eating commercial pet foods that don't contain natural digestive enzymes makes your pet's body work harder," says Dr. DeHaan. Over time, this additional stress can cause the pancreas to stop working efficiently. He recommends giving dogs and cats a high-quality, all-natural food like Innova, Flint River, or Wysong, available in some pet supply stores and from mail-order companies. Better yet, give pets a natural diet made at home, he says. Switching your pet to a more wholesome food may help prevent pancreatitis in the future. For more information on preparing natural diets at home, see page 61.

**Give the pancreas some help.** Vets have found that giving pets supplemental digestive enzymes, such as FloraZyme LP powder, can help the pancreas "rest" during flare-ups of pancreatitis, making the condition easier to control, says Dr. DeHaan. Give dogs weighing under 15 pounds and cats one-half teaspoon per meal. Dogs 15 to 50 pounds can take one to two teaspoons per meal, and dogs over 50 pounds can take one tablespoon per meal.

**Give them live-culture yogurt.**
Pets love the taste of yogurt, and the bacteria it contains act as a natural digestive aid. Dr. DeHaan recommends giving cats up to one teaspoon of yogurt three to five days a week. Dogs can take one to two tablespoons, depending on their size.

**Strengthen the pancreas with herbs.** There are a number of herbal remedies that appear to help the pancreas repair itself. Dr. DeHaan recommends a nonprescription product called P-14, which combines 14 different herbs and is available through mail order and from some pet supply stores and veterinarians. For cats, mix one-quarter to one-half of a capsule into moist food once a day. Give dogs weighing under 15 pounds one capsule a day. Dogs 15 to 50 pounds can take two capsules, and larger dogs can take three capsules daily. You can give the capsules once a day for a month, then every other day thereafter to keep the pancreas healthy. When giving pets a new supplement, it is a good idea to start out with half the usual dose to make sure that they are not sensitive to it, he says.

**BEST BET!** **Protect them with vitamins.** "Antioxidants like vitamin E and vitamin C may reduce the severity and frequency of pancreatitis attacks and may even speed recovery

---

## Meet the Experts

**Roger L. DeHaan, D.V.M.,** is a holistic veterinarian in private practice in Frazee, Minnesota. He is certified in chiropractic.

**Jory Olsen, D.V.M.,** is a veterinary internal-medicine specialist in private practice in Marietta, Georgia.

**Susan G. Wynn, D.V.M.,** is a veterinarian in Atlanta and co-editor of *Complementary and Alternative Veterinary Medicine*.

---

from a severe episode," says Dr. Olsen. He recommends giving pets a product called Cell-Advance, available from veterinarians, which contains a variety of antioxidants. Cats and dogs under 20 pounds can take one 440-milligram capsule once a day. Give larger dogs an 880-milligram capsule for every 20 pounds of weight, he advises.

**Keep them away from chemicals.** Holistic veterinarians believe that exposure to chemicals such as pesticides or herbicides can damage the pancreas, possibly bringing on an attack of pancreatitis. It is worth doing everything you can to protect your pet from unnecessary exposure to chemicals, says Dr. Olsen, by using natural flea-control products, for example, or keeping him inside after you have had the yard treated.

# PORCUPINE QUILLS

## The Signs
- Quills are stuck in or near your pet's mouth and nose.
- His skin is red and inflamed.
- Pieces of quill are stuck under the skin, causing swelling or an abscess.

## The Cause

Most pets are pretty curious about those unusual spiky fellows that they will occasionally spot ambling along a road. Porcupines, however, don't appreciate nosy strangers. When they feel threatened, they will lash out. And with approximately 30,000 loosely attached quills, they can deliver some instant acupuncture, and not the healing kind.

Porcupine quills don't always cause a lot of pain at first, but they can cause serious damage, says Jan Facinelli, D.V.M., a holistic veterinarian in private practice in Denver. The quills have overlapping barbs that allow the quills to penetrate deeply into the skin. In addition, the puncture wounds may get painfully infected, she says.

The conventional veterinary approach is to remove the quills, clean the wounds, and send your pet on his way. Holistic veterinarians, on the other hand, believe it is also important to treat the emotional trauma that accompanies a physical attack. So if your pet has been on the receiving end of a porcupine's tail, here are a few ways to help him recover after the spines are out.

## The Solutions — FOR DOGS & CATS

**Soothe the skin with an herbal wash.** A natural way to reduce inflammation and clean puncture wounds is with concentrated tinctures of calendula (*Calendula officinalis*) and St. John's wort (*Hypericum perforatum*). Put no more than two drops of each tincture in one-half cup of water and use the solution to gently bathe the wounds, Dr. Facinelli advises. It is best to use tinctures that are alcohol-free because alcohol may be harmful for cats.

**Provide puncture protection.** Infection is the main risk of puncture wounds. A homeopathic strategy to prevent infection is with Ledum 30C—three pellets given three times a day for up to three days. Some pets will swallow the pellets whole if you put them on their tongues. If your pet isn't a cooperative pill-taker, you can crush the pellets and put them in a teaspoon

## Call the VET

The same barbs that make it easy for porcupine quills to penetrate the skin also make it very difficult to get them out. It is possible to remove quills at home with a pair of pliers, but this can be excruciatingly painful. Most pets won't hold still for it.

"If your pet is lucky enough to get away with just one or two quills, you may be able to remove them yourself," says Michael W. Lemmon, D.V.M., a holistic veterinarian in Renton, Washington, and past president of the American Holistic Veterinary Medical Association. The spurs can be removed by gripping them close to the skin with a pair of pliers and pulling them straight out. It makes more sense, however, to take your pet to the vet, who will probably use an anesthetic to numb the pain.

Don't wait too long before getting help, Dr. Lemmon adds. Porcupine quills can rapidly work their way into the body, and once they are lodged in place, natural muscle contractions pull them in deeper.

of milk, says Dr. Facinelli. Most pets will lap it right up.

**Reduce the pain.** A safe, drug-free way to relieve the pain of porcupine punctures is to give Hypericum homeopathically. Dr. Facinelli recommends giving dogs and cats three pellets of Hypericum 30C, and then repeating the dose up to three times as needed. It is not a good idea to mix homeopathic remedies, she adds, so only give Hypericum after you have stopped using Ledum.

**Push out the barbs with Silica.** Even after porcupine quills are removed, small barbs may remain under the skin, causing swelling or an abscess. A homeopathic remedy called Silica will help push the barbs out of the skin, says Michael W. Lemmon, D.V.M., a holistic veterinarian in Renton, Washington, and past president of the American Holistic Veterinary Medical Association. He recommends giving one pellet of Silica 6X two to four times a day. Keep giving the pellets for one to two weeks.

**Reduce anxiety with Bach Rescue Remedy.** A combination of five flower essences, Bach Rescue Remedy will help pets relax after they have had a prickly encounter and will ease pain and swelling, says Dr. Lemmon. He recommends giving two to four drops of the essence as often as necessary. "The main idea is to give

Bach Rescue Remedy to your pet often—as much as every 5 to 20 minutes if he is really suffering. Then taper the treatment down to two or three times a day," he says.

To enhance the calming effects of Rescue Remedy, it is a good idea to massage the drops onto your pet's gums, ears, or around the quill wounds. Or you can add the drops to his food or water, he adds.

**Speed healing with vitamins.** Vitamins C and E are antioxidant nutrients that help stressed-out pets recover more quickly. Dr. Lemmon recommends giving dogs and cats weighing under 15 pounds between 50 and 100 international units (IU) of vitamin E once a day. Pets 15 to 40 pounds can take 200 to 300 IU a day,

---

### Meet the Experts

**Jan Facinelli, D.V.M.,** is a holistic veterinarian in private practice in Denver. She is certified in acupuncture and homeopathy.

**Michael W. Lemmon, D.V.M.,** is a holistic veterinarian in Renton, Washington, and past president of the American Holistic Veterinary Medical Association.

---

and larger dogs can take 400 IU a day. For vitamin C, give pets under 15 pounds 250 milligrams a day. Larger pets can take up to 1,000 milligrams of vitamin C a day. If your pet starts having diarrhea, you are giving too much vitamin C, and you will want to scale back the amount.

# PROSTATE PROBLEMS

### The Signs
- Your pet has blood in his urine.
- He is urinating more than usual.
- He has become constipated.

### The Cause

It is one of nature's strange plot twists. Testosterone, the hormone that makes young males aggressive and sexy, later turns them into flustered, middle-aged guys who have trouble with the most basic bodily function.

The problem with testosterone is that it causes the prostate—the gland that supplies the fluid that transports sperm—to gradually swell. If the gland gets large enough, it can also put pressure on the rectum, causing constipation.

Swelling isn't the only problem afflicting this unfortunate gland. Prostate infections are fairly common. And in older males, prostate cancer is always a risk. Any problem with the prostate gland is potentially serious and needs to be treated by a vet, says John M. Simon, D.V.M., a holistic veterinarian in private practice in Royal Oak, Michigan.

The usual treatment for prostate problems is to give medications, although in some cases pets need to be neutered, which lowers testosterone levels. Both medications and surgery can have serious side effects, which is why holistic veterinarians tend to be cautious about picking up a scalpel or prescription pad. It is often possible, they say, to use natural remedies to stop infection and discomfort and even to reverse the effects of testosterone on the gland. Here is what veterinarians advise.

## The Solutions FOR DOGS & CATS

**BEST BET!** **Give him saw palmetto.** This herbal remedy has been used to shrink swollen prostate tissue in men, and it appears to work equally well for pets, says Dr. Simon. Available in pill or capsule form in health food stores, saw palmetto (*Serenoa repens*) is very safe, although you need to use it under a veterinarian's supervision. Cats and dogs weighing under 15 pounds can take 5 to 10 milligrams of saw palmetto a day. Pets 15 to 50

pounds can take 20 milligrams, and larger dogs can take 30 to 40 milligrams. The quickest way to give the medication is to pop it down your pet's throat, although it will go down easier when you coat it with oil or butter first.

**Flush the tissue.** Pets with prostate problems often have an accumulation of fluids and toxins in the gland. To keep the tissue clean and healthy, use an herbal supplement called PR, advises Michelle Tilghman, D.V.M., a holistic veterinarian in private practice in Stone Mountain, Georgia. "It's a combination of herbs that help clean and flush the prostate." Pets weighing under 15 pounds can take one capsule once a day. Pets 15 to 50 pounds can take two capsules once a day, and larger dogs can have two capsules twice a day.

**Reduce swelling with vitamin C.** A natural anti-inflammatory, vitamin C can help shrink the prostate to its normal size, says Maria H. Glinski, D.V.M., a holistic veterinarian in private practice in Glendale, Wisconsin. She recommends mixing a little powdered vitamin C with water and squirting it in your pet's mouth with a needleless syringe. It is best to use a buffered form of vitamin C, such as sodium ascorbate, because it is less likely to irritate the stomach, she adds. Cats and dogs under 15 pounds can take 250 milligrams of powdered vitamin C twice a day. Pets 15 to 50 pounds can take 500 milligrams twice a day, and larger dogs can have 1,000 milligrams twice a day. Vitamin C may cause diarrhea, but reducing the dose will usually firm things up again.

**Stop infection with vitamin E.** "Vitamin E is great for immune enhancement and the health of mucous membranes," says Dr. Glinski. Cats and dogs with prostate problems who weigh under 15 pounds should take 100 international units (IU) of vitamin E a day. Those 15 to 50 pounds can take 200 IU, and large dogs can have 400 IU a day. You can give them vitamin E capsules or open a capsule and squeeze the oil on their food, she advises.

**Strengthen immunity.** The herbs echinacea (*Echinacea purpurea* or *Echinacea angustifolia*) and goldenseal (*Hydrastis canadensis*), often found together in combination supplements, stimulate the immune system and help stop infections throughout the body, says Dr. Simon. He recommends using a combination herbal tincture, available in health food stores. You will have to adjust the recommended human dose to your pet's size, assuming the full dose is for a 150-pound person. A 30-pound dog, for example, would take about one-quarter to one-half of the human dose once a day for two weeks. It is best to use tinctures that are alcohol-free because alcohol may be harmful for cats.

Some pets hate the taste of goldenseal, he adds. If your pet won't touch it, it is fine to give echinacea by itself.

**Nourish the gland.** "Zinc and magnesium are both good for the overall health of the prostate gland," says Dr. Simon. Give five milligrams of magnesium and two milligrams of zinc for every pound of weight once a day for about a month.

**Keep him away from temptation.** It is natural for the prostate gland to swell when dogs and cats are around females in heat, says Dr. Glinski. For pets that already have prostate pain, the swelling can be doubly uncomfortable. It is best to keep them out of smelling distance of receptive females, she says.

**Keep him regular.** Since pets with swollen prostate glands may have trouble passing stools, it is a good idea

---

## Meet the Experts

**Maria H. Glinski, D.V.M.,** is a holistic veterinarian in private practice in Glendale, Wisconsin. She is certified in acupuncture.

**John M. Simon, D.V.M.,** is a holistic veterinarian in private practice in Royal Oak, Michigan. He is certified in acupuncture and chiropractic.

**Michelle Tilghman, D.V.M.,** is a holistic veterinarian in private practice in Stone Mountain, Georgia. She is certified in acupuncture.

to give them a mild laxative such as psyllium seeds, says Dr. Glinski. Cats and dogs weighing under 15 pounds can take one-quarter teaspoon of psyllium once or twice a day. Pets 15 to 50 pounds can take three-quarters to one teaspoon, and larger dogs need about one teaspoon once or twice a day. Psyllium doesn't have a lot of taste, so it is easy to hide in their food, she says.

**BEST BET!** **Have him neutered.** Probably the best solution for prostate problems—both to treat and prevent them—is to have your pet neutered, which stops the production of testosterone. "When testosterone is no longer produced, the prostate gland has no need to be activated, and the likelihood of swelling and inflammation virtually disappears," says Dr. Tilghman.

# RINGWORM

## The Signs

- Your pet has bald patches that are spreading.
- The fur is breaking off close to the skin.
- He has crusty or scaly sores.

## The Cause

Ringworm is a fungus that makes itself at home in the outer layers of the skin, nails, and hair. It is not uncommon for healthy cats to carry around the fungus and not get symptoms as long as their immune systems keep it in check. (Dogs with ringworm invariably have symptoms.) When ringworm temporarily gets the upper hand, however, it gives off toxins that can damage the skin and hair, causing bald patches on the head, paws, or back.

Ringworm is highly contagious, both to pets and people, so it is important to call your vet when you suspect that your pet is infected, says Robert Kennis, D.V.M., a veterinary dermatologist at Texas A&M University College of Veterinary Medicine in College Station. More common in cats than dogs, ringworm usually isn't serious, although it may spread over the entire body and cause crusty sores.

The traditional treatment for ringworm is to give an oral drug such as griseofulvin. The medication is very effective, but it may cause dangerous side effects, says Dr. Kennis. Most holistic veterinarians feel that it is better to soothe the discomfort and fight the ringworm naturally, without using drugs, until it goes away on its own. Here is what they advise.

## The Solutions FOR DOGS & CATS

**Soothe the sores.** The herb calendula (*Calendula officinalis*) is a natural antibiotic that relieves inflammation and can help ringworm sores heal more quickly, says Michelle Tilghman, D.V.M., a holistic veterinarian in private practice in Stone Mountain, Georgia. She recommends applying calendula tincture to the sores every day until they heal, using a cotton swab. Or apply goldenseal (*Hydrastis canadensis*) tincture to the sores two or three times a day, using a cotton ball. It is best to use tinctures that are alcohol-free because alcohol may be harmful for cats.

**Wash away fungal food.** Dousing your pet with apple cider vinegar will clear away skin cells that are ringworm's main source of nourishment, says Joanne Stefanatos, D.V.M., a holistic veterinarian in private practice in Las Vegas. A vinegar rinse (two tablespoons of apple cider vinegar in one quart of water) helps relieve itching as well. Repeat once a week, after shampooing as needed.

If you don't like the smell of vinegar, you can substitute a product called MalAcetic shampoo, available from veterinarians. It contains vinegar and other ringworm-fighting ingredients, says Steven A. Melman, V.M.D., a veterinarian with practices in Potomac, Maryland, and Palm Springs, California, and author of *Skin Diseases of Dogs and Cats*.

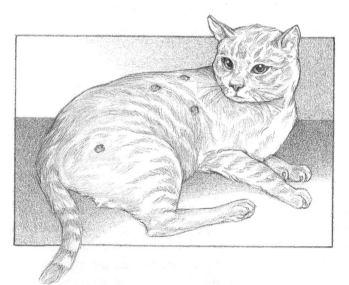

Pets with ringworm will have one or more bald (or sparsely furred) patches on their coats. The skin will look irritated, and there may be scales or crusty sores.

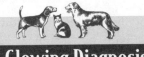

## A Glowing Diagnosis

Ringworm could be called the great pretender because it resembles many other skin problems, such as allergies, mange, and skin infections. This is why veterinarians have developed a special test for ringworm: They turn out the lights.

When patches of ringworm damage are illuminated with a type of black light (called a Wood's lamp) in a dark room, they will sometimes glow in the dark, making dogs and cats look a little like furry fireflies. "It's a nice, quick screening tool," says Robert Kennis, D.V.M., a veterinary dermatologist at Texas A&M University College of Veterinary Medicine in College Station.

The light only works, however, on certain strains of ringworm, he adds, so some pets may be infected even when they don't have the glow.

**BEST BET!** **Bleach it away.** Ringworm spores can survive anywhere in the house and are capable of reinfecting pets for up to a year after they have been treated. To get rid of the spores, Dr. Kennis recommends wiping counters, floors, and other areas in the house with household bleach. Straight bleach is best, although you can dilute 1 part bleach in 10 parts water when you are washing delicate surfaces like linoleum or wood.

**Keep him confined.** Until your pet is completely healed, it is a good idea to keep him confined to one area in the house, says Dr. Kennis. This will make it easier to control and eliminate ringworm spores that are constantly drifting off his coat. Some veterinarians recommend keeping pets in a stainless-steel cage until the ringworm is gone, although keeping them in a small room with a tile floor that is easily cleaned will also help contain the fungus.

**Clean the carpets.** Sucking up contaminated hairs and spores can help prevent your pet from getting reinfected, so it is a good idea to vacuum the house every day and to remove the vacuum bag and seal it inside a plastic garbage bag. "You can also steam-clean carpets, upholstery, drapes, and the like," says Alexander Werner, V.M.D., a veterinary dermatologist in private practice in Studio City, California.

**Update your pet's wardrobe.** When pets with ringworm start scratching, the spores go flying. Dressing your pet in an old T-shirt and putting socks on his feet will help control the fungus and prevent him from nibbling and scratching the sore spots, says Dr. Stefanatos. Washing the clothes in bleach and drying them thoroughly can also be helpful be-

## Meet the Experts

**Robert Kennis, D.V.M.,** is a veterinary dermatologist at Texas A&M University College of Veterinary Medicine in College Station.

**Steven A. Melman, V.M.D.,** is a veterinarian with practices in Potomac, Maryland, and Palm Springs, California, and the author of *Skin Diseases of Dogs and Cats*.

**Joanne Stefanatos, D.V.M.,** is a holistic veterinarian in private practice in Las Vegas. She is certified in acupuncture and chiropractic.

**Michelle Tilghman, D.V.M.,** is a holistic veterinarian in private practice in Stone Mountain, Georgia. She is certified in acupuncture.

**Alexander Werner, V.M.D.,** is a veterinary dermatologist in private practice in Studio City, California.

**Susan G. Wynn, D.V.M.,** is a veterinarian in Atlanta and co-editor of *Complementary and Alternative Veterinary Medicine*.

thoroughly with bleach, followed by a rinsing with hot, soapy water. Pets with ringworm should always be kept away from young children or people who are already ill because they are more vulnerable to the fungus than those whose immune systems are strong.

**Treat all your pets.** Since ringworm is readily passed from pet to pet, it is important to treat all your pets, even those that aren't yet infected, says Dr. Melman. If you don't, the spores are sure to survive and cause trouble all over again.

## The Solutions — FOR CATS

**Give extra support.** Some cats have weakened immune systems that allow ringworm to hang on even when they are getting medical treatment. Reishi mushroom (*Ganoderma lucidum*) and astragalus (*Astragalus membranaceus*), taken together, strengthen the immune system and help cats with chronic ringworm battle the infection while they are taking medication, says Susan G. Wynn, a veterinarian in Atlanta and co-editor of *Complementary and Alternative Veterinary Medicine*. She recommends giving three drops of each tincture once a day, either by mixing the tinctures in broth or butter or by adding them to your cat's food.

cause the bleach will kill the spores. "It can decrease itchiness by 50 percent or more," she says.

**Protect yourself.** The ringworm fungus is contagious, so you don't want to handle your pet too much until he has recovered. Dr. Kennis advises wearing a smock when you are treating the sores or even cuddling your pet. Afterward, wash your hands

# SHEDDING

## The Signs

- Hair comes loose when you stroke your pet.
- Knots of loose fur hang in your dog's coat.
- There are wads of fur clinging to furniture or carpets.
- Your pet's coat tangles or mats.

## The Cause

Fur that's beautiful when it is attached to your pet isn't so attractive when it is clinging to clothes or furniture. During shedding season especially, your house may start resembling a barbershop. "It's not unusual to fill an entire garbage bag with shed fur," says Lowell Ackerman, D.V.M., a veterinary dermatologist in Mesa, Arizona, and author of the *Guide to Skin and Haircoat Problems in Dogs*.

All cats and dogs shed, even the nearly hairless breeds like Mexican Hairless dogs and Sphynx cats. They shed most during spring and summer when longer daylight hours (the temperature doesn't matter) stimulate the body to let go of old hairs as new ones push their way through. There is an emotional component to shedding as well. Cats that are frightened will sometimes shed handfuls of fur as their skin tightens and pulls out loose hairs.

Shedding is more of a housecleaning problem than a health problem, although large amounts of dead fur next to the skin can cause hot spots or skin infections. Cats tend to get most of their hair balls during shedding season, Dr. Ackerman adds, because they will swallow more loose hair during grooming.

Nothing can beat a thorough brushing for keeping stray hair to a minimum. There are also many natural treatments that promote healthy skin and fur. Here is what to do when the fur is flying.

## The Solutions *FOR DOGS & CATS*

**Shine the coat with fatty acids.** Holistic veterinarians have found that the omega-3 and omega-6 fatty acids found in some fish and plant oils are very helpful for keeping fur and skin in top condition. It is fine to give your pets cooked boneless fish, but they really need supplements to get the full benefits of fatty acids. "I prefer Eskimo Oil because pets like

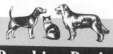

# Brushing Basics

Dogs and cats need a lot of grooming during the shedding season. Brushes and combs aren't interchangeable, however. It is important to choose the right grooming tools for your pet's breed and coat type. Here is what to look for.

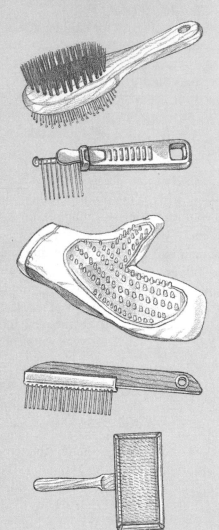

**Combination bristle/pincushion brush.** Recommended for pets with short coats, these usually have wire bristles on one side for removing large amounts of fur and softer bristles on the other side for smoothing and shining the coat.

**Slicker brush.** These have bent wire bristles that help remove hair from the thick under-coat. They come in many different sizes and are good for all coat types.

**Grooming glove.** This is a brush that slips over your hand. Some have nubby rubber teeth that feel good to your pet. Grooming gloves will remove substantial amounts of hair, and most pets won't even realize that they are being groomed. They work for all coat types, but are best for pets with short or only moderately thick coats.

**Combs.** These come in many different tooth sizes. Pets with very fine coats can be groomed with a fine-toothed comb. Pets with heavier coats will need larger-toothed combs.

**Mat splitter.** These are designed to cut through and separate hair mats, including mats that lie next to the skin.

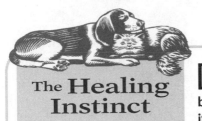

## The **Healing Instinct**

Dogs and cats often get itchy during shedding season. Since they can't use a hairbrush to remove loose fur, they deal with itching in their own way: by turning the whole house into a rubbing post. That is why you will often find clumps of fur on couches or carpets, says Lowell Ackerman, D.V.M., a veterinary dermatologist in Mesa, Arizona, and author of the *Guide to Skin and Haircoat Problems in Dogs*.

This perpetual rubbing and flank-friction does more than make them comfortable, he adds. Rubbing away the matted undercoat allows air to circulate next to the skin, which helps prevent skin infections. It also makes pets less vulnerable to parasites such as fleas and ticks because these pests like to nest in matted fur.

the flavor, it doesn't need refrigeration, and it is easy to give," says Donna M. Starita, D.V.M., a holistic veterinarian in private practice in Boring, Oregon.

Available from veterinarians, Eskimo Oil can be squirted in your pet's mouth with a needleless syringe. Since dogs and cats like the taste, however, it makes more sense to add the oil to their food. Cats can take one-eighth teaspoon of Eskimo Oil once a day, says Dr. Starita. Dogs under 50 pounds can take one-quarter teaspoon twice a day, and larger dogs can have one-half teaspoon twice a day.

**BEST BET!** **Feed the fur naturally.** Hair is made of protein, and the quality of the protein in your pet's diet will affect how her hair looks. Unfortunately, some commercial foods use poor-quality protein as well as ar-

tificial additives and preservatives. This can cause an increase in loose, brittle fur, says Nancy Scanlan, D.V.M., a holistic veterinarian in private practice in Sherman Oaks, California.

One of the easiest ways to make hair healthier is to give pets an all-natural food—one that contains no artificial ingredients, says Carolyn Blakey, D.V.M., a holistic veterinarian in private practice in Richmond, Indiana. Foods like Innova and Wysong contain high-quality ingredients that will help prevent shedding, she says. You can buy all-natural foods in some pet supply stores and through mail order.

**Balance the skin with herbs.** Shedding usually increases when the skin isn't as healthy as it should be, says Dr. Scanlan. An excellent way to

## Meet the Experts

**Lowell Ackerman, D.V.M.,** is a veterinary dermatologist in Mesa, Arizona, and the author of the *Guide to Skin and Haircoat Problems in Dogs*.

**Carolyn Blakey, D.V.M.,** is a holistic veterinarian in private practice in Richmond, Indiana. She is certified in acupuncture.

**Nancy Scanlan, D.V.M.,** is a holistic veterinarian in private practice in Sherman Oaks, California. She is certified in acupuncture and chiropractic.

**Donna M. Starita, D.V.M.,** is a holistic veterinarian in private practice in Boring, Oregon.

**Susan G. Wynn, D.V.M.,** is a veterinarian in Atlanta and co-editor of *Complementary and Alternative Veterinary Medicine*.

improve skin health is to give dogs and cats a Chinese herbal combination called Skin Balance, available from veterinarians. Give pets weighing under 15 pounds one-half tablet three times a day. Pets 15 to 50 pounds can take one to two tablets three times a day, and dogs over 50 pounds can have two tablets three times a day.

**BEST BET! Brush away the hair.** Regular brushing is the easiest way to rid your pet—and your sofa—of excess hair. Brush your pet once a day, using a brush that's right for her coat, says Susan G. Wynn, D.V.M., a veterinarian in Atlanta and co-author of *Complementary and Alternative Veterinary Medicine*. Move the brush in the same direction as the hair grows, she adds.

# SKIN CHEWING

## The Signs

- Your pet licks or nibbles her skin for more than a few seconds at a time.
- Her skin has darkened or turned red.
- She has bare patches in her fur.
- There is a reddish stain on the fur or front feet.

## The Cause

Dogs and cats spend a lot of time grooming—everything from licking their bellies to nibbling their toes. But when their skin is itchy or irritated, they won't leave it alone. They will act as though their paws, tails, or flanks are corn on the cob, chewing so vigorously and for so long that they will wear away the fur or even damage the skin.

## Call the VET

**M**ost dogs and cats will occasionally have itchy spells. Within a day or two, they should be feeling better and will turn their attention—and their teeth—to more interesting things, like rubber balls or catnip mice.

Itching that doesn't go away fairly quickly should always be seen by a veterinarian, says Steven A. Melman, V.M.D., a veterinarian with practices in Potomac, Maryland, and Palm Springs, California, and author of *Skin Diseases of Dogs and Cats*. There are a number of serious conditions, from hard-to-treat emotional problems to internal illnesses, that can cause constant chewing. Some dogs and cats will go so far as to chew their skin raw, he adds.

"If you find yourself using a home treatment like a cool-water bath more often than once a day for three or four days, you have to see your vet," says Dr. Melman.

Chewing usually begins when pets are sensitive to something in the environment, like pollen, fleas, or chemicals in their food, says Steven A. Melman, V.M.D., a veterinarian with practices in Potomac, Maryland, and Palm Springs, California, and author of *Skin Diseases of Dogs and Cats*. Even when the original problem is gone, dogs and cats may keep chewing out of habit, especially when they are stressed or bored.

Skin problems can be complicated to treat, so it is a good idea to talk to your vet when problems begin. In the meantime, here are a few natural, drug-free ways to take a bite out of chewing.

## The Solutions FOR DOGS & CATS

**Apply a soothing ointment.** Hypericum, the active ingredient in St. John's wort, may help reduce itching that causes skin chewing, says Susan G. Wynn, D.V.M., a veterinarian in Atlanta and co-editor of *Complementary and Alternative Veterinary Medicine* Apply it to your pet's skin twice a day, she says. The ointment is available in health food stores.

**BEST BET!** **Counter the itch with a Chinese cure.** Specialists in traditional Chinese medicine sometimes recommend a product called Armadillo Counter-Poison Pill. "It combines several herbs, and it works as well as antihistamines to soothe itchy skin," says Michelle Tilghman, D.V.M., a holistic veterinarian in private practice in Stone Mountain, Georgia. She recommends giving pets under 15 pounds one tablet twice a day. Pets 15 to 50 pounds can take two tablets twice a day, and larger pets can take three tablets twice a day.

**Calm the skin with an herbal blend.** A product called Hokamix, available from veterinarians and mail-order catalogs, contains a variety of herbs that reduce skin inflammation and help the body fight allergies that can cause chewing, says Nancy Scanlan, D.V.M., a holistic veterinarian in private practice in Sherman Oaks, California. Mix the Hokamix with their food, following the directions that come in the box. Most pets like the taste, so you won't have to work to disguise it, she adds.

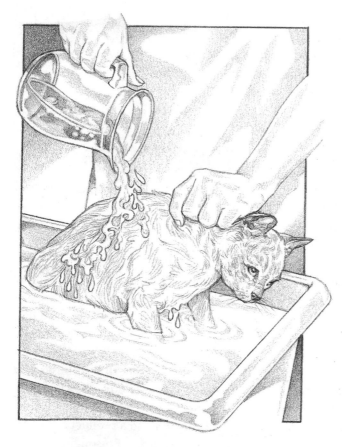

Cats hate being sprayed with water even more than they hate baths, so the best way to rinse pollen and other allergens off your cat's coat is to slowly lower her (one hand supporting her bottom, the other beneath the chest) into a sink half filled with water. Restrain her firmly by the back of the neck and ladle water over her with a cup. Putting a small towel in the bottom of the sink will give her traction so that she is less likely to slip.

**Soothe the emotions.** It is very common for dogs and cats to chew their skin during times of stress, says Carolyn Blakey, D.V.M., a holistic veterinarian in private practice in Richmond, Indiana. To help them feel more tranquil, she recommends giving four drops of the flower essence crab apple. You can put the drops directly in their mouths or into their water bowls once a day.

**BEST BET!** **Rinse away problems.** Rinsing pets with cool water once a day will wash away dust, pollen, and other substances that may cause itching and skin chewing, says Dr. Melman. You can gently spray dogs with a garden hose or a spray nozzle in the bathtub. It is especially helpful to wash their feet after they have been outside. Cats aren't thrilled about water in any form, but they particularly hate being sprayed. So you may have to bathe them with water instead, he says.

**BEST BET!** **Use a natural shampoo.** When a plain water rinse doesn't stop the itch, you may want to try a soothing all-natural shampoo made with oatmeal, says Dr. Blakey. Make sure that the shampoo doesn't contain dyes, fragrances, or animal proteins, which can trigger allergic reactions, Dr. Melman adds. And rinse out the soap thoroughly when you are done. Even small amounts of residual suds will cause itching when they dry.

## Meet the Experts

**Carolyn Blakey, D.V.M.,** is a holistic veterinarian in private practice in Richmond, Indiana. She is certified in acupuncture.

**Steven A. Melman, V.M.D.,** is a veterinarian with practice in Potomac, Maryland, and Palm Springs, California, and the author of *Skin Diseases of Dogs and Cats*.

**Nancy Scanlan, D.V.M.,** is a holistic veterinarian in private practice in Sherman Oaks, California. She is certified in acupuncture and chiropractic.

**Michelle Tilghman, D.V.M.,** is a holistic veterinarian in private practice in Stone Mountain, Georgia. She is certified in acupuncture.

**Susan G. Wynn, D.V.M.,** is a veterinarian in Atlanta and co-editor of *Complementary and Alternative Veterinary Medicine*.

**Use a homeopathic combo.** Health food and pet supply stores stock a variety of homeopathic remedies for stopping itch-related chewing, such as HomeoPet Hot Spot Dermatitis or HomeoPet Skin and Seborrhea. "They are typically low-potency pills that contain a combination of remedies, and at least one of the ingredients is likely to help," says Dr. Blakey. Dogs can take 10 drops and cats can have 3 drops, both three times a day. Call your vet if your pet keeps chewing, she says.

**BEST BET!** **Feed them naturally.** The artificial dyes and flavorings in many commercial pet foods often cause itchy skin, says Dr. Blakey. Most holistic veterinarians recommend giving pets all-natural diets—either diets made from scratch or commercial foods such as Wysong or Innova. You can buy all-natural foods in some pet supply stores and through mail order. For more information on natural diets, see page 61.

**Soothe the skin with fish-oil supplements.** Fish oil contains omega-3 fatty acids, which help relieve irritation that can lead to skin chewing, says Dr. Wynn. Give cats and dogs weighing under 20 pounds 500 milligrams a day, she says. Pets 20 to 50 pounds can take 1,000 to 2,000 milligrams. Dogs 51 to 80 pounds can take 3,000 milligrams, and larger dogs can have 4,000 milligrams. Oils made from the whole fish, like salmon oil, are a good choice because they contain more omega-3 fatty acids than those made from just a part of the fish, like cod-liver oil.

# SPRAYING

## The Signs

- Your cat is urinating on walls or furniture, probably near windows or doors.
- He stands with his back legs straight, shuffles his back feet, and quivers his tail when he wets.
- The urine is yellow or clear, with a very strong smell.

## The Cause

Like urban graffiti, a cat's urine spray is meant to grab attention. It helps attract mates and drive away male competition. "For most cats, spraying is like the mark of Zorro—a dramatic gesture that says, 'I was here, I'm virile, and not to be messed with,'" says Nicholas Dodman, B.V.M.S. (bachelor of veterinary medicine and surgery, a British equivalent of D.V.M.), professor of behavioral pharmacology and director of the behavior clinic at Tufts University School of Veterinary Medicine in North Grafton, Massachusetts. Spraying is most common in males, although females sometimes do it, too.

Spraying isn't always a sign of cocky vigor. Some cats spray in order to boost their confidence when they are feeling insecure and anxious. Unfortunately, spraying can make the human members of the family even more anxious as they try to figure out where the overpowering smell is coming from.

Once your cat starts spraying, it can be difficult to make him stop. Although spaying or neutering will reduce the hormones that can trigger spraying, and mood-altering drugs can make cats calmer and more secure, there are also some natural ways to keep your pet's urine in the box and off the walls.

## The Solutions

**BEST BET!** **Calm them with good scents.** A cat's urine is filled with pheromones, natural chemicals that convey signals of anxiety, anger, or aggression. The pheromones in the facial glands, by contrast, convey messages of peace and contentment. Because cats won't spray in "happy" places, you can often control spraying by overwriting the urine marks with a product called Feliway, which contains chemicals similar to those in the facial glands, says Alison Clarke, V.M.D., a re-

## Call the VET

Spraying is usually caused by emotional upsets, but there are a number of physical problems, such as diabetes or urinary tract infections, that can cause cats to lift their tails in the wrong places. It is always worth taking him to the vet for a checkup before you try to treat the problem at home, says Gary Landsberg, D.V.M., a veterinary behaviorist in private practice in Thornhill, Ontario, Canada.

Even if your cat gets a clean bill of health, there is one physical "problem" that often causes spraying: Unneutered pets are much more likely to spray than their fixed counterparts. Having your cat spayed or neutered may be all it takes to stop the misbehavior.

Don't waste time when your pet starts spraying, Dr. Landsberg adds. Some cats, once they get in the habit, have a hard time giving it up. "Take that first spray very seriously," he says. "It's wise to whisk him right off to the vet to see if there is a physical problem and to nip the habit in the bud."

tired veterinarian in Leonardtown, Maryland. After washing the urine marks, she recommends spraying them with the pheromones twice a day for about a month, then once or twice a week thereafter. Feliway is available from veterinarians.

**Soothe anxiety.** Since spraying cats are often anxious cats, it may be helpful to treat them with flower essences, which will make them calmer and more secure, says Arthur Young, D.V.M., a holistic veterinarian in private practice in Stuart, Florida. He recommends putting a drop of the essence Bach Rescue Remedy on the skin on the inner part of each earflap four times a day. In addition, you may want to mix flower essences in your cat's drinking water. Put two drops each of Bach Rescue Remedy, chestnut bud, vervain, and vine in his water each day, he advises.

**Stroke away bad feelings.** We all have amazing healing powers in our hands, says Dr. Clarke. She recommends using a technique called Tellington Touch (TTouch) in which you use your fingertips to rub firm, gentle, clockwise circles all over your cat's body for about five minutes once a day. TTouch allows you to pass soothing energy into your cat, she explains. It doesn't matter which part of the body you focus on, she adds, although the ears and the surrounding areas tend to be most effective.

**BEST BET!** **Battle it with boxes.** Anxiety sometimes begins at the litter box, especially if you live in a

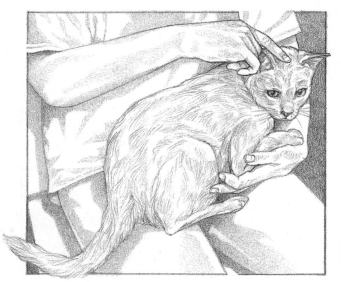

The GV20 point can help ease anxiety. To find the point, feel for the depression just in front of the bump on top of the head between the ears.

multiple-cat household. Giving each cat his own box will help keep them all content, says Dr. Clarke. "You absolutely need at least one litter pan per cat. Anything less often causes cats to spray."

It is also helpful to put the litter boxes in different parts of the house rather than all lined up in a row. This gives each cat privacy and reduces the possibility of squabbles over squatting rights.

**Clean naturally.** Cats dislike chemical smells, and using household cleaners on the litter box will often make spraying worse. Ammonia-based cleaners are especially offensive because, to cats, they smell like the urine of another cat. Your pet may start spraying in order to warn off the phantom intruder. "I've never found anything better than plain soap and water for basic cleaning," says Dr. Clarke.

**BEST BET!** **Neutralize the smell.** Cats that get in the habit of spraying often return to the same spots for a bit of urine renewal. Scrubbing will remove most of the smell, but invariably a few molecules will be left behind. Dr. Clarke recommends soaking the area with an odor neutralizer, such as Nature's Miracle. Odor neutralizers contain natural enzymes or bacteria that break down the chemicals in the urine.

**Press for comfort.** Deeply massaging the acupressure point GV20 will open energy channels in the body, which can help keep pets more self-assured, says Judith Rae Swanson, D.V.M., a holistic veterinarian in private practice in Chicago. The point is located in a pinpoint depression in front of the bump on top of the head between the ears. She recommends gently sinking your fingernail into the point and massaging for about 20 seconds, three or four times a day.

## Meet the Experts

**Alison Clarke, V.M.D.,** is a retired veterinarian in Leonardtown, Maryland.

**Nicholas Dodman, B.V.M.S**, is a professor of behavioral pharmacology and director of the behavior clinic at Tufts University School of Veterinary Medicine in North Grafton, Massachusetts. He is the author of *The Cat Who Cried for Help* and *The Dog Who Loved Too Much*.

**Gary Landsberg, D.V.M.,** is a veterinary behaviorist in private practice in Thornhill, Ontario, Canada.

**Judith Rae Swanson, D.V.M.,** is a holistic veterinarian in private practice in Chicago. She is certified in acupuncture.

**Arthur Young, D.V.M.,** is a holistic veterinarian in private practice in Stuart, Florida. He is certified in homeopathy.

**Give him some peace.** Cats are solitary animals, and they often feel better when they are keeping their own company. "If your cat is spraying, try giving him a room of his own with his own litter pan, toys, and food and water dishes," says Dr. Clarke. "Most act happier immediately."

Every cat reacts differently to his environment, she adds, so you may have to try different living arrangements until you find one that seems to make your cat most content. In some cases, providing a large, pleasant box or cage where he can retreat to will reduce his tendency to spray, she says.

**BEST BET!** **Treat your cat kindly.** Cats don't spray out of spite but merely to obey powerful physical or emotional needs, says Gary Landsberg, D.V.M., a veterinary behaviorist in private practice in Thornhill, Ontario, Canada. It doesn't help to punish cats by yelling or stamping your feet. In fact, getting angry will make your cat even more insecure—and more likely to spray. The best approach is to give him all the love and attention you can and reward him with a treat or a few strokes whenever he uses his box instead of the wall, he advises.

# STUD TAIL

## The Signs
- Fur on the top side of your pet's tail is oily and matted.
- He has a bald, waxy spot on his tail.
- There is a brown, oily discharge next to his skin.

## The Cause

Even though your pet's skin usually feels dry and smooth, oils are constantly being pumped to the surface. One of the main oil-producing glands is located on the top side of the tail near where it attaches to the body. During their normal grooming, dogs and cats distribute this oil, which lubricates the skin and coat.

"When your pet's system gets out of balance, the tail gland can over-secrete oil, creating a greasy mess," says David McCouggage, D.V.M., a holistic veterinarian in Longmont, Colorado, and editor in chief of the *Journal of the American Holistic Veterinary Medical Association*. This condition, called stud tail, occurs almost exclusively in unneutered male cats, although male dogs can get it, too. Sometimes it is merely messy and will go away on its own. But if the oil irritates the skin or bacteria colonize the area, pets can get painful sores.

The main treatment for stud tail is to remove the excess oil and clean the area thoroughly to prevent infection. But holistic veterinarians go a little further. They believe that the best approach (apart from neutering) is to correct imbalances that may be causing the body to churn out so much oil.

## The Solutions FOR DOGS & CATS

**Get rid of the oil.** Once your pet develops stud tail, you need to get rid of the irritating oil right away by washing the infected area. Regular pet shampoos aren't always effective at cutting through heavy grease, so veterinarians often recommend using a high-power degreaser, containing chemicals such as benzoyl peroxide. A more natural and equally effective approach is to use a shampoo that contains natural salicylic acid (which is derived from willow bark), oatmeal, or tea tree oil.

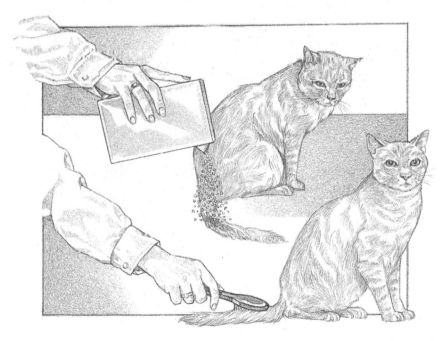

To remove excess oil from pets that hate the water, give them a "dry bath" by dusting the base of the tail with cornstarch. It is incredibly absorbent and will blot up a lot of the oil.

Use a brush to work the cornstarch through the fur and over the skin. Always brush in the direction the fur grows. Then dust the area again with cornstarch and repeat until most of the oil has been absorbed.

Groomers often use a shampoo called D'Grease, which is available from some wholesale distributors.

"For more severe cases, gently wipe the area with alcohol-soaked cotton balls," says Dr. McCouggage. You don't want to use alcohol too often because it irritates the skin, he adds. Make sure to keep your pet from licking until the alcohol dries.

**Blot the oil.** Since it is a rare cat that will sit patiently for bathing, you may want to try dusting the oily area once a day with a little bit of cornstarch. It can absorb tremendous amounts of oil and is safe for long-term use. Sprinkle it on the area, then use a brush to distribute it through the fur, Dr. McCouggage advises.

**Give extra love.** Dogs and cats that are depressed or lonely tend to stop grooming, which allows oils to stay in place and irritate the skin. Making your pet feel like an appreciated member of the family will help keep both his emotions and his skin in top condition, says Dr. McCouggage. "Pets that are happy and living in a healthy environment are much less likely to develop stud tail."

**Improve the skin with fish oils.** There are two types of fatty acids, omega-3's and omega-6's, that are essential for healthy skin, says Joanne Stefanatos, D.V.M., a holistic veteri-

narian in private practice in Las Vegas. She recommends giving cats or dogs with stud tail a liquid supplement called Omegaderm. Available from veterinarians, it contains a healthful mix of these fatty acids. You can give cats and dogs under 25 pounds a teaspoon of the oil twice a day, while larger pets can take up to a tablespoon.

**Have him neutered.** The most effective treatment for stud tail is neutering, says Susan G. Wynn, D.V.M., a veterinarian in Atlanta and co-editor of *Complementary and Alternative Veterinary Medicine*. Stud tail is caused by hormonal problems, so the removal of hormones through neutering is an excellent remedy, she says.

# SUNBURN

## The Signs

- Your pet's nose, ears, or tummy is red and tender.
- The edges of his ears are dry, cracked, or curling.

## The Cause

Many pets, especially cats, love nothing more than napping in puddles of light. Since cats can sleep 16 hours or more a day, in six years they could potentially doze away four years of their lives in the sun. All of this sunny warmth may be good for contentment, but it isn't so good for the skin.

Your pet's coat provides some protection from the sun, but the nose, rims of the ears, and sparsely furred tummy get the full blast. White pets are most susceptible to sunburn, as are those that live at high altitudes and in sunny parts of the country, says Lowell Ackerman, D.V.M., a veterinary dermatologist in Mesa, Arizona, and author of the *Guide to Skin and Haircoat Problems in Dogs*.

Veterinarians sometimes recommend treating sunburn with over-the-counter spray-on anesthetics. These medications can ease the pain, but they don't help the burn heal. A better approach is to use soothing natural remedies that not only cool the skin but also help the burn heal more quickly.

## The Solutions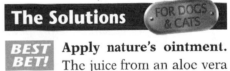

**BEST BET!** **Apply nature's ointment.** The juice from an aloe vera plant contains natural substances

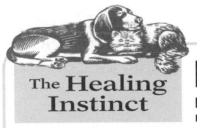

## The Healing Instinct

Even though dogs and cats love the sun, they don't do so well in the heat, which is probably why they don't get sunburned more often than they do. "They'll lie under the porch and get out of the sun in order to stay cool," says Lowell Ackerman, D.V.M., a veterinary dermatologist in Mesa, Arizona, and author of the *Guide to Skin and Haircoat Problems in Dogs*.

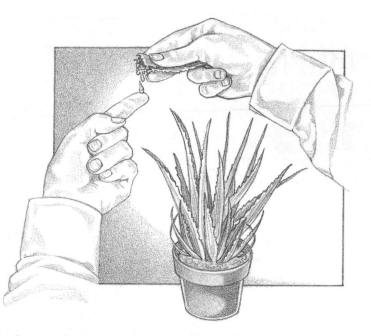

Gel from the aloe vera plant is perhaps the best medicine for healing sunburn. Break off one of the fleshy leaves and squeeze it near the end. A thick, almost-transparent gel will come out. Dip your finger in the gel and spread on the burned area.

called aloins, which help reduce infection and scarring and help speed healing. Aloe is one of the best remedies for sunburn, says Carin A. Smith, D.V.M., a veterinary consultant in the state of Washington and author of *101 Training Tips for Your Cat*. If you have an aloe vera plant at home, break off a leaf, squeeze out the gel, and spread it on the sore spots, she advises. Or you can use an aloe-based cream, available at health food stores.

**Help healing with vitamin E.** "Applying vitamin E to sunburned noses will help keep them from scarring," says Dr. Ackerman. He recommends removing the oil from a vitamin E capsule and spreading it on your pet's nose once or twice a day.

**BEST BET! Moisturize the skin.** Pets that get too much sun lose tremendous amounts of moisture from their skin, making it dry and sore. Applying a moisturizer to burned areas will help restore the skin's natural moisture balance, says Dr. Ackerman. He recommends applying a moisturizer containing coconut or jojoba oil two or three times a day. Plain petroleum jelly works, too, he adds.

**Put out the fire.** The quickest way to ease the pain of sunburn is to spray the area with a mist of cool water, suggests Dr. Ackerman. Of course, cats hate getting wet even more than they hate sunburn. One solution is to sneak up behind them and give their ears a quick spray.

Or you can soak a cloth in cold water, wring it out, and drape over the burned areas, says Dr. Smith. (Just make sure that you leave room for him to breathe.) When the cloth warms up, rewet it and apply it again.

**Cool it with witch hazel.** This is an herbal extract that evaporates as quickly as rubbing alcohol. It will cool inflamed skin but without the sting of alcohol, says Dr. Ackerman. He recommends applying witch hazel with a cotton ball three or four times a day.

**BEST BET!** **Offer some shade.** Some pets love the sun so much that they will put up with anything, including sunburn, to get a little more of it. The only solution is to make sure that they don't overdo it. "Shade the dog's run or keep him in a fenced, shaded part of the yard," says Alexander Werner, V.M.D., a veterinary dermatologist in private practice in Studio City, California. "And try to keep cats inside."

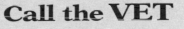

# Call the VET

Sunburn usually stops hurting in a day or two and doesn't cause serious problems. Pets that have been badly burned, however, may get blisters or skin infections. "Call your vet if your pet's sunburn is developing scabs or is oozing or if he stops eating," says Carin A. Smith, D.V.M., a veterinary consultant in the state of Washington and author of *101 Training Tips for your Cat*.

Some conditions that look like sunburn actually aren't—and are a lot more serious, adds Robert Kennis, D.V.M., a veterinary dermatologist at Texas A&M University College of Veterinary Medicine in College Station. For example, some pets—especially dogs with white noses, like collies—may get an immune system disorder called lupus that can cause nose-color changes that resemble sunburn. And a sunburn that won't heal could actually be the beginning of cancer.

Don't wait more than a few days for a sunburn to heal, Dr. Kennis adds. If it is not getting better quickly, there is a good chance that something else is wrong, and you will need to see your vet.

**Pull the curtains.** The sun that comes through glass doors and windows can be just as intense as the sun outside, which is why cats that sleep on sunny windowsills sometimes get a little pink. You may need to keep the blinds or drapes closed during the brightest parts of the day, says Dr. Werner.

**BEST BET!** **Apply a little sunscreen.** "The daily use of sunblock is a very effective way to reduce sun damage to your pet's skin," says Dr. Werner. Use a sunscreen with a sun protection factor (SPF) of 15 or higher and apply it to exposed areas, such as the ears and nose. It is fine to use human sunscreens on pets as long as they don't contain zinc oxide or PABA, which can be harmful if your pet licks them off. Or you can use a sunscreen made for pets, available in pet supply stores. When using a sunscreen, keep your pet busy for a few minutes. This will allow the sunscreen to dry and soak into the skin before your pet licks it off.

| Meet the Experts |
| --- |
| **Lowell Ackerman, D.V.M.,** is a veterinary dermatologist in Mesa, Arizona, and the author of the *Guide to Skin and Haircoat Problems in Dogs*. |
| **Robert Kennis, D.V.M.,** is veterinary dermatologist at Texas A&M University College of Veterinary Medicine in College Station. |
| **Carin A. Smith, D.V.M.,** is a veterinary consultant in the state of Washington and the author of *101 Training Tips for Your Cat*. |
| **Alexander Werner, V.M.D.,** is a veterinary dermatologist in private practice in Studio City, California. |

**Update his wardrobe.** Dogs and cats with very thin fur or those that have been shaved to keep them comfortable in summer can burn very quickly. You can help keep them safe by putting them in T-shirts before they go outside, says Dr. Ackerman.

# TEETHING

## The Signs
- Your puppy or kitten is chewing everything in sight.
- Her gums look red and sore.

## The Cause

When your new shoes fall victim to your puppy's nonstop chewing, or your kitten gnaws through the paperback on your nightstand, you will probably disagree with veterinarians who say that teething isn't a problem. Like it or not, every pet goes through a teething stage, and it is not a comfortable process—for your pet or for you, says Christina Chambreau, D.V.M., a holistic veterinarian in Sparks, Maryland, and education chairperson for the Academy of Veterinary Homeopathy.

The teething age of puppies and kittens is usually between four and eight months, when their permanent teeth replace the baby, or deciduous, teeth. To relieve the pain and pressure, pets often chew and gnaw. You can buy medications to relieve teething pain, but there are other, more natural solutions that are just as effective. Here is what holistic veterinarians recommend.

## The Solutions · FOR DOGS & CATS

**Pour some aloe vera.** The juice from this medicinal plant is available in a drinkable form, and it is a great way to help sore gums recover more quickly, says Dr. Chambreau. You can pour some in a bowl for your pet to lap up, or you can freeze it to a slushy consistency and rub it directly on her gums. Another way to give your pet the juice is to take a needleless syringe

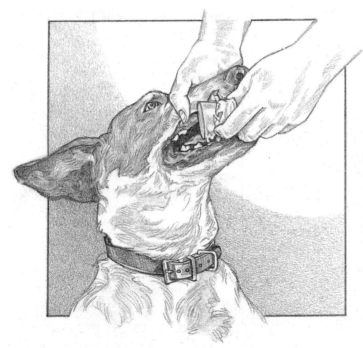

Aloe vera juice not only helps sore gums recover more quickly, but, if you freeze it to a slushy consistency and sponge it on the gums, it will also help numb the pain from teething almost instantly. Or you can freeze it in a paper cup, peel back the cup's edge and rub the frozen juice on the gums.

and squirt it into her mouth, she says. You can buy drinkable aloe vera juice in health food stores and some major supermarkets.

**BEST BET!** **Give them something to chew.** Just as birds gotta fly and fish gotta swim, teething puppies and kittens gotta chew. A chew toy, available in pet supply stores, will relieve pressure on their gums before they turn their attention to your Italian loafers. Two good choices are Nylabones and Kong toys, says Charlene Kickbush, D.V.M., a dog breeder and holistic veterinarian in private practice in Watkinsville, Georgia.

**Put cold to work.** Holistic veterinarians often recommend that teething pets chew cold things—anything from ice chips to aloe vera slushies. The cold will help numb gum pain, says Jeffrey Feinman, V.M.D., a holistic veterinarian in private practice in Fairfield County in Connecticut. One of his favorite solutions is to soak a rope toy in water, freeze it, and then let your pet chew it. Or give your pet an occasional fruit-flavored popsicle, adds Dr. Kickbush.

**Pour a little tea.** Chamomile tea is a natural way to help teething pets be less fretful and anxious, says Susan G. Wynn, D.V.M., a veterinarian in Atlanta and co-editor of *Complementary and Alternative Veterinary Medicine*. Soak a tablespoon of dried chamomile in a cup of hot filtered water. Strain the tea and let it cool to room temperature. Then squirt a little in your pet's mouth with a needleless syringe, she advises.

Another effective way to use chamomile is with homeopathy. Dr. Chambreau recommends slipping three to five homeopathic Chamomile pellets (12X or 30X potency) in a small piece of paper, crushing them to a powder, and then putting the powder in your pet's mouth. You can give this remedy two or three times a day, she says.

**Stop the inflammation.** Homeopathic Ulmus fulva is very effective for

## Meet the Experts

**Christina Chambreau, D.V.M.,** is a holistic veterinarian in Sparks, Maryland, and education chairperson for the Academy of Veterinary Homeopathy.

**Jeffrey Feinman, V.M.D.,** is a holistic veterinarian in private practice in Fairfield County in Connecticut.

**Charlene Kickbush, D.V.M.,** is a dog breeder and holistic veterinarian in private practice in Watkinsville, Georgia. She is certified in acupuncture and chiropractic.

**Susan G. Wynn, D.V.M.,** is a veterinarian in Atlanta and co-editor of *Complementary and Alternative Veterinary Medicine*.

easing gum irritation and inflammation, says Dr. Kickbush. She recommends giving two 12X pellets three or four times a day. When using the liquid form, put 10 to 15 drops in your pet's water each day.

**Calm her with essences.** Flower essences can help relieve teething pain and irritability, says Dr. Chambreau.

Effective essences include walnut flowers, vervain, morning glory, pale pink rose, and Bach Rescue Remedy (a combination designed to relieve stress, pain, and anxiety). Mix two drops of any one of these essences in an ounce of pure water. Shake the bottle, then give your pet a dropperful once or twice a day.

# TICKS

## The Signs

- You keep pulling tick "balloons" off your pet.
- Your pet suddenly has lost his appetite.

## The Cause

Ticks are like vampires, only without sex appeal. They lie in wait for pets (or people) to pass by then leap on board and begin enjoying a good blood meal.

Although ticks are ugly to behold, their bites usually aren't painful and don't cause itching. But they can transmit serious diseases like Rocky Mountain spotted fever or Lyme disease, so it is worth doing everything you can to keep them away. This is especially important for dogs because they get ticks much more often than cats do. "Cats are very sensitive to things on their coats and usually get rid of ticks quickly by licking or scratching them off," says Lori Tapp, D.V.M., a holistic veterinarian in private practice in Asheville, North Carolina.

To keep the critters away, mainstream veterinarians sometimes recommend using tick collars or, more recently, medications that can be applied to the coat or taken orally. Even though the medications used to control ticks are usually safe, they are essentially pesticides that stay in (or on) your pet's body for a long time. Most holistic veterinarians favor a more natural approach not only because it is better for your pet's overall health but also because it can help strengthen his natural defenses, making ticks less likely to cause diseases, says Christina Chambreau, D.V.M., a holistic veterinarian in Sparks, Maryland, and education chairperson for the Academy of Veterinary Homeopathy.

## The Solutions  FOR DOGS & CATS

**Boost immunity with echinacea.** Pets are much less likely to get infected with tick-borne illnesses when their immune systems are working well. The herb echinacea (*Echinacea purpurea* or *Echinacea an-*

*gustifolia*) has been shown to strengthen the immune system, says Michele Yasson, D.V.M., a holistic veterinarian in private practice in New York City and Rosendale, New York. "Use one-quarter of the recommended human dose for cats and dogs that weigh less than 20 pounds." Pets 20 to 50 pounds can take one-half of the human dose, and dogs over 50 pounds can take the full human dose. You can give echinacea for about two weeks at a time.

The easiest way to give echinacea is to open the capsules and sprinkle the powder in your pet's food. When

## Call the VET

The tick that causes Lyme disease is much smaller than the usual "dog ticks." Many dogs get bitten—and infected—and their owners never even see the culprit. That is why it is essential to recognize the signs of tick-borne infections as soon as they become visible.

"If your dog's appetite falls off and he gets listless and lethargic, or if you notice he has pain, swelling, or heat in any of the joints, take him to a vet as soon as possible," says Lori Tapp, D.V.M., a holistic veterinarian in private practice in Asheville, North Carolina. Other warning signs of tick infections include diarrhea, vomiting, limping, or difficulty breathing.

You will also want to call your vet when you know your pet has been bitten by a tick, even if he seems to be fine. Illnesses caused by ticks are much easier to treat when you catch them early, and they are diagnosed with simple blood tests, says Dr. Tapp.

using liquid echinacea, put a few drops in water and mix the solution in the food, she advises. Don't use liquid echinacea that contains alcohol because pets dislike the taste, she adds.

**Repel ticks with essential oils.** "The combination of cedarwood and citronella essential oils seems to be an effective tick repellent," says Jeffrey Levy, D.V.M., a holistic veterinarian in private practice in Williamsburg, Massachusetts. He recommends mixing equal amounts of the two oils together and diluting them with rubbing alcohol, using 1 part oil to 10 parts alcohol. Shake up the mixture and apply a small amount to your pet's lower legs before he goes outside. Some pets will insist on licking the oils off, in which case you will want to try another remedy instead.

Even though it is safe to apply diluted essential oils externally, they may interfere with some homeopathic treatments, Dr. Levy adds. "If your pet is getting homeopathy, check with your vet before using the oils."

**Keep them away with garlic.** Vampires aren't the only bloodsuckers that don't like garlic—ticks avoid it, too. But stringing garlic around your pet's neck won't suffice; he will have to eat it. Garlic contains compounds that are secreted through the skin, and ticks and fleas find it distasteful, says Dr. Tapp.

She recommends giving your pet fresh raw garlic (powdered doesn't work) every day. Cats can have about one-eighth teaspoon of fresh garlic a day for no more than two weeks since too much garlic can cause a certain type of anemia. Dogs over 50 pounds can have as much as two teaspoons a day, and smaller dogs can have one-quarter to one-half teaspoon. Most dogs like the taste, so you can just stir some in their food, says Dr. Tapp.

**BEST BET!** **Check for ticks often.** It takes ticks quite a bit of time to penetrate the skin and start feeding, and a lot longer—more than 24 hours in some cases—before they can transmit diseases. When you pick ticks off your pet within a few hours after they climbed on, they are unlikely to be a problem. "You can often find ticks by feeling your pet well with your hands or using a flea comb," says Dr. Yasson. Flea combs are small-toothed combs that readily pick up even small ticks. She recommends doing a tick patrol at least once a day during the warm months, especially when your pet has been spending time outside.

**Remove the critters.** It is no one's favorite job, but removing feeding ticks promptly will help prevent them from passing diseases, says Dr. Levy. It is best to use tweezers, although you can remove ticks with your fingers as long as you wear gloves or grip the tick with a small piece of plastic wrap. "Grab the tick as close to the skin as possible, then

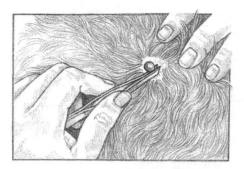

Ticks have a curved, anchorlike jaw that enables them to hold on tight for the day or two it takes them to feed. To remove embedded ticks, grip them with tweezers as close to the skin as possible. Gently, but firmly, pull them straight out. Don't try to twist them out because this will often cause the head to break off and remain in the skin.

pull gently and slowly," he says. In most cases, the head will pull out of the skin, and you can discard the tick in a small jar of rubbing alcohol. Don't worry if the head stays in the skin, he adds. It will fall out on its own over time.

**Soothe the wound.** After you remove the tick, you might see a bump or some redness on your pet's skin. "I recommend applying a natural herbal salve such as a comfrey ointment to the tick bite," says Dr. Yasson.

Or apply a little tea tree oil, adds Beatrice Ehrsam, D.V.M., a holistic veterinarian in private practice in New Paltz, New York. "It's a good antiseptic. Dilute a few drops in one ounce of water and apply it with a cotton ball." Don't let your pet lick the area until the salve has soaked into the

skin. (Avoid using tea tree oil on cats, which can be dangerous.)

**BEST BET!** **Clear the underbrush.** Ticks thrive in many parts of the country, and you will never get rid of them all. Ticks live a foot or two off the ground in scrub and grasses, Dr. Tapp explains. "Keep your pet from running in areas where ticks tend to frequent and get rid of underbrush and low branches in your yard." It is also a good idea to keep your grass mowed short. Pets that play on well-mowed lawns are much less likely to get ticks, she says.

## Meet the Experts

**Christina Chambreau, D.V.M.,** is a holistic veterinarian in Sparks, Maryland, and education chairperson for the Academy of Veterinary Homeopathy.

**Beatrice Ehrsam, D.V.M.,** is a holistic veterinarian in private practice in New Paltz, New York. She is certified in acupuncture.

**Jeffrey Levy, D.V.M.,** is a holistic veterinarian in private practice in Williamsburg, Massachusetts.

**Lori Tapp, D.V.M.,** is a holistic veterinarian in private practice in Asheville, North Carolina. She is certified in homeopathy.

**Michele Yasson, D.V.M.,** is a holistic veterinarian in private practice in New York City and Rosendale, New York. She is certified in acupuncture.

# ULCERS

## The Cause

He is not a hard-boiled corporate executive. He doesn't fret over the ups and downs of the stock market or perform emergency surgery. So why does your pet have an ulcer?

Although stress may play a role in causing ulcers, most dogs and cats get them when they are taking anti-inflammatory medications for arthritis or other long-term problems, says Henry Pasternak, D.V.M., a holistic veterinarian in private practice in Pacific Palisades, California. Aspirin and similar drugs inhibit a hormonelike substance that protects the stomach lining. In addition, these drugs irritate the stomach, and the combination can lead to ulcers.

Pets that are generally healthy are much less likely to get ulcers than those with underlying problems, adds Christina Chambreau, D.V.M., a holistic veterinarian in Sparks, Maryland, and education chairperson for the Academy of Veterinary Homeopathy. "Stomach ulcers are a sign that the dog or cat is weak overall," she says.

Holistic veterinarians usually attack ulcers on two fronts: by improving nutrition and other factors that play a role in overall health and by treating the ulcers with gentle, natural remedies instead of medications. Here is what they advise.

## The Solutions · FOR DOGS & CATS

**Feed them more often.** Ulcers tend to flare when there are long gaps between meals, which allow harsh stomach acids to irritate the stomach. Feeding pets more often will help buffer the acids that can lead to ulcers. Divide your pet's food into two meals a day if he currently is having only one, or into three meals if he is having only two, says Anne Lampru, D.V.M., a holistic veterinarian in private practice in Tampa, Florida.

**Soothe the stomach with aloe vera.** Putting aloe vera juice in your pet's water every day will help prevent nausea and help ulcers heal more quickly, says Dr. Lampru. She recommends giving one teaspoon of aloe vera juice a day to cats and to small dogs under 15 pounds and two tablespoons or more a day to larger dogs. "Make sure that you use aloe vera that is specifically meant for drinking," she says. "You don't want to use the gel." You can buy aloe vera juice at health food stores.

**BEST BET!** **Slip them some slippery elm.** The bark from slippery elm trees has long been used to soothe sore throats, and it appears to work for sore stomachs as well, says Robin Cannizzaro, D.V.M., a holistic veterinarian in private practice in St. Petersburg, Florida. She recommends using powdered slippery elm (*Ulmus rubra*), which you can mix with warm water to form a pudding-like paste. Pets under 15 pounds can take one-half teaspoon of slippery elm at a time, and larger pets can take up to one tablespoon. It is a good idea to give the slippery elm three or four times a day between meals.

Some pets will lick slippery elm off the spoon, but most won't be so obliging. You may have to spoon the mixture into your pet's mouth, says Dr. Cannizzaro. If you can't find the powdered form of slippery elm, it is fine to buy capsules and empty the contents into water to form the paste.

**Coat the intestines with pectin.** Used in jellies and jams as well as in Kaopectate, pectin binds to irritated surfaces in the intestinal tract and helps them heal, states Beatrice Ehrsam, D.V.M., a holistic veterinarian in private practice in New Paltz, New York. She recommends giving dogs and cats 50 milligrams of pectin for every 20 pounds of weight once a day. You can buy pectin in supermarkets and natural food stores.

**Give them bland meals.** Even though dogs and cats need a lot of protein to stay healthy, many protein sources are slightly acidic, which can irritate already-tender tummies. "Reduce protein to about 20 percent of the diet for dogs and 50 percent for cats," says Dr. Ehrsam.

Pets with ulcers shouldn't be snacking on rich leftovers either. "Give your pet bland, easily digested food like rice, chicken, cottage cheese, boiled potatoes, and hard-boiled eggs," says Dr. Pasternak.

**Speed healing with glutamine.** An amino acid called L-glutamine, available in health food stores, is recommended for healing mucous membranes throughout the body, including those in the intestinal tract, says Dr. Ehrsam. Pets over 15 pounds can take 100 milligrams of L-glutamine a day, while smaller pets can take 50 milligrams.

**BEST BET!** **Protect the stomach with licorice.** Licorice root (*Glycyrrhiza glabra*) extract stimulates the production of prostaglandins, the hormonelike substances that help protect the stomach's walls, says Dr. Pasternak. He suggests using the deglycyrrhizinated form of licorice extract, available in health food stores. Dogs over 50 pounds can take between 300 and 600 milligrams, spread out between

## Meet the Experts

**Robin Cannizzaro, D.V.M.,** is a holistic veterinarian in St. Petersburg, Florida. She is certified in acupuncture and homeopathy.

**Christina Chambreau, D.V.M.,** is a holistic veterinarian in Sparks, Maryland, and education chairperson for the Academy of Veterinary Homeopathy.

**Beatrice Ehrsam, D.V.M.,** is a holistic veterinarian in private practice in New Paltz, New York. She is certified in acupuncture.

**Anne Lampru, D.V.M.,** is a holistic veterinarian in private practice in Tampa, Florida. She is certified in acupuncture and homeopathy.

**Jeffrey Levy, D.V.M.,** is a holistic veterinarian in private practice in Williamsburg, Massachusetts.

**Henry Pasternak, D.V.M.,** is a holistic veterinarian in private practice in Pacific Palisades, California. He is certified in acupuncture.

**Sandra Priest, D.V.M.,** is a holistic veterinarian in private practice in Knoxville, Tennessee. She is certified in chiropractic.

two meals. Pets 15 to 50 pounds can take 100 to 300 milligrams, and smaller pets can take 100 to 200 milligrams. Licorice is entirely safe, but it is best not to give it for more than a week without checking with your vet.

**BEST BET!** **Avoid the painkillers.** Even though buffered aspirin is easier on the stomach than regular aspirin, it can still lead to ulcers in dogs, says Jeffrey Levy, D.V.M., a holistic veterinarian in private practice in Williamsburg, Massachusetts. (Aspirin can be toxic for cats, and they should never take it.) If your dog has arthritis or another condition for which he needs long-term pain relief, ask your vet if there are other, gentler remedies that you can try.

**Reduce the stress in your pet's life.** Stress doesn't cause ulcers in pets, but it can make existing ulcers worse. "Create a loving environment," says Sandra Priest, D.V.M., a holistic veterinarian in private practice in Knoxville, Tennessee. "Spend lots of time with your pet and try to keep him relaxed."

# URINARY TRACT INFECTIONS

## The Signs

- There is blood in your pet's urine.
- Your pet cries or strains when urinating.
- The urine has a bad smell.
- Your pet wants to go out more often or is having accidents in the house.

Urinary tract infections are just as uncomfortable for pets as they are for people, and they get them nearly as often. Caused by bacteria in the bladder or urethra (the tube through which urine flows), urinary tract infections can make it very painful to urinate. And if the infections aren't caught early, they can spread upward to the kidneys, causing serious problems.

Both holistic and mainstream veterinarians treat urinary tract infections with antibiotics, but holistic vets go a little bit further. They use a variety of natural remedies to strengthen the immune system so that it is better able to resist the infection. In addition, they feel that it is important to correct imbalances in the body that allow bacteria to thrive, says Bob Ulbrich, V.M.D., a holistic veterinarian in private practice in Portland, Oregon.

## The Solutions — FOR DOGS & CATS

**Reduce irritation with herbs.** An herbal tincture called Goldenrod Horsetail Compound, which contains corn silk, goldenrod, horsetail, pipsissewa leaf, and juniper berry, can help soothe and support an irritated urinary system, says Dr. Ulbrich. Dogs weighing under 15 pounds can have half a dropperful of the tincture twice a day until they are feeling better. Larger dogs can take between one and two droppersful a day. The easiest way to give the tincture is to mix it in your pet's food, he says.

Alcohol tinctures aren't safe for long-term use in cats, so an herbal tea is a better choice. Look for a combination of goldenrod, horsetail, parsley, marsh mallow root, and elderberry called Urinary Tea Blend, says Dr. Ulbrich. Cats can take one teaspoon of the cooled tea three times a day until symptoms have cleared up, he says. You can find both products in some health food stores or at veterinarian offices.

**BEST BET!** **Relieve pain with Cantharis.** The homeopathic remedy Cantharis will quickly ease discomfort in pets that are straining to urinate, says Maria H. Glinski, D.V.M., a holistic veterinarian in private practice in Glendale, Wisconsin. It is most effective when there is also blood in the urine. She recommends giving two or three 30C pellets at the first sign of infection and repeating the treatment once an hour for three hours. Your pet doesn't have to swallow the pellets. Just put them in her mouth, where they will be absorbed by the mucous membranes. If your pet isn't getting better within 12 hours, you will want to call your vet, she says.

**BEST BET!** **Stop infection with cranberry.** "Cranberry stops bacteria from adhering to the surface of the bladder, and it acidifies the urine," says Michelle Tilghman, D.V.M., a holistic veterinarian in private practice in Stone Mountain, Georgia. Bacteria don't thrive in an acid environment, she explains. It would take a lot of cranberry juice to make a difference, however, and most pets dislike the taste, so Dr. Tilghman recommends using the cranberry supplement CranActin, available in health

## Call the VET

Most urinary tract infections will go away fairly quickly once they are treated with antibiotics. But they can also get worse, sometimes very quickly. "The infection can ascend into the kidney and cause very serious problems," says Maria H. Glinski, D.V.M., a holistic veterinarian in private practice in Glendale, Wisconsin.

If you suspect that your pet has an infection—she may be urinating very often or crying when she urinates, or the urine will contain blood or have a foul smell—it is fine to wait for a day before calling your vet. But if she isn't getting better by then and seems to be in pain, you will need to make an appointment right away.

An exception to this wait-and-see rule is if your pet is straining to urinate, but nothing is coming out. Pets that can't urinate could have a stone blocking the urethra. Especially common in male cats, this is an emergency that needs immediate treatment.

food stores. You can give one capsule for every 20 pounds of pet.

**Boost immunity with DMG.** A powerful antioxidant, dimethylglycine (DMG) is an amino acid that strengthens the immune system and helps it fight infections, says John M. Simon, D.V.M., a holistic veterinarian in private practice in Royal Oak, Michigan. It is available in liquid form in health food stores. You will want to give your pet a fraction of the full human dose, based on a 150-pound person. A 10-pound cat, for example, would take about one-fifteenth of the full human dose once a day.

**Strengthen the body with vitamin C.** "It is also great for the lining of the bladder because it is a natural anti-inflammatory," says Dr. Glinski. She recommends giving pets under 15 pounds about 250 milligrams of vitamin C twice a day. Pets 15 to 50 pounds can have 500 milligrams twice a day, and larger dogs can take 1,000 milligrams twice a day. Use a buffered form of vitamin C, such as sodium ascorbate, because it is less likely to irritate the digestive tract. Since vitamin C can cause diarrhea, you may have to cut back the dose until you find an amount that your pet will tolerate.

**Restore the body's balance.** The problem with antibiotics is that they kill beneficial bacteria along with those that cause infection. To restore a healthful bacterial balance when your pet is taking antibiotics for an infection, you may want to give supplements containing *Lactobacillus bifidus*, says Gerald Buchoff, B.V.Sc.A.H. (bachelor of veterinary science and animal husbandry, the Indian equivalent of D.V.M.), a holistic veterinarian in private practice in North Bergen, New Jersey. "Give pets under 20 pounds one-eighth teaspoon twice a day. Larger pets can take one-quarter teaspoon twice daily. But wait an hour or two after your pet takes the antibiotic."

**Switch to a chemical-free food.** The chemical additives, preservatives, and artificial colors in some commercial pet foods may weaken immunity and make pets more vulnerable to infections, says Dr. Glinski. "Stick with home cooking or with high-quality, all-natural commercial foods." For more on natural and homemade diets, see page 61.

**BEST BET!** **Give additional fluids.** Dogs and cats that don't drink a lot also don't urinate a lot, and this allows bacteria to stay inside the bladder and urinary tract, says Dr. Tilghman. You can't force pets to drink, but you can increase their fluid intake by giving them moist foods or by moistening dry food with a little bit of water or broth, she says.

**Provide clean water.** "The chemicals in some drinking water can deter pets from drinking," says Dr. Tilghman. "This makes them more susceptible to infection because their urine gets very concentrated." She recommends giving dogs and cats filtered or spring water not only to help relieve but also to prevent urinary tract infections.

**Provide plenty of breaks.** When dogs and cats are recovering from urinary tract infections, you want to encourage them to urinate as often as possible, says Dr. Tilghman. Frequent urination will prevent urine in the bladder from getting too concentrated, she explains.

## The Solutions FOR DOGS

**Keep her clean.** Females that were spayed at an early age sometimes develop loose tissue that allows urine to pool around the urethra. "In females, the urethra is very short, and bacteria can ascend very quickly to the bladder," says Dr. Tilghman. If your pet gets infections frequently, you may be able to prevent problems by giving her bottom a quick wipe with a baby wipe whenever she urinates. This will remove bacteria before they get a chance to move upstream, she explains.

# VISION PROBLEMS

## The Signs

- Your pet seems clumsy or disoriented.
- He bumps into things.
- His pupils are dilated, even in bright light.
- His eyes are bloodshot or cloudy.
- He has trouble finding you when you call.

## The Cause

Maybe your dog occasionally bumps into furniture or brushes your leg when he is walking by. Or your cat looks out the window but doesn't seem to be focusing on anything. Or you toss a toy on the carpet, and your pet can't find it. Dogs and cats don't depend on sight as much as people do, so it is not always obvious when their vision is starting to fade. But vision problems are very common, especially in older pets, and they can make it difficult for them to get around.

The most common vision problem in pets is aging lenses, or lenticular sclerosis, which makes the eyes a little cloudy. A more serious problem is cataracts, which are fairly common in older pets, says Michele Yasson, D.V.M., a holistic veterinarian in private practice in New York City and Rosendale, New York. "Glaucoma also causes problems, especially in cats that have high blood pressure." Another serious vision problem is retinal degeneration, which may cause blindness.

Serious eye problems are rare, however, and most dogs and cats with minor vision problems get along just fine as long as you help them adjust and take a few simple steps to protect their eyes from further harm.

## The Solutions FOR DOGS & CATS

**Give spirulina.** Age-related vision problems may be caused by a deficiency of micronutrients, says Sandra Priest, D.V.M., a holistic veterinarian in private practice in Knoxville, Tennessee. An excellent way to supplement your pet's diet is with spirulina, an algae that is packed with trace minerals that aren't always easy to get from diet alone. Dr. Priest recommends giving cats and dogs weighing under 15 pounds about 125 milligrams of spirulina a day. Pets 15 to 50 pounds can take 250 milligrams, and larger dogs can take 500 milligrams. Veterinarians recommend giving it for about three months, then stopping it for a month.

Spirulina may affect the balance of blood sugars in the body, she adds. You don't want to give it to pets with diabetes or Cushing's disease without checking with your veterinarian first.

**BEST BET! Improve circulation with bilberry.** Holistic veterinarians often use the herb bilberry (*Vaccinium myrtillus*) for treating vision problems because it appears to stimulate blood circulation to the eyes. "It's good for a lot of eye problems, including cataracts and retinal degeneration," says Dr. Priest. Give 20 mil-

ligrams of bilberry twice a day to dogs and cats under 15 pounds. Pets 15 to 50 pounds can take 25 milligrams twice a day, and dogs over 50 pounds can take 30 milligrams twice a day.

**Give your pet the best food you can find.** Common commercial diets don't always provide all the nutrients that dogs and cats need, which can hasten age-related vision problems, says Dr. Priest. She recommends giving pets high-quality natural diets that don't contain chemical preservatives or additives. Home-cooked diets can be superb, but commercial natural foods like Wysong, available at some pet supply stores and through mail-order companies, are also a good choice, she says.

## Call the VET

Many dogs and cats lose at least some of their vision as they get older, and it is usually not a problem. But there are a number of serious conditions, including glaucoma and tumors in the eye or brain, that can also cause vision loss. Quick treatment may save your pet's sight, so you need to call your vet at the first sign of problems.

Symptoms to watch for include bloodshot eyes, whiteness on the cornea, or eyes that are suddenly larger than usual. "If he has glaucoma, he can lose his vision within 36 to 48 hours, so you need to see your vet right away," says Anne Lampru, D.V.M., a holistic veterinarian in private practice in Tampa, Florida.

**ALTERNATIVE**

## 🐾 SUCCESS

# A SIGHT TO REMEMBER

Some dogs adjust to changes in their vision just fine, but Chuck, a seven-year-old Chesapeake Bay retriever with retinal degeneration, was having a terrible time.

"He was almost completely blind," says Lori Tapp, D.V.M., a holistic veterinarian in private practice in Asheville, North Carolina. "He was afraid to go anywhere without his owner. He didn't dare go out in the fields like he used to. He couldn't even see well enough to know it was time to lift his feet when he got to the bottom of the stairway."

Chuck's usual veterinarian felt that medications wouldn't help, but Dr. Tapp thought natural medicines might do the trick. She recommended that Chuck be taken off his commercial diet and given fresh, natural foods. She also started giving Chuck a glandular supplement along with a variety of homeopathic remedies. "At different points in his treatment, he required everything from superficial remedies like Apis to very deep, long-acting remedies like Sulfur," she says.

Improvement didn't come all at once, but over a period of months Chuck started getting better. He still can't see at night, Dr. Tapp says, but he is now able to get around during the day. "He can do a lot of the things he used to do," she says. "He goes out in the fields now, and he runs up to the bottom of the stairs, and he knows right when to pick his feet up."

**BEST BET!** **Stop eye damage with vitamins.** As dogs and cats get older, harmful oxygen molecules called free radicals gradually damage cells throughout the body, including the lens of the eye. Giving pets vitamins A, C, and E will help block the damaging effects of free radicals, says Dr. Priest. She recommends using a supplement that includes a mix of these nutrients. Cats need about 50 milligrams of vitamin C, 100 international units (IU) of vitamin E, and 500 IU of vitamin A each day. Dogs can take between 250 and 500 milligrams of vitamin C, 100

---

## Meet the Experts

**Beatrice Ehrsam, D.V.M.,** is a holistic veterinarian in private practice in New Paltz, New York. She is certified in acupuncture.

**Anne Lampru, D.V.M.,** is a holistic veterinarian in private practice in Tampa, Florida. She is certified in acupuncture and homeopathy.

**Sandra Priest, D.V.M.,** is a holistic veterinarian in private practice in Knoxville, Tennessee. She is certified in chiropractic.

**Lori Tapp, D.V.M.,** is a holistic veterinarian in private practice in Asheville, North Carolina. She is certified in homeopathy.

**Michele Yasson, D.V.M.,** is a holistic veterinarian in private practice in New York City and Rosendale, New York. She is certified in acupuncture.

---

to 200 IU of vitamin E, and 1,000 IU of vitamin A.

**Keep your pet company.** Even though most pets easily adjust to slight losses of vision, some get confused and anxious. Plan on giving your pet extra attention and reassurance, says Beatrice Ehrsam, D.V.M., a holistic veterinarian in private practice in New Paltz, New York. You may even want to add another pet to the family. "They take care of each other," she explains. "You will often see the new pet guarding a companion who is losing his vision."

**Safeguard the steps.** Dogs and cats are surefooted, but they do make mistakes, especially when they can't see where they are going. "Put up a baby gate at the top of the stairs," suggests Dr. Priest.

**BEST BET!** **Keep things predictable.** There is nothing wrong with redecorating, but you don't want to start shoving furniture around when your pet is struggling with serious vision problems. "Most animals that are losing vision compensate very well," says Dr. Ehrsam. "They know how many steps it is from the doorway to the litter box or the food bowl, and they get around fine." When you shift the furniture, however, once-familiar rooms can seem like a maze.

It is worth taking a little time to guide your pet around when you shift the furniture, Dr. Ehrsam advises. Show him where the couch is and help him find the path that is easiest to navigate. Once you have shown him where things are, he will quickly learn to find his way around.

# VOMITING

## The Signs
- Your pet is retching.
- You are finding messes on the floor.

## The Cause

Dogs and cats have many ways of detoxifying their bodies, and one of the quickest is vomiting. It is not good for your carpets, but it is a very efficient way to remove irritating substances from the digestive tract or at least to let you know that something is wrong, says Susan G. Wynn, D.V.M., a veterinarian in Atlanta and co-editor of *Complementary and Alternative Veterinary Medicine*.

Vomiting that lasts more than a day always needs to be checked by your vet. But vomiting usually isn't serious, and you can stop it fairly quickly with natural remedies that will help soothe your pet's stomach. Here are some tips that you may want to try.

## The Solutions FOR DOGS & CATS

**Soothe the stomach with chamomile.** A popular remedy in aromatherapy, essential oil of chamomile can calm an upset stomach fairly quickly, says Donna M. Starita, D.V.M., a holistic veterinarian in private prac-

tice in Boring, Oregon. She recommends putting the undiluted oil in a nebulizer, a small heating unit that vaporizes the oil and fills the air with the scent. Let your pet breathe the scent for several hours, she advises. If you don't have a nebulizer, you can dilute the oil half-and-half with vegetable oil and apply it to the tips of your pet's ears once a day for a few days.

**Press away nausea.** Dogs and cats have three acupressure points that you can stimulate to relieve nausea: ST36, located on the outside of the hind leg just below the knee; LIV14, located at a slight bump in the middle of the eighth rib counting back from the shoulders; and PC8, located near the dewclaw about one-half inch above the wrist pad on the front foot, says Joanne Stefanatos, D.V.M., a holistic veterinarian in private practice in Las Vegas. She recommends pressing each point for about 60 seconds twice a day.

**BEST BET!** **Clear out the toxins with Nux vomica.** A homeopathic remedy used for a variety of digestive problems, Nux vomica helps detoxify the body, reducing the need to vomit, says Kathleen Carson, D.V.M., a holistic veterinarian in private practice in Hermosa Beach, California. She recommends diluting 20 drops of Nux vomica 6C in an ounce of water and giving your pet half a dropperful three times a day for two to three days.

**Reduce stress with Bach Rescue Remedy.** Vomiting is stressful because dogs and cats may feel as though they are losing control of their bodies, and the stress of vomiting can make them feel even sicker. A quick way to relieve stress is with a flower essence called Bach Rescue Remedy, says Dr. Carson. This essence is particularly effective when combined with the essence crab apple, which helps detoxify the body. She recommends putting six to eight drops of each essence in an ounce of spring water. Give your pet between a quarter and half a dropperful at least four times a day, she advises.

**Ease nausea with peppermint tea.** A classic remedy for digestive problems in humans, peppermint tea works for dogs and cats as well. "Give them strong peppermint tea, as much as they want," suggests Dr. Starita.

 **Plan some recovery time.** Putting pets on a food fast for 24 hours will help stop vomiting and give the stomach a chance to recover. It is also a good idea to reduce the amount of water they drink. "Give them ice cubes to lick," says Dr. Starita. Most pets like ice, which will help keep them hydrated without overloading the body with water.

**BEST BET! Give her bland foods.** Even when your pet is starting to feel better, you don't want to overwhelm the stomach with rich foods or large meals. Eating too much causes the body to release large amounts of digestive juices, which can irritate the stomach all over again. After your pet has fasted for a day, give her tiny amounts of bland foods—a mixture of nonfat cottage cheese, rice, and diced boneless chicken breasts, for example—several times a day. It is easier for the body to handle a mouthful of food than large amounts all at once, says Dr. Starita.

**Encourage slow eating.** It is usually not a problem in cats, but dogs sometimes gobble their food in a hurry, causing it to come back up just as fast, says Anne Lampru, D.V.M., a holistic veterinarian in private practice in Tampa, Florida. One way to encourage your pet to eat more slowly is to put a large object—a tennis ball, for example—in her food dish. She will have to pick around the ball to get at her food, she explains.

**Give your pets warm food.** Food straight from the refrigerator isn't very appealing to dogs and cats. For one thing, cold food doesn't release all the aromas they need to feel hungry. It can also irritate their stomachs, Dr. Lampru explains. It is best to give them food that is at room temperature, she advises.

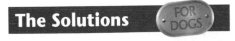
**The Solutions** FOR DOGS

**Coat the stomach with bismuth.** The main ingredient in Pepto-Bismol, bismuth is a white, chalky substance that coats the stomach walls and reduces inflammation, keeping the stomach calm. You can buy bismuth in drugstores and supermarkets, but it is easier just to give Pepto-Bismol when your dog first starts getting sick, says Dr. Starita. She recommends giving dogs weighing under 15 pounds one-half teaspoon of Pepto-Bismol two or three times a day. Dogs 15 to 50 pounds can take one to two teaspoons, and larger dogs can take two tablespoons two or three times a day.

Even though Pepto-Bismol is safe for dogs, it contains aspirin, which can be dangerous for cats, Dr. Starita adds. So check with your veterinarian before giving Pepto-Bismol to your cat.

---

### Meet the Experts

**Kathleen Carson, D.V.M.,** is a holistic veterinarian in private practice in Hermosa Beach, California.

**Anne Lampru, D.V.M.,** is a holistic veterinarian in private practice in Tampa, Florida. She is certified in acupuncture and homeopathy.

**Donna M. Starita, D.V.M.,** is a holistic veterinarian in private practice in Boring, Oregon.

**Joanne Stefanatos, D.V.M.,** is a holistic veterinarian in private practice in Las Vegas. She is certified in acupuncture and chiropractic.

**Susan G. Wynn, D.V.M.,** is a veterinarian in Atlanta and co-editor of *Complementary and Alternative Veterinary Medicine.*

---

# WOOL SUCKING

## The Signs
- Your cat is always chewing on wool, cotton, or other materials.

## The Cause

It was cute when your cat starting sucking on an old pair of socks. It was less amusing when she destroyed your wool gloves, the slipcovers on the couch, and your new angora sweater.

Veterinarians aren't sure why, but some cats become almost obsessed with sucking and chewing on fabrics, a condition known as wool sucking. Some cats may do it because they were abandoned or left the nest too early, and sucking on fabric reminds them of the comfort of nursing. Emotional stress or nutritional deficiencies may play a role. And since cats look entirely blissful while chewing on wool (or any other fabric), it may be nothing more than an act of pure pleasure.

Wool sucking is really more of a people problem than a pet problem since the main threat is to your belongings. But sucking sometimes turns to chewing, and chewing can turn to swallowing—and that is when it starts getting dangerous. Veterinarians will sometimes treat wool sucking with medications, such as fluoxetine (Prozac), which help curtail many types of compulsive behavior. Before turning to powerful drugs, however, you may want to try a few simpler and safer approaches.

## The Solutions

**BEST BET!** **Upgrade her diet.** Some cats may start sucking or chewing material because their diets aren't providing all the nutrients they need. "They could have a need for trace minerals," says Michael W. Lemmon, D.V.M., a holistic veterinarian in Renton, Washington, and past president of the American Holistic Veterinary Medical Association.

He recommends changing your cat's diet, giving her 75 percent organic raw meat and 25 percent raw vegetables, such as carrots. In addition, you should mix in her food one-quarter to one-half teaspoon of powdered sea vegetables, such as kelp or dulse, which are rich in trace minerals. Try the diet for about a month. If your cat becomes less materially inclined, she probably just needs a higher-quality food, he says. For more information on healthful, natural diets, see page 61.

**Give her more fiber.** Cats need dietary fiber just as much as people do, and they may start gnawing material to replace fiber that is missing in their diets, says Dr. Lemmon. He recommends mixing a teaspoon of oat bran, wheat bran, or flaxseed in your cat's food every day.

**Calm her nerves with homeopathy.** There are a number of homeopathic remedies that can help ease the anxiety that can lead to wool sucking. For example, Silica 6X, given twice a day for seven days, can help stop wool sucking in cats that are also nervous or shy, says Robin Cannizzaro, D.V.M., a holistic veterinarian in private practice in St. Petersburg, Florida. The usual dose is two or three drops of liquid Silica or four to five pellets. If your cat isn't getting better within a week, call a holistic veterinarian for advice, she advises.

**Relieve her anxiety.** Since cats may turn to wool during times of tension, you may want to give her calming herbs, such as St. John's wort (*Hypericum perforatum*) or kava kava (*Piper methysticum*), says Dr. Cannizzaro. "You can use a product that combines the two herbs, or you can

**ALTERNATIVE**

## SUCCESS

### CHANGING TASTES

Karlee had an insatiable appetite for fabrics. She preferred wool but in a pinch would chew on cotton and acrylic. Karlee's owner, tired of discovering holes in her sweaters and wet spots on her socks, finally took her to Jeffrey Levy, D.V.M., a holistic veterinarian in private practice in Williamsburg, Massachusetts.

Dr. Levy discovered that Karlee, a domestic short-hair who was one year old at the time, chewed fabrics only at night. And when she was caught in the act, she seemed unaware that she was doing anything wrong. Dr. Levy realized that her behavior was similar to cats with mild seizure disorders.

He decided to treat Karlee with homeopathic Belladonna. The results were all he hoped for. Within six weeks, Karlee had quit chewing fabrics entirely, and, Dr. Levy learned later, she never started again.

give them separately." St. John's wort may cause side effects in some pets, however, so talk to your vet before using it at home. If it is going to work, you should see results in about two weeks, she adds.

**Try healing essences.** Flower remedies can be very helpful for cats that are sucking wool if they are nervous or upset, says Christina Chambreau, D.V.M., a holistic veterinarian in Sparks, Maryland, and education chairperson for the Academy of Veterinary Homeopathy. "A cat who is tense and anxious, for example, might need vervain," she says. "One who is fearful and timid might need aspen and mimulus. A cat who starts wool sucking after another animal is added to the household may need holly for jealousy." You may want to try chestnut bud as well since it is a common remedy for stopping repetitious behavior.

To prepare the remedies, put two drops of an essence in a one-ounce dropper bottle filled with pure water. Shake it 10 to 20 times and give your cat one dropperful three or four times a day. You can put the drops in her mouth

## Meet the Experts

**Robin Cannizzaro, D.V.M.,** is a holistic veterinarian in private practice in St. Petersburg, Florida. She is certified in acupuncture and homeopathy.

**Christina Chambreau, D.V.M.,** is a holistic veterinarian in Sparks, Maryland, and education chairperson for the Academy of Veterinary Homeopathy.

**Michael W. Lemmon, D.V.M.,** is a holistic veterinarian in Renton, Washington, and past president of the American Holistic Veterinary Medical Association.

**Jeffrey Levy, D.V.M.,** is a holistic veterinarian in private practice in Williamsburg, Massachusetts.

or in her drinking water. "You should notice some improvement within two weeks," says Dr. Chambreau. "It is a good idea to continue giving it for a month or two, then resume it later if the behavior starts to recur."

**Soothe her with massage.** One way to calm anxious cats is with massage. "Cradle one ear in each hand and massage them gently between your fingers," says Dr. Cannizzaro. "You don't want to pull hard or yank on the ears, but just use gentle pressure." If your cat doesn't enjoy all this ear attention, you can massage a spot in the center of the head. "Just in front of the pointy crest is a tiny indentation," she says. "A gentle massage on that spot can be very calming."

**BEST BET!** **Put away temptation.** Sometimes the best remedies are also the simplest. When your cat won't leave your belongings alone, try to make her favorite targets unavailable. "Store the items out of reach," says Dr. Lemmon.

**BEST BET!** **Change the flavor.** Some of the perennial favorites among wool-sucking cats—like carpets and curtains—can't be stuffed in a drawer. "Apply a flavor or odor that your cat doesn't like," advises Dr. Lemmon. Sprinkling black pepper on your cat's object of choice may be all it takes to keep her away. Or you can dissolve black pepper in hot water, let it cool, then spray it in places where you don't want her to go. "Your cat will taste it and think, 'Hey, this isn't so good after all,'" he says.

# WORMS

## The Signs
- Your pet is vomiting or has diarrhea.
- He has been scooting his bottom across the floor.
- There are small fragments or whole worms in the stool.
- He is thin, though he eats well.
- He seems tired.

## The Cause

Many puppies and kittens are born with intestinal worms or get them soon after birth. Adult pets also get worms, which cause symptoms ranging from diarrhea to an itchy bottom.

Many types of worms don't cause serious problems, but they should still be taken seriously because pets tend to get worms when their immune systems aren't as strong as they should be, says Michele Yasson, D.V.M., a holistic veterinarian in private practice in New York City and Rosendale, New York. "Healthy dogs and cats run up against worms all the time, but their bodies just spew them out. They don't become a problem unless the environment in the body actually encourages them to thrive."

Pets with worms are usually given oral medications. The medications, available over the counter and from vets, are very effective, but you don't want to use them again and again, says Christina Chambreau, D.V.M., a holistic veterinarian in Sparks, Maryland, and education chairperson for the Academy of Veterinary Homeopathy. That is why holistic veterinarians prefer to use a preventive approach. A stronger and healthier pet is much less likely to get worms in the first place.

## The Solutions FOR DOGS & CATS

**Add bran to his diet.** One way to get worms out of the intestinal tract is to give your pet oat or wheat bran, says Dr. Chambreau. She recommends adding a little bit of bran—one-half teaspoon for cats and dogs under 15 pounds and two teaspoons for larger pets—to their regular food every day.

**Eliminate worms with herbs.** An herbal combination called Para-L, sold as a liquid, will help remove worms from the body, says Dr. Chambreau. Ask your vet how much to give and the best way to use it safely.

**Add garlic to his food.** This pungent herb helps clean and tonify the intestines, possibly killing some of the worms, says Dr. Chambreau. Dogs over 50 pounds can have as much as two teaspoons of garlic a day, and smaller dogs can have one-quarter to one-half teaspoon a day. Cats shouldn't be given more than one-eighth teaspoon of garlic a day for about two weeks. You can chop or mince the garlic and add it directly to your pet's food. Or you can puree it in a little water, along with some fresh vegetables.

**Give him some sweet potatoes.** Pets with worms sometimes have digestive troubles such as diarrhea. A tasty way to soothe their stomachs is with sweet potatoes, says Beatrice Ehrsam, D.V.M., a holistic veterinarian in private practice in New Paltz, New York. "Give your pet cooked sweet potatoes every day," she suggests. Pets under 15 pounds can have two teaspoons of sweet potatoes a day, and larger pets can have a tablespoon or more, she says.

**Put some spice in his food.** Cayenne pepper and hot-pepper sauces such as Tabasco create an inhospitable environment in the intestines, and some worms may simply pack up and leave, says Dr. Chambreau. "Start with a few drops or sprinkles and increase the amount

## Call the VET

Some types of worms, such as tapeworms, are visible in the stool, but others stay out of sight in the intestines, quietly removing blood and essential nutrients. As the worm populations increase, your pet may get increasingly tired and weak. He may be vomiting and have diarrhea, and his belly may be distended as well.

Worms pose another danger. Children who play in areas where infected dogs have been may get infected themselves.

Worms sometimes go undetected because the symptoms can be caused by a variety of problems. It is worth asking your vet to check for worms during your pet's annual checkup. (Be sure to bring along a fresh stool sample, which is used to detect worms.) In the meantime, if your pet suddenly seems tired and lethargic and he doesn't get better within a few days, make an appointment to see your vet.

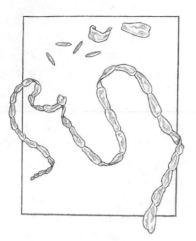

Tapeworms don't cause obvious physical symptoms, but you can often see the rice-like worm segments around your pet's rear end or in his stool.

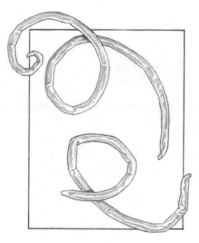

Roundworms may cause vomiting, diarrhea, a potbelly, or a dull coat. Look for beige, spaghetti-like worms in the stool, especially in puppies and kittens.

until your pet lets you know he doesn't like it anymore. Then back off."

**Put him on a rich diet.** Worms that live in the intestines can rob your

pet of essential nutrients. To keep him well-nourished while he is being treated, give him a diet that is high in both protein and fat, says Lori Tapp, D.V.M., a holistic veterinarian in private practice in Asheville, North Carolina. For dogs with worms, about 40 percent of the diet should come from meat or eggs; for cats, protein should make up 60 percent or more of the diet. To increase the amount of fat in the diet, you can add a little butter or canola or olive oil to his food, she says. Or you can temporarily switch your pet to puppy or kitten food, which is much richer than foods that are made for adults. If your pet is sensitive to changes in his diet, however, or has

## Meet the Experts

**Christina Chambreau, D.V.M.,** is a holistic veterinarian in Sparks, Maryland, and education chairperson for the Academy of Veterinary Homeopathy.

**Beatrice Ehrsam, D.V.M.,** is a holistic veterinarian in private practice in New Paltz, New York. She is certified in acupuncture.

**Lori Tapp, D.V.M.,** is a holistic veterinarian in private practice in Asheville, North Carolina. She is certified in homeopathy.

**Michele Yasson, D.V.M.,** is a holistic veterinarian in private practice in New York City and Rosendale, New York. She is certified in acupuncture.

had pancreatitis in the past, it is best not to change his diet even temporarily.

**Increase the iron with raw liver.** Some intestinal parasites remove large amounts of blood from the intestines, causing a drop in iron. Giving your pet raw organic liver once a day for two to four weeks will quickly restore the iron that is lost, says Dr. Tapp. "Liver should make up no more than 15 percent of the meat in his diet."

**BEST BET!** **Improve digestion with enzymes.** To help your pet get the most nutrition from his food, it is a good idea to give him digestive enzymes, such as Prozyme, says Dr. Ehrsam. You can give one-quarter teaspoon of the enzyme for every cup of food. Keep giving the enzyme until your pet is free of worms, she advises. Another way to maximize nutrition is to give your pet acidophilus, which contains beneficial bacteria that improve digestion, says Dr. Ehrsam. She recommends giving one capsule twice a day to dogs weighing 15 pounds or more and half a capsule twice a day smaller pets.

# WOUNDS

## The Signs
- Your pet has been cut, scraped, or bitten.
- The wound is bleeding heavily or won't stay closed.
- The area is red or swollen.

## The Cause

The skin protects your pet's body from the harsh world outside. It blocks toxins and bacteria and admits oxygen that nourishes tissues throughout the body. But when pets are wounded and the skin is broken, bacteria and other harmful organisms crowd their way inside, often causing infection. Most wounds heal on their own, but they can disrupt the body's protective energy, making your pet more vulnerable to a variety of health threats, says Carvel Tiekert, D.V.M., executive director of the American Holistic Veterinary Medical Association and a holistic veterinarian in Bel Air, Maryland.

Veterinarians have traditionally relied on bandages or stitches to stop bleeding and on antiseptics and antibiotics to fight infection. The goal of alternative medicine is somewhat different. Rather than merely treating the wound, holistic veterinarians try to strengthen and balance your pet's natural healing powers to help wounds

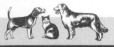

## After the Fight

Wounds caused by fights can be worrisome because bacteria-laden saliva or tiny bits of claw may get trapped under the skin, causing a painful, swollen, pus-filled infection called an abscess.

Cats usually get abscesses on the head, front legs, or at the base of the tail, while dogs sometimes get them between the toes, on the hind legs, or near the ears. Abscesses are potentially serious, and you will need to call your vet if your pet seems lethargic or has lost his appetite or if the abscess has ruptured and formed an even larger wound, says Susan G. Wynn, D.V.M., a veterinarian in Atlanta and co-editor of *Complementary and Alternative Veterinary Medicine*. In most cases, however, abscesses are easy to treat at home.

- Rinse the area well with warm water, then apply a warm, moist compress for 10 to 15 minutes, two or three times a day. Applying moist heat increases blood flow and softens the skin, which will help the abscess drain, Dr. Wynn explains.

- Give a dose of homeopathic Hepar sulphuris, using a 30X potency. This will help the abscess rupture and drain, says Dr. Wynn. Pets under 15 pounds can take two pellets of Hepar sulphuris, and those 15 pounds and over can take three pellets.

heal more quickly and to prevent infections and other problems. Here is what they advise.

## The Solutions  FOR DOGS & CATS

**Stop the flow.** The first step with any wound is to stop the bleeding. A Chinese remedy called yunnan pai yao, available through mail order, will stop bleeding fairly quickly when it is sprinkled into a cut or scrape, says Dr. Tiekert. At first, the bleeding will increase and the blood will turn a brighter red. This is normal, he says. Just wait a few minutes, then sprinkle in a little more of the powder. The bleeding will usually stop right away.

**BEST BET!** **Wash away the risks.** Wounds with dirt inside take longer to heal and often get infected. The easiest way to clean a wound is to flush it well with a saline solution, available at grocery stores and drugstores, says Dr. Tiekert. Flush the wound thoroughly with the saline until it looks clean. If you don't have saline solution, go ahead and use tap water, he adds. "A clean water rinse from a hose is fine for first-aid."

**Trim the area.** Stray fur that dangles into a wound is sure to slow healing and promote infection. It is a good idea to trim the fur surrounding a wound right away, Dr. Tiekert says. He recommends dipping the scissors in mineral oil before cutting the hair. This will cause the fur to stick to the scissors instead of falling into the wound.

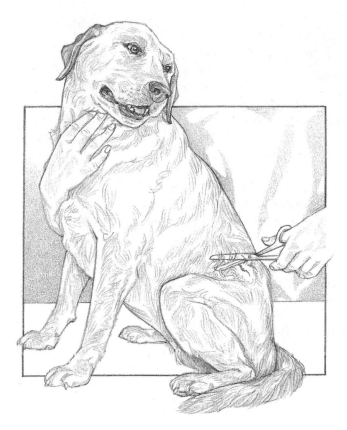

To improve air flow and keep fur out of a wound, trim the surrounding area with a pair of blunt-nosed scissors, creating a border of about two to three inches. Dipping the scissors in mineral oil will cause the fur clippings to stick to the scissors instead of falling into the wound. After trimming around a wound, put a little KY jelly on a piece of gauze and press it to the wound. When you remove it, loose hair clippings will come up with it.

**Keep it moist.** Wounds heal most quickly when they are kept slightly moist. A good way to trap moisture is to apply a little calendula (*Calendula officinalis*) ointment three times a day, says Elayne Williams, D.V.M., a holistic veterinarian in private practice in Fort Collins, Colorado. Or you can smear calendula ointment on a nonstick pad and tape it over the wound. Changing the bandage once a day will help the wound heal more quickly, she says.

**Feed the healing process.** The body needs extra nutrients for wounds to heal properly. Dr. Tiekert recommends giving dogs and cats vitamin C and bioflavonoid supplements. Cats and dogs under 15 pounds can take 250 milligrams each of vitamin C and bioflavonoids twice a day for two to five days, he says. Pets 15 to 50 pounds can take 500 milligrams of each twice a day, and larger dogs can have 1,000 milligrams of each supplement twice a day. Vitamin C in large doses may cause diarrhea, so you may have to scale back the amount until your pet is comfortable again.

Dr. Tiekert also recommends

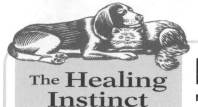

## The Healing Instinct

Dogs and cats don't think twice about licking their wounds. They do it as naturally and automatically as they breathe—and with good reason. Researchers have found that dog and cat saliva contains chemicals that can block bacteria and reduce the risk of infection. In fact, laboratory studies have found that when dog saliva is pitted against harmful bacteria, it works nearly as well as antibiotics.

Licking isn't always helpful, adds Elayne Williams, D.V.M., a holistic veterinarian in private practice in Fort Collins, Colorado. Some pets—especially dogs—will lick wounds so much and for so long that the constant friction actually makes them worse. But as long as your pet isn't licking the wound for more than about 10 minutes at a time several times a day, he is probably doing himself some good.

giving pets pancreatic enzymes, which will help them digest their food more thoroughly and get more micronutrients into the bloodstream. The supplements are available in health food stores and may be labeled as "pancrezyme," "pancreatin," or "raw pancreas." Give dogs one tablet of the enzyme once a day, he advises. Cats can take half a tablet once a day. In addition, you may want to give your pet a little cheese, egg, or cooked meat because the body needs a lot more protein when wounds are healing.

**Strengthen his immunity.** The herb echinacea (*Echinacea purpurea* or *Echinacea angustifolia*), available in bulk and powdered forms, stimulates the immune system so that it is better able to fight infection. "It's pretty easy to give since pets don't

mind the taste," says Dr. Williams. She suggests opening up an echinacea capsule and mixing the contents in your pet's food. Or you can pop the capsule down the hatch. Dogs over 50 pounds can take the full human dose. Pets 15 to 50 pounds should take half that amount, and those under 15 pounds should take about one-quarter of the human dose.

**Ease the bruising.** When wounds are accompanied by a lot of bruising, which often occurs with bite wounds, homeopathic Arnica can be very helpful. Dr. Tiekert recommends giving dogs two pellets of Arnica 30C once or twice on the day of the injury. Cats should be given one pellet, he says.

**Clear the wound with Silica.** A 30C dose of homeopathic Silica, given

## Meet the Experts

**Lynda Clark, N.D., D.V.M.,** is a naturopathic doctor and holistic veterinarian in private practice in Christiansted, St. Croix, Virgin Islands. She is certified in acupuncture and homeopathy.

**Alison Clarke, V.M.D.,** is a retired veterinarian in Leonardtown, Maryland.

**Carvel Tiekert, D.V.M.,** is executive director of the American Holistic Veterinary Medical Association and a holistic veterinarian in Bel Air, Maryland. He is certified in acupuncture and chiropractic.

**Elayne Williams, D.V.M.,** is a holistic veterinarian in private practice in Fort Collins, Colorado. She is certified in acupuncture.

**Susan G. Wynn, D.V.M.,** is a veterinarian in Atlanta and co-editor of *Complementary and Alternative Veterinary Medicine.*

twice a day for one to three days, will help the body remove debris from wounds and help prevent scar tissue from forming. "It's great for healing," says Lynda Clark, N.D., D.V.M., a naturopathic doctor and holistic veterinarian in private practice in Christiansted, St. Croix, Virgin Islands.

**BEST BET!** **Use magnets for tough wounds.** Deep or slow-to-heal wounds often respond to magnet therapy, which increases the flow of electricity and blood through the body. "This would be great to try for pets with pressure sores or stubborn wounds," says Alison Clarke, V.M.D., a retired veterinarian in Leonardtown, Maryland. You can buy magnetic sleeping pads from pet supply catalogs and some holistic veterinarians. They are simple to use, she says. All you have to do is encourage your pet to take a nap on the pad.

# Alternative Healing Resource Guide

## NATURAL AND HOLISTIC VETERINARY ASSOCIATIONS

You can send a self-addressed, stamped envelope to receive a list of practitioners in your area.

**Academy of Veterinary Homeopathy**
751 NE 168th Street
North Miami, FL 33162

**American Academy of Veterinary Acupuncture**
AAVA
P.O. Box 419
Hygiene, CO 80533-0419

**American Holistic Veterinary Medical Association**
2214 Old Emmorton Road
Bel Air, MD 21015

**American Veterinary Chiropractic Association**
623 Main Street
Hillsdale, IL 61257

**Florida Holistic Veterinary Medical Association**
751 Northeast 168th Street
North Miami Beach, FL 33162

**Georgia Holistic Veterinary Medical Association**
334 Knollwood Lane
Woodstock, GA 30188

**Great Lakes Holistic Veterinary Medical Association (mostly Ill. and Wis.)**
9824 Durand Avenue
Sturtevant, WI 53177

**International Association for Veterinary Homeopathy**
Sonnhaldenstr. 18
CH-8370 Sirnach
Switzerland

**International Veterinary Acupuncture Society**
P.O. Box 1478
Longmont, CO 80502

**Rocky Mountain Holistic Veterinary Medical Association**
311 South Pennsylvania Street
Denver, CO 80209

## NATURAL HEALTH ORGANIZATIONS

**American Massage Therapy Association**
820 Davis Street, Suite 100
Evanston, IL 60201

**Canadian Herb Society**
Van Dusen Botanical Display Garden
5251 Oak Street
Vancouver, British Columbia
Canada V6M 4H1

**Flower Essence Society**
P.O. Box 459
Nevada City, CA 95959

**Office of Alternative Medicine Clearinghouse**
National Institutes of Health
P.O. Box 8218
Silver Spring, MD 20907

**Linda Tellington-Jones**
TEAM and TTouch Trainings
P.O. Box 3793
Santa Fe, NM 87501

## PUBLICATIONS

**Best Friends Magazine**
Best Friends Animal Sanctuary
5001 Angel Canyon Drive
Kanab, UT 84741

**Dr. Bob and Susan Goldstein's Love of Animals Natural Care and Healing for Your Pets**
606 Post Road East
Westport, CT 06880

**The Enchanted Connections Review**
18 Josephine Lane
Ft. Salonga, NY 11768

**Natural Cat and Dog**
Fancy Publications
P.O. Box 6050
Mission Viejo, CA 92690

**Natural Rearing Newsletter**
Ambrican Enterprises Ltd.
P.O. Box 1436
Jacksonville, OR 97530

**North Star's Healthy Pets Naturally!**
148 Channel Road
Tinmouth, VT 05773

**PetSage**
4313 Wheeler Avenue
Alexandria, VA 22304

## AROMATHERAPY AND ESSENTIAL OILS

**Aura Cacia**
P.O. Box 399
Weaverville, CA 96093

**Oshadhi USA**
1340 G. Industrial Avenue
Petaluma, CA 94952

**Young Living Essential Oils**
250 South Main Street
Payson, UT 84651

## FLOWER ESSENCES

**Alaskan Flower Essence Project**
P.O. Box 1369
Homer, AK 99603
Specializes in flower, gem, and environmental essences.

**Flower Essences Services**
P.O. Box 1769
Nevada City, CA 95959

**Global Health Alternatives**
193 Middle Street, Suite 201
Portland, ME 04101

**Green Hope Farm Flower Essences**
P.O. Box 125
Meriden, NH 03770

**The Source**
2501 71st Street
North Bergen, NJ 07047
Specializes in flower remedies.

## GLANDULARS, NUTRICEUTICALS, AND SUPPLEMENTS

**The Botanical Animal**
Equilite, Inc.
20 Prospect Avenue
Ardsley, NY 10502

**Natural Animal Nutrition**
2109 Emmorton Park Drive
Edgewood, MD 21040

**Nutramax Laboratories, Inc.**
5024 Campbell Boulevard
Baltimore, MD 21236

**Nutritech Inc.**
5000 West Oakey Boulevard, Unit D-13
Las Vegas, NV 89146

**Nutrition Now, Inc.**
6350 Northeast Campus Drive
Vancouver, WA 98661

**Prozyme Products Ltd.**
6600 North Lincoln Avenue
Lincolnwood, IL 60645

**Vita Plus Industries, Inc.**
953 East Sahara Avenue, Suite 21B
Las Vegas, NV 89104

## HERBS

**Animals' Apawthecary**
P.O. Box 212
Conner, MT 59827
Specializes in glycerine-based herbal preparations.

**Azmira Holistic Animal Care**
2100 N. Wilmot Road, Suite 109
Tucson, AZ 85712
Specializes in Western herbs.

**Essiac International**
P.O. Box 23155
Ottawa, Ontario
Canada K2A 4E2

**Essiac (U.S. distributor)**
3869 Mallard Way
Little River, SC 29566
Specializes in Essiac tea.

**Frontier Natural Products Co-op**
3021 78th Street
P.O. Box 299
Norway, IA 52318

**Harmany Veterinary Products**
3065 Center Green Drive, Suite 140
Boulder, CO 80301

**Healing Herbs for Pets**
4292-99 Fourth Avenue
Ottawa, Ontario
Canada K1S 5B3
Specializes in Chinese herbal remedies for dogs and cats

**Herb Pharm**
P.O. Box 116
Williams, OR 97544
  Specializes in organic
  herbs and tinctures.

**Herb Research Foundation**
1007 Pearl Street, Suite 200
Boulder, CO 80302

**Merritt Naturals**
P.O. Box 532
Rumson, NJ 07760

## HOMEOPATHIC REMEDIES

**Arnica, Inc.**
144 East Garry Avenue
Santa Ana, CA 92707

**Boiron**
P.O. Box 559
6 Campus Boulevard,
Building A
Newtown Square, PA 19073

**Dr. Goodpet**
P.O. Box 4547
Inglewood, CA 90309
  Specializes in combina-
  tion homeopathic
  remedies.

**Dolisos America, Inc.**
3014 Rigel Avenue
Las Vegas, NV 89102

**Hahnemann Laboratories, Inc.**
1940 Fourth Street
San Rafael, CA 94901

**Heel BHI**
11600 Cochiti Road Southeast
Albuquerque, NM 87123

**Homeopathic Educational Services**
2124 Kittredge Street
Berkeley, CA 94704

**Standard Homeopathic Company**
154 West 131st Street
Los Angeles, CA 90061

## MAGNET THERAPY

**Magnetic Field Therapy**
IBS Systems Corp.
4754 East Flamingo Road #453
Las Vegas, NV 89121

**Magnetic Wellness Products**
3500 Parkdale Avenue,
Building A
Baltimore, MD 21211

**Magnet Sales and Manufacturing, Inc.**
11248 Playa Court
Culver City, CA 90230

**Norfields Magnets**
632¾ North Doheny Drive
Los Angeles, CA 90069

## PET SUPPLY COMPANIES

You can write to these
companies to request a
product catalog.

**Advanced Biological Concepts**
301 Main Street
P.O. Box 27
Osco, IL 61274
  Specializes in nutritional
  and herbal products.

**Alta Health Products**
2137 East Summersweet
Drive
Boise, ID 83716

**BioEnergetics Inc.**
P.O. Box 127
Sandy, OR 97055

**Cat Faeries**
584 Castro, Room 545
San Francisco, CA 94114
  Specializes in flower
  remedies (custom
  blending is available),
  gifts for cats, and hand-
  made catnip toys filled
  with wild-crafted
  catnip.

**DermaPet**
8909 Iverleigh Court
P.O. Box 59713
Potomac, MD 20854
  Specializes in natural
  skin- and ear-care
  products.

**Doctors Foster and Smith**
2253 Air Park Road
P.O. Box 100
Rhinelander, WI 54501

**The Dog's Outfitter**
The Home Pet Shop
Humboldt Industrial Park
1 Maplewood Drive
Hazleton, PA 18201

**Earthwise Animal Products**
P.O. Box 654
Millwood, NY 10546

**Halo Purely for Pets**
3438 East Lake Road #14
Palm Harbor, FL 34685
 Specializes in herbal dip,
 ear wash, nutritional supplements, homemade
 stew for dogs and cats,
 and bird food.

**Holistic Pet Center:
The Health Food Store
for Pets**
15599 Southeast 82nd Drive
P.O. Box 1166
Clackamas, OR 97015

**Jeffers Pet Catalog**
P.O. Box 948
West Plains, MO 65775

**Morrills' New
Directions**
21 Market Square
Houlton, ME 04730

**Natural Animal, Inc.**
P.O. Box 1177
St. Augustine, FL 32085
 Specialize in products for
 natural flea control.

**The Natural Pet Care
Company**
All the Best Care
8050 Lake City Way
Seattle, WA 98115

**North Star Natural Pet
Products**
148 Channel Road
Tinmouth, VT 05773

**PetSage**
4313 Wheeler Avenue
Alexandria, VA 22304

**P.O.R.G.I.E. Natural Pet
Supply**
2023 Chicago Avenue, Suite
B-22
Riverside, CA 92507

**Pro-Tec Pet Health**
P.O. Box 23676
Pleasant Hill, CA 94523

**R. C. Steele**
1989 Transit Way
P.O. Box 910
Brockport, NY 14420

**Solid Gold Health Prod-
ucts for Pets, Inc.**
1483 North Cuyamaca Street
El Cajon, CA 92020

**Springtime, Inc.**
10942-J Beaver Dam Road
P.O. Box 1227
Cockeysville, MD 21030
 Specializes in supple-
 ments, food concentrates,
 herbal extracts, and vitamins and minerals.

**Whiskers**
235 East Ninth Street
New York, NY 10003

**The Whole Pet, Natu-
rally! Inc.**
44 Coachlight Square
Montrose, NY 10548

## NATURAL PET FOODS

These manufacturers
use premium ingredi-
ents and do not use ar-
tificial preservatives or
additives. Write for in-
formation on products
and the names of local
distributors.

**The Robert Abady Dog
Food Company**
Nutra-vet Research
Corporation
201 Smith Street
Poughkeepsie, NY 12601

**Animal Food Services**
675 East State Street
Iola, WI 54945

**California Natural**
Natura Pet Products
1101 South Winchester
Boulevard, Suite J225
San Jose, CA 95128

**Flint River Ranch**
1243 Columbia Avenue,
Suite B-6
Riverside, CA 92507

**Fromm Family Foods
(Fromm Dog and Cat
Foods)**
P.O. Box 365
Mequon, WI 53092

**Green Foods
Corporation**
320 North Graves Avenue
Oxnard, CA 93030

**Iams Company**
7250 Poe Avenue
Dayton, OH 45414
 Manufactures both Iams
 and Eukanuba cat and
 dog foods

**Innova**
Natura Pet Products
1101 South Winchester
Boulevard, Suite J225
San Jose, CA 95128

**Natural Life**
1601 West McKay
Frontenac, KS 66763

**Nature's Menu**
847 Madison Street
Madison, WI 53711

**Nature's Recipe**
341 Bonnie Circle
Corona, CA 91720

**Nutro Natural Choice**
Nutro Products, Inc.
445 Wilson Way
City of Industry, CA 91744

**PetGuard, Inc.**
P.O. Box 728
Orange Park, FL 32067

**PHD Products, Inc.**
P.O. Box 8313
White Plains, NY 10602

**Precise Pet Products**
P.O. Box 630009
Nacogdoches, TX 75963

**Sensible Choice**
Pet Products Plus
5600 Mexico Road
St. Peters, MO 63376

**Sojourner Farms**
1 19th Avenue South
Minneapolis, MN 55454

**Solid Gold**
Solid Gold Health Products for
Pets, Inc.
1483 North Cuyamaca Street
El Cajon, CA 92020

**Wysong**
1880 North Eastman Road
Midland, MI 48642

# Index

Underscored page references indicate boxed text.
**Boldface** page references indicate illustrations.

## A

Abscesses, <u>430</u>
Accidents, bathroom, 304–10
  calling the vet about, <u>305</u>
Aches and pains, from fever, 250
Acidophilus, for treating
  cancer, 175–76
  flatulence, 257, <u>258</u>
  worms, 429
Acne, 103–5, **103**
Acupressure, 30–31, 34
  effects of, 5, 22–23, 24
  how to use, 34–35
  meridians in, 30–31, <u>32–33</u>, **32–33**
  for preventing dehydration, 209
  for treating
    aggression, 253
    allergies, 121
    anemia, 129
    appetite loss, 132
    arthritis, 135
    back problems, 141–42
    bladder-control problems, 155
    car sickness, 181
    constipation, 201–2
    diarrhea, 222–23
    drooling, 229
    dung eating, 230
    energy imbalance, 23
    epilepsy, 22
    eye irritation, 241–42
    feline immunodeficiency virus, 247
    fever, 249
    hearing problems, 280
    heart disease, 285–86, <u>285</u>
    hip dysplasia, 296

    house soiling, 306–7, **306**, **307**
    inflammatory bowel disease, **314**, 315
    lameness, 340
    liver problems, 353
    nail-bed infections, 193
    nausea, 420
    pad cracks, 371–72
    spraying, **394**, 395
Acupuncture
  acupressure as alternative to, 30
  effects of, 5, 24
  for heart problems, <u>286</u>
Additives, food, health affected by, 10, 16
Adolph's meat tenderizer, for preventing dung eating, 231
Aggression, 105–11
  alternative treatment for, <u>107</u>
  of cats, <u>108</u>
  cause of, 105–6
  fighting from, 253–55
  immediate attention for, <u>106</u>
  jealousy and, <u>329</u>
  solutions for, 106–11
Agility, loss of, with aging, 116–17
Aging, 112–17
  alternative care for, <u>113</u>
Agrimony, for treating
  barking, 150
  hives, 299–300
  jealousy, 329–30
Alcohol, rubbing
  as antiseptic, 99
  for fever, 247
Alfalfa, for treating
  bad breath, 145–46
  hip pain, <u>54</u>

**439**

# B

# J

# K